NEW RESEARCH ON CERVICAL CANCER

NEW RESEARCH ON CERVICAL CANCER

GEORGE Z. ROLLAND
EDITOR

Nova Science Publishers, Inc.
New York

For permission to use material from this book please contact us:
Telephone 631-231-7269; Fax 631-231-8175
Web Site: http://www.novapublishers.com

LIBRARY OF CONGRESS CATALOGING-IN-PUBLICATION DATA
Available upon request.

ISBN 13 978-1-60021-300-7
ISBN 10 1-60021-300-6

Published by Nova Science Publishers, Inc. ✦ New York

Contents

PREFACE

Cervical cancer is a malignancy of the cervix. Worldwide, it is the second most common cancer of women. It may be present with vaginal bleeding but symptoms may be absent until the cancer is in advanced stages, which has made cervical cancer the focus of intense screening efforts. Most scientific studies point to human papillomavirus (HPV) infection responsible for 90% of the cases of cervical cancer. There are 7 most common types of HPV - 16, 18, 31, 33, 42, 52 and 58. Types 16 and 18 being the most common cause of the cancer. Treatment is with surgery (including local exicision) in early stages and chemotherapy and radiotherapy in advanced stages of the disease. This book presents cutting edge research in this field. This involves programs for cancer screening, alternative approaches to cervical cancer prevention, HPV/Co-Infections and Host Genetic Profiles, Small Cell Carcinoma of the Uterine Cervix, Indicators of HPV-induced carcinogenesis, functional genomics as a tool for understanding cervical cancer, histone deacetylase inhibitors, Chinese women and cervical cancer and cervical cancer in Northeastern Thailand.

Chapter 1 discusses a hospital based community outreach program to increase cervical cancer screening among women in Taiwan. This case study, "*Love Yourself before You Take Care of Your Family*", describes a comprehensive process of the development and evaluation of a cancer screening intervention program for Chinese women. Three major phases of the study are presented in the following order: (1) Measurement development and the assessment of factors influence screening utilization; (2) Intervention development using a framework called Intervention Mapping (IM); an innovative process of designing effective intervention, and (3) Program evaluation using a controlled-randomized intervention trial. The primary outcome was to receive a cervical cancer screening (Pap smear test) after the intervention. A secondary outcome was to advance knowledge and beliefs concerning cervical cancer screening. The intervention lasted for three months. Female family members of inpatients who were admitted into a major teaching hospital in Taichung, Taiwan were asked about their cervical cancer screening history. Women who had not had a cervical cancer screening in the past 12 months were identified as non-adherent and thus the were eligible to participate in the control-randomized intervention trial. IM helped ensure that theory and evidence guided (a) the identification of psychosocial and environmental determinants related to cancer screening behavior, and (b) the selection of the most appropriate methods and strategies to address the identified determinants. The program used methods such as information transmission, modeling, persuasion, and facilitation. Strategies used included direct mail campaigns, role model stories and testimonials, as well as phone intervention. Women in the intervention group reported a higher rate of receiving a cervical cancer screening than women did in the comparison group. Currently, theory- and evidence-based health promotion intervention programs targeting Chinese women, or Asian women in general, to increase cancer screening is scarce. This case study serves as an excellent model to assist researchers and practitioners in planning, implementing, and evaluating health promotion programs in cancer screening. The validated research instrument, with an English-Chinese side-by-side translation, is enclosed at the end of the chapter.

Cervical screening is acknowledged as currently the most effective approach for cervical cancer control. To date, there is extensive and strong evidence that cytology-based screening programs have been effective in reducing the incidence of and mortality from the disease in developed countries. However, conventional Papanicolaou (Pap) smears have inherent methodological shortcomings. New developments in cytology, such as liquid-based techniques and automated reading, seem to effectively overcome some of these limitations and have the potential to improve sensitivity and specificity of cytology both in diagnosis of and screening for cervical pre-cancer and cancer.

The recognition that cervical cancer is a consequence of an acquired infection with a few types of oncogenic human papillomaviruses (HPV) has led to novel opportunities for screening based on the use of HPV-tests. Current HPV testing systems are able to detect the presence of viral DNA in exfoliated cervical epithelial cells in close to 100% of invasive cervical cancer and up to 90% of its precursors. Thus, in terms of public health and also for practical purposes, all cervical cancer cases should be considered to be caused by HPV infection. A number of clinical studies have also demonstrated HPV testing to be more sensitive for the detection of clinically relevant pre-invasive cervical disease than cytology alone and the combination of HPV tests and cytology may achieve a negative predictive value of >97% in detecting high grade intraepithelial neoplasia and cervical cancer.

However, in most women, cervical HPV infections remain asymptomatic and are transient, becoming undetectable in 1-2 years even by the most sensitive genetic tests. This is also true for high-risk HPV (HR-HPV) types. It is the long term persistence of certain HR-HPV genotypes that is strongly associated with cervical carcinogenesis in permissive cases. Therefore, discrimination between transient and persistent infections with a certain HPV genotype is essential for risk-adapted screening protocols, which can only be defined by genotyping of two consecutive probes.

Nevertheless, even the highly sensitive test combination of cytology and HR-HPV genotyping cannot predict the biological potential of prevalent cervical pre-cancers towards progression or regression. This can only be assessed by using an adequate biomarker of neoplastic transformation, e.g. DNA aneuploidy, in combination with morphological and HPV tests.

Chapter 2 focuses on the clinical utility of conventional, ancillary and experimental methods for cervical screening and possible future directions for enhanced screening accuracy and prognostication using risk-adapted multimodal protocols.

Over the past years, the knowledge on natural history and epidemiology of the *Human Papillomavirus* (HPV) infection has advanced tremendously. Besides numerous ongoing efforts to understand the biological basis of complex traits as cervical cancer, many questions concerning the interaction of the virus with its host remain unanswered. Worldwide, HPV is one of the most prevalent sexual transmitted agents and, at the same time, cervical cancer is the rare consequence of HPV infection. Despite the prominent role of HPV in genital cancer development, other genetic, epigenetic and environmental factors have also been involved. The aim of the present study in chapter 3 was to evaluate in a multifactorial fashion the HPV (genotyping, viral load), *Herpes Simplex Virus* and *Chlamydia trachomatis* infections combined with *k-ras*, *c-myc* and *c-erbB-2* oncogene status, as co-factors in cervical carcinogenesis in a set of 304 preneoplastic and neoplastic cervical cancer tissue. Furthermore, genetic polymorphisms belonging to the HLA-DQA1 gene and the tumor suppressor gene p53 were also evaluated, in order to define their role in cervical cancer development. Principal component analysis (PCA) was employed to perform an integrative multifactorial analysis and to view the overall trend of the data. In addition, genome-wide expression profiling obtained by DNA microarray platform was downloaded from public available databases. The authors' statistical analysis identified 167 transcript differentially expressed between normal cervical tissue and invasive carcinomas ($p<0.01$). Finally, *Single Nucleotide Polymorphisms* (SNPs) analysis in cervical cancer research were also discussed.

Small cell carcinoma is a unique type of neuroendocrine tumor. It occurs most commonly in the lungs and is only rarely seen in extrapulmonary sites including the uterine cervix. Irrespective of anatomic location, the diagnosis of this highly aggressive malignant neoplasm is usually based on its classic histopathologic features. Sometimes, immunohistochemical stains, and occasionally, electron microscopic examination, may be needed to confirm the diagnosis. No specific biomarkers have been identified to distinguish small cell lung carcinoma (SCLC) from its extrapulmonary counterparts. However, primary small cell carcinoma of the uterine cervix (SCCC) is distinct in that it typically occurs in middle-aged women and is etiopathogenetically associated with high risk types of human papillomavirus (HPV), particularly type 18. This is in contrast with SCLC, which is typically seen in older individuals and associated with cigarette smoking. SCCC also differs from SCLC in chromosomal alterations as well as molecular mechanisms that regulate the expression of tumor suppressor genes, in particular, *Rb* and *p53*. In SCCC, these two tumor suppressors are likely inactivated at the protein level via interaction with HPV oncoproteins, whereas in SCLC they are inactivated at the genetic level through gene mutations. Furthermore, c-kit proto-oncoprotein and bcl-2 anti-apoptotic protein that may bear therapeutic significance are frequently overexpressed in SCLC but infrequently in SCCC. Chapter 4 discusses current understanding of the etiology, pathogenesis and clinicopathologic features for SCCC and emphasizes the distinction from SCLC.

The protein $p16^{INK4a}$, an inhibitor of cycline-dependent kinases CDKs 4/6, is encoded by the tumor suppressor gene *INK4a.* In various tumors its control function over a cell passing through G1/S check-point is broken due to mutational or epigenetic events. Cervical carcinomas stay by themselves with this respect. Owing to the pRb inactivation by the HPV E7 oncoprotein cells uncontrollably pass to the S- cell cycle stage. In the *RB* signal pathway $p16^{INK4a}$ acts upstream of pRb. In cells of HPV-positive cervical dysplasia and carcinomas it looses the role of the G1/S check-point controller. The content of $p16^{INK4a}$ increases drastically. The feed-back loop between pRb inactivation by the oncoprotein E7 and the sharp growth of the $p16^{INK4a}$ amount had been demonstrated in in vitro systems. However details of this feed-back loop in primary dysplasia and carcinoma remain not quite clear. Nonetheless, the given phenomenon was taken as the basis of the proposal to use detection of p16^{INK4a} for early diagnostics of cervical cancer. In chapter 5, the authors had demonstrated formerly that the share of p16^{INK4a}-positive cells increases in the following row: LSIL → HSIL → invasive carcinoma. However in line with the communications of other research groups they had registered some samples of HSIL and invasive squamous carcinomas either containing very small numbers of p16^{INK4a}-positive cells or fully lacking them (the "negative" samples). Thus in the present study correspondence of expression of the HPV E7 oncogene and cellular gene *INK4a* was evaluated in squamous cervical carcinomas at two levels. The virus oncogene expression was studied by two methods: RT-PCR and immunochemistry with HPV16 E7-specific antibodies. To study an expression of the gene *INK4a* two kinds of experiments were performed: semi-quantitative RT-PCR including the development of the PCR product by Southern blot hybridization with the radio-active probe; immunochemistry with the p16^{INK4a}-specific antibodies. For RNA isolation both total tumor samples and tumor cell populations enriched by microdissections were used. Expression levels of the HPV *E7* oncogene greatly varied from sample to sample; in most carcinomas they were accompanied with the 3-30-fold rise of the *INK4a* m-RNA amount in comparison with that in normal tissue. So transcription of the gene *INK4a* contributes to the cervical cancer-specific overexpression of its protein product p16^{INK4a}. The gene *INK4a* transcription in specimens with a predominantly cytoplasmic location of p16^{INK4a} was not less active than that in the carcinomas expressing p16^{INK4a} in majority of nuclei. Thus both variants of staining with p16^{INK4a}-specific antibodies are to be regarded as positively stained. The results obtained are in accordance with the notion that the HPV *E7* oncogene has some influence on the gene *INK4a* transcription activation. However in "negative" samples some different links of the feed-back loop seem to be disturbed. There exist rare cervical carcinomas harboving HPV DNA and expressing the oncogene E7 at both the m-RNA and the protein level while fully lacking the *INK4a* expression at the both levels.

Cervical cancer (CC) is the second cause of cancer deaths in women worldwide. High risk human papillomavirus (HPV) infection is the major initiating event in cervical carcinogenesis, of the two most common HPV types (HPV16 and 18), which are present in more than 60-70% of invasive CC. The progressive histopathologic changes that occur during cervical carcinogenesis can be divided in distinctive multiple stages, ranging from low to high grade lesions, which, nevertheless, still do not carry 100% risk of progression, indicating that some additional factors are involved in CC tumorigenesis. In the recent years, the discovery of a number of disease biomarkers, including p16^{INK4a}, through immunohistochemical and mRNA studies, has enhanced the diagnostic accuracy of both cervical cytology and histology. More recently, development of high-throughput technologies, such as single nucleotide polymorphism (SNP) analysis, comparative genomic hybridization (CGH) and gene expression profiling using SAGE and cDNA microarrays, has significantly increased the potential for biomarker discovery. As discussed in chapter 6, over the past few years, the authors have used this technology including matrix CGH, SAGE, cDNA expression and tissue microarrays in CC samples at different stages from early to cancer and CC cell lines. Theirr findings indicate some differences in gene expression between cell lines and tissue samples, regardless of having the same HPV type. Also, genes overexpressed in other cancers are also present in CC. Moreover, some genes encoding proteins related to tumorigenesis are overexpressed in CC, as well as CC cell lines, regardless of the presence or absence of HPV and its particular types. In addition these techniques have facilitated an increased understanding of the pathogenesis for cervical cancer.

The objective of chapter 7 was an investigation by the authors of the effect of a variety of histone deacetylase inhibitors (HDACIs) [suberoyl anilide bishydroxamine, valproic acid, trichostatin A, and sodium butyrate] on three cervical cancer cell lines. Cervical cancer cells were treated with various concentrations of HDACIs, and their effects on cell growth, cell cycle, apoptosis, and related measurements were investigated.

The results indicated the 3-(4,5-dimethylthiazol-2-yl)-2,5-diphenyltetrazolium bromide assays showed that all cervical cancer cell lines were sensitive to the growth inhibitory effects of HDACIs. Cell cycle analysis indicated that their exposure to HDACIs decreased the proportion of cells in the S-phase and increased the proportion in the G0/G1 phases of the cell cycle. Induction of apoptosis was confirmed by annexin V staining of externalized phosphatidylserine and loss of the transmembrane potential of mitochondria. This induction occurred in concert with altered expression of genes related to cell growth, malignant phenotype, and apoptosis. Furthermore, HDACIs treatment of these cell lines increased acetylation of H3 and H4 histone tails.

These results raise the possibility that HDACIs may prove particularly effective in the treatment of cervical cancers.

Chapter 8 will draw on empirical work conducted in South East Asia that depict a contemporary picture of women's health behaviors, beliefs and attitudes about cervical screening and cancer. Compared with other regions, South Asia has a relatively high rate of cervical cancer, much of this morbidity should be avoidable with cervical screening, but uptake rates remain low. This chapter will be approached from a socio- cultural basis and then aligned to inform the provision of appropriate preventive health strategies.

A particular focus will be on marginalized women, isolated by circumstances of poverty, migration and race; this will include domestic workers and new migrants. The discussion will draw how socio -cultural beliefs pose barriers to medically based health preventative behaviors and the intersection of these themes. Socio-cultural issues of fatalism, embarrassment, modesty, and cancer as a contagion will be elaborated upon. In addition, the structural reality of long working hours, workplace stigmatization, illegal status and financial impoverishment will be examined in respect to how these influence screening attendance patterns. Lay-professional interactions that eclipse negotiating engendered relationships will also provide a lenses from which to interpret women's' perceptions of pain, embarrassment, fertility, associations with promiscuity and other risk factors.

The conclusion will highlight the importance of mainstreaming gender, society and culture into the more traditional and medicals health care education and service provision systems that exist in SE Asia.

As discussed in chapter 9, cervical cancer remains the most common cancer among Thai women even though its incidence has decreased according to the age-standardized rate. Contrariwise, other data suggest the incidence rate of this cancer gradually increased in Northeast Thailand between 1992 and 2000. HPV infection is the major cause of cervical cancer and has been confirmed as a critical risk factor for the development of cancer in this region. The prevalence of HPV-16 infection was prominent, followed by HPV-18. The number of sexual partners and passive smoking history were identified as risks for HPV infection. As for passive smoking, tobacco specific carcinogens/mutagens may exist in the cervical mucus through smoking and/or in the semen of tobacco smoking partners. Cervical exposure to such carcinogens can reduce cervical immunity resulting in the persistence of HPV infection and also generating DNA lesions. It is hypothesized that certain genetic backgrounds, such as chemical metabolizing enzyme genes, may play roles in the development of this cancer.

In: New Research on Cervical Cancer
Editor: George Z. Rolland, pp. 1-46
ISBN 1-60021-300-6

Chapter I

USING INTERVENTION MAPPING IN PROGRAM DEVELOPMENT TO PROMOTE CERVICAL CANCER SCREENING AMONG CHINESE WOMEN: FROM NEEDS ASSESSMENT, INTERVENTION DEVELOPMENT, TO PROGRAM EVALUATION

Su-I Hou*
Department of Health Promotion and Behavior, College of Public Health,
University of Georgia, Athens, GA 30602, USA

ABSTRACT

This chapter discusses a hospital-based community outreach program to increase cervical cancer screening among women in Taiwan. This case study, "*Love Yourself before You Take Care of Your Family*", describes a comprehensive process of the development and evaluation of a cancer screening intervention program for Chinese women. Three major phases of the study are presented in the following order: (1) Measurement development and the assessment of factors influence screening utilization; (2) Intervention development using a framework called Intervention Mapping (IM); an innovative process of designing effective intervention, and (3) Program evaluation using a controlled-randomized intervention trial. The primary outcome was to receive a cervical cancer screening (Pap smear test) after the intervention. A secondary outcome was to advance knowledge and beliefs concerning cervical cancer screening. The intervention lasted for three months. Female family members of inpatients who were admitted into a major teaching hospital in Taichung, Taiwan were asked about their cervical cancer screening history. Women who had not had a cervical cancer screening in

* Correspondence concerning this article should be addressed to Su-I Hou, DrPH, RN, CHES. Department of Health Promotion and Behavior, 309 Ramsey Center, University of Georgia, Athens, GA 30602, USA. 706-542-8206 (phone); 706-542-4956 (fax); *shou@uga.edu* (email).

the past 12 months were identified as non-adherent and thus the were eligible to participate in the control-randomized intervention trial. IM helped ensure that theory and evidence guided (a) the identification of psychosocial and environmental determinants related to cancer screening behavior, and (b) the selection of the most appropriate methods and strategies to address the identified determinants. The program used methods such as information transmission, modeling, persuasion, and facilitation. Strategies used included direct mail campaigns, role model stories and testimonials, as well as phone intervention. Women in the intervention group reported a higher rate of receiving a cervical cancer screening than women did in the comparison group. Currently, theory- and evidence-based health promotion intervention programs targeting Chinese women, or Asian women in general, to increase cancer screening is scarce. This case study serves as an excellent model to assist researchers and practitioners in planning, implementing, and evaluating health promotion programs in cancer screening. The validated research instrument, with an English-Chinese side-by-side translation, is enclosed at the end of the chapter.

Keywords: cervical cancer, screening, Chinese women, measurement development, intervention mapping, program evaluation

INTRODUCTION

Cervical cancer is the second most common cancer among women worldwide. Although cervical cancer mortality has decreased during the past decades, recent epidemiological data from the U.S. cancer registry (Ries et al., 2000) indicates that cervical cancer disproportionately affects Asian women. Asian women have a higher incidence of cervical cancer (8.9/100,000) as compared to Caucasian women (8.7/100,000). Asian women also have a higher mortality rate of cervical cancer (2.7/100,000) than whites (2.5/100,000) (American Cancer Society, 2006a).

Although Pap smear tests have been proven to be an effective screening method of detecting cervical cancer at early stage, existing data suggest that close to 30% of the Asian women 18 years and over do not have regular screenings. The prevalence of cervical cancer screening among Asian women in the United States is close to 68%, as compared to 80%, 82%, and 75% among White, African American, and Hispanic or Latina women, respectively (American Cancer Society, 2006b). Screening rates, however, differ among different Asian ethnic groups. For example, the proportions of women reporting at least one Pap smear test ranged from 36% - 81% among Chinese Americans and 37-76% among Vietnamese Americans (Lee-Lin & Menon, 2005).

Among Chinese women in Taiwan, the few existing studies reported similar low rates of cervical cancer screening utilization, around 60% (Lee, Kuo, & Chou, 1997; Wang & Lin, 1996). In Taiwan, the National Health Insurance Plan (NHIP, 1996) provides free health care coverage of an annual cervical cancer screening for women age 30 years and older. Married women under 30 are also entitled to this benefit with a small co-payment. The implementation of NHIP has significantly lowered the cost barrier. Screening utilization might, therefore, have been improved. However, the annual screening rate is still far below satisfactory. Recent data from the Bureau of Health Promotion in the Department of Health in

Taiwan showed an average screening rate of 28% in 1999 among eligible women (Table I). Similarly, baseline data collected in the current case study showed that about 70% of the female family members we approached (n= 656 out of 969) reported not having a Pap smear test in the past 12 months (Hou, Fernandez, Baumler, & Parcel, 2002).

Table I. Pap smear screening rates among women age 30 and older in Taiwan

Year	1996	1997	1998	1999
Total screened women	875,606	1,147,672	1,424,809	1,602,000
Women age 30 and older	5,298,993	5,435,899	5,587,000	5,728,798
Screening rate (%)	16.5	21.1	25.5	28.0

Source: Department of Health, R.O.C., Taiwan

In 1990, there were 6.9 million Asians living in the United States. Between 1990 and 2000, the Asian population grew by 3.3 million to 10.2 million. This represents a growth of 48% compared to 13% for the total U.S. population (U.S. Census Bureau, 2003). About a quarter of the U.S. Asian population was of Chinese origin (U.S. Census Bureau, 2005). It is important to understand factors influencing cervical smear utilization among this population in order to develop appropriate and effective screening promotion programs. It is also important to develop and validate a Chinese version of the screening instrument so that culturally and linguistically appropriate measurements of screening belief can be obtained.

This chapter discusses a hospital-based community outreach program to increase cervical cancer screening among women in Taiwan. This case study, "*Love Yourself before You Take Care of Your Family*", describes a comprehensive process of the development and evaluation of the screening intervention program. Three major phases of the study are presented in the following order: (1) Phase I: Needs assessment - Measurement development and assessment of factors influence screening utilization (Hou, S., Fernandez, M., Baumler, E., Parcel, G & Chen, P, 2003), (2) Phase II: Intervention development using a framework called Intervention Mapping (IM), an innovative process of designing effective intervention (Hou, S., Fernandez, M., & Parcel, G, 2004); and (3) Phase III: Program evaluation using a controlled-randomized trial (Hou S, Fernandez M, Baumler E, & Parcel GS, 2002). Each phase is presented with the same structure outlines: overview, significance, methods, results, and discussion and recommendations. Accompanied tables and figures are also included. The validated research instrument on screening related psychosocial measurement, with English-Chinese side-by-side translation (Hou, S. & Luh, W, 2005), is enclosed at the end of the chapter.

Phase I: Needs Assessment - Measurement Development and Assessment of Factors Influence Cancer Screening Utilization Among Chinese Women

Overview

The purpose of this phase was to develop a theory-based measurement to assess psychosocial beliefs and related factors influencing cervical cancer screening utilization among Chinese women in Taiwan (n=125). Theoretical constructs examined included: perceived benefits, perceived barriers, norms towards cervical cancer screening, and perceived risk of cervical cancer. The reliabilities of the scales showed good internal consistence (Chronbach alpha ranged 0.68-0.88). Results indicated that 30% of the participants in the study had never received a Pap smear test, and only 58% reported having received a recent Pap smear test (within the past three years). Intention to have a Pap smear test in the coming year was higher among screened women (90% vs. 58%). Multiple logistic regression analysis revealed significant associations between recent screening uptake and women's knowledge, perceived pros, cons, and norms of a Pap smear test. In addition to identifying screening associated factors, this study also provided a basis for measuring important theory-based constructs. Although some scale items were developed for Chinese culture, data showed that psychosocial factors were universally relevant. Intervention efforts tailoring these factors could potentially impact cancer screening for women in other populations.

Significance

Although cervical cancer screenings can save lives, existing data suggest that Asian women tend not to have regular screenings. It is important to identify factors influencing screening utilization to develop intervention programs that could be effective and culturally sensitive for reaching Chinese women. This study examined the relationships between several psychosocial factors and cervical cancer screening behavior among women in Taiwan.

According to the National Breast and Cervical Cancer Early Detection Program (NBCCEDP) reported by the CDC, general problems for women concerning cervical cancer screening included fear, embarrassment, cost, transportation, communication barriers, lack of physician referral, lack of child care, and lack of time. Reasons why that Asian women fail to seek cervical cancer screening may be somewhat different since the Asian population constituted only about 2~3% in the sample of the NBCCEDP report. Cultural differences could limit generalization of the identified barriers. In recent years, there have been only a few studies which addressed factors that hinder Asian women from obtaining a cervical cancer screening. While Asian women had some concerns similar to women in the U.S. (access, communication, and embarrassment), the few existing studies suggested that other barriers were more prominent among this population and included marital status, sexual behavior, perceived risk, language barriers, and gender of physicians (Yi, 1994; Yu, Kim, Chen, & Brintnal, 2001; Jackson et al, 2000; Taylor et al, 2002; Hou, S. & Lessick, M, 2002).

In Taiwan, the National Health Insurance Plan (NHIP, 1996) provides free health care coverage for a Pap smear test to women aged 30 and over. Married women under 30 are also entitled to this benefit with a small co-payment. Despite universal coverage for these women, most women do not obtain regular screenings. Wang and Lin (1996) examined cervical cancer screening service utilization among women aged 20 and older in Taiwan in 1993. Their data indicated that 40% of the sampled women in Taipei had never had a Pap smear test. Given the high incidence and mortality rate of cervical cancer in Taiwan, the low screening prevalence, and the availability of an inexpensive screening method, it is important to understand the psychosocial factors that influence women's cervical cancer screening behavior. This phase of the study describes the results from a pilot study conducted in spring 1999 in Taichung, Taiwan (Hou S, Fernandez E, Baumler E, Parcel G & Chen P, 2003). This needs assessment was conducted to: (a) identify factors associated with cervical cancer screening behavior in order to inform the design of effective intervention in Phase II, and (b) test the scale reliabilities of the research measurement and refine the preliminary survey instrument for a prospective controlled-randomized trial in Phase III.

Methods

Target Group Selection

The target group of the research was female family members of inpatients who were admitted to one of the major teaching hospitals in Taiwan. Female family members of inpatients were chosen as the target group because this group was considered more similar to women in the community compared with female patients. Women visiting outpatient center were originally considered as the target group. However, feedback from stakeholder interviews suggested that outpatient clinic was usually busy in its nature, and the hectic environment might present many barriers for women to participate in the research survey. On the other hand, female family members of inpatients usually had more time while they were visiting or accompanying the hospitalized family members or friends. A self-administered questionnaire, consisting of 73 items, was distributed to a convenient sample of 160 female family members of inpatients who were admitted to one of the major teaching hospitals in Taichung, Taiwan in spring 1999. These women were asked to return the questionnaire to the nurse's station after they completed the survey. The response rate was 78% (125/160). Those who declined participation gave reasons such as they were not interested or had a low literacy level.

Measurement Development to Assess Psychosocial Beliefs towards Screening

The survey consisted of items in six major categories: (1) prior screening experience; (2) perceived pros and cons of a cervical cancer screening; (3) perceived norms of screening; (4) perceived risk (susceptibility) to cervical cancer; (5) knowledge related to cervical cancer and its screening; and (6) demographic variables. The categories described above represented constructs derived from existing health behavioral theories and models. These included perceived pros/cons from the Transtheoretical Model (Prochaska, Norcross, & DiClemente, 1994), perceived norms from the Theory of Planned Behavior (Ajzen & Fishbein, 1980), and perceived risk (susceptibility) from the Health Belief Model (Rosenstock, 1974). In addition to the theoretical foundation, these constructs were chosen based upon evidence from

Table 1.1. Why women do not get screened - Determinants of cervical cancer screening

Determinants (Theories [a])	Description	Prioritiy	Empirical Evidence from Literature
Personal determinants			
Knowledge	Knowledge of cervical cancer, Pap screening, and guideline	More important More changeable	Neilson, 1998 Kelly, 1996 Pham, 1992 Huang, 1994
Beliefs			
Perceived susceptibility (HBM)	Perceived risk of cervical cancer	More important Less changeable	Neilson, 1998 Seow, 1995
Perceived benefits or pros (HBM, TTM)	Early detection	Less important More changeable	Neilson, 1998 CDC, 1998
Perceived barriers or cons (HBM, TTM)	Fear of procedure & detecting cancer	More important Less changeable	Neilson, 1998 CDC, 1998
	Embarrassment and discomfort	More important Less changeable	Kelly, 1996 Pham, 1992
	Physicians' sex	More important Less changeable	Seow, 1995
	Culture value of sexual activity	More important Less changeable	Yi, 1994; 1998 Buller, 1998
Attitudes toward cancer (TPB)	Little one can do Can't be prevent	More important More changeable	Pham, 1992 Seow, 1995
Self-efficacy expectation (HBM, SCT)	Communication	Less important Less changeable	Buller, 1998 CDC, 1998
Perceived norms (TPB)	Perceived norms of screening	More important Less changeable	Gotay, 1998
Demographics	Age, marital status	More important Less changeable	Yi, 1994, 1998
External determinants			
Accessibility Affordability	Accessibility & affordability to screenings	More important More changeable	Neilson, 1998 Marcus, 1998 Straton, 1995 Mandelblatt, 1993
Social support	Significant other support a screening	More important Less changeable	Burnett, 1995 Mickey, 1995 Suarez, 1994 Guidry, 1996 Gotay, 1998
Advise / feedback of health care professionals	Recommendation from physicians	More important More changeable	Pham, 1992 Yi, 1994

Notes: [a] Theories: HBM – Health Belief Model (Janz et al, 2002); TTM – Transtheoretical Model (Prochaska, et al., 1994); TPB – Theory of Planned Behavior (Ajzen, 1988); SCT – Social Cognitive Theory (Bandura, 1986).

existing literature that suggest their significant association with screening behaviors (see Table 1.1). Some pros/cons items were adapted from previous studies examined breast cancer screenings (Pearlman *et al.*, 97; Rakowski *et al.*, '92, '93, '97), with additional items developed from the focus groups conducted among women in Taiwan. Some of the knowledge items were adapted from an unpublished thesis by Huang (1994) from National Taiwan University. The remainder of knowledge items, susceptibility and perceived norms items were developed by the principal investigator, based on social and behavioral theories as well as focus group findings obtained from Chinese women. Scale items were developed in English, translated into Chinese, and back translated. Items on the two English versions were checked for discrepancies of meaning.

Pilot Testing the Preliminary Measurement

Before the pilot survey was administered, three focus groups were conducted to ensure the appropriateness and clarity of the items as well as to validate the specific constructs selected in the preliminary questionnaire. Based on the feedback from the focus group, appropriate revisions of the survey items were made. The final version of the needs assessment survey instrument consisted of 11 pros scale items, 11 cons scale items, 4 perceived norms scale items, 2 perceived risk items, and 17 knowledge scale items.

Scoring of the Scales

The items making up the perceived pros/cons, perceived norms, and susceptibility scales were 5-point Likert scale items. Item responses ranged from 1 (strongly disagree) to 5 (strongly agree). The total score calculated for each particular scale was the sum of the item scores in that scale. Knowledge scale items were scored one (1) if correct response were answered, and were scored zero (0) when an incorrect or "do not know" response were indicated.

Data Analysis

Chronbach alpha was used to calculate the internal consistencies of the various scales related to screening beliefs. Items with discrimination (corrected-item-total correlation CITC) less than 0.2 were re-evaluated for their appropriateness. Item difficulty (mean) was also used to evaluate knowledge scale items. Item means that fell in the range of 0.3~0.7 were considered moderately difficult items. Scales with Chronbach alpha above 0.70 were considered good reliabilities (Nunnally & Bernstein, 1994). Women who had never had a Pap smear test, had not had one in the past three years, or could not remember when their last Pap smear test was, were classified as screening non-participants. To help identify determinants of recent screening participation, demographic and screening beliefs were compared among screening participants vs. non-participants. Categorical variables were analyzed by cross-tabulations using chi-square statistics. Continuous variables were analyzed using t-tests in two-group comparisons. Variables with significant associations were included in the multivariate model. Logistic regression modeling was used to analyze the effect of each factor on screening participation, after adjusting for the confounding variables.

Results

Sample Characteristics

A total of 125 women completed the needs assessment survey. The mean age was 37.93 (SD=10.45). Most women in the sample were married (90%). About 62% of the women worked full time, and 32% of the women had college education level or higher (Fig. 1.1). There were no significant differences between screening participants and non-participants in age, employment status, or education. Marital status was the only variable that showed a significant association with recent cervical cancer screening participation (p=0.033). Screening non-participants were more likely to be women who reported themselves as "never-been married" (17.31% vs. 5.48%).

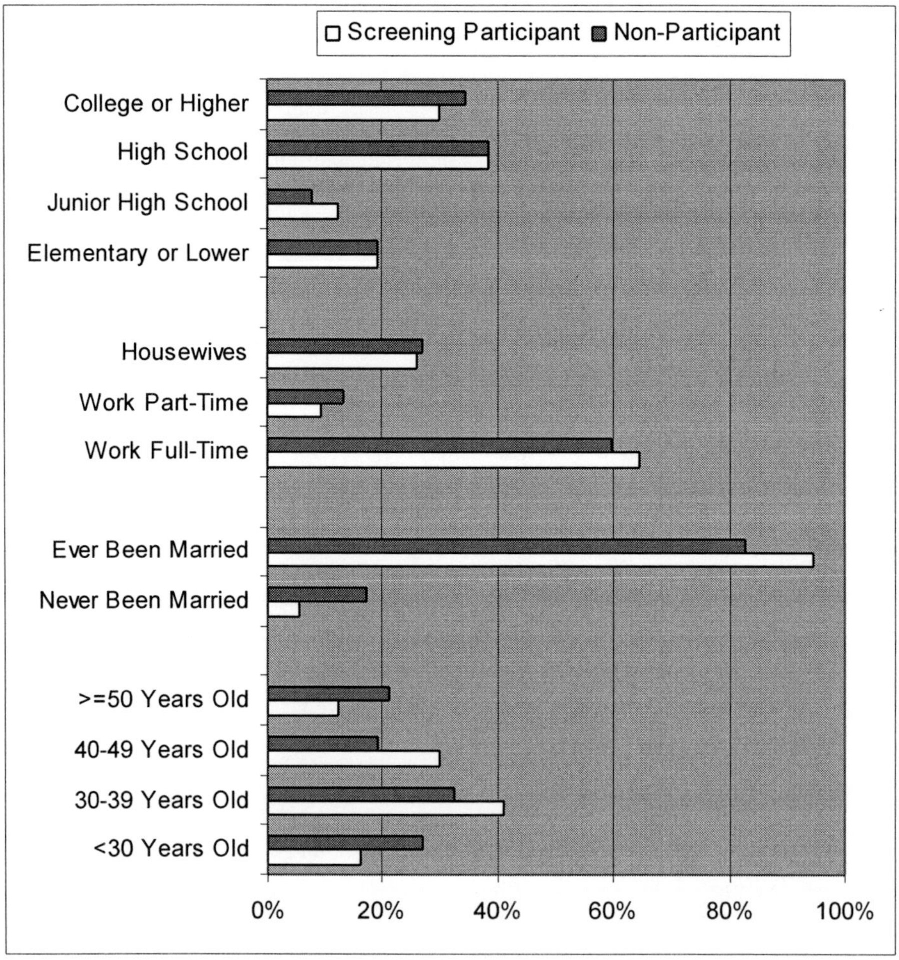

Fig. 1.1. Demographics of the women participated in the needs assessment survey (n=125). Notes: [a] Age was analyzed by t-test, marital status, employment, and education were analyzed by chi-square tests. [b] Ever Been Married: including married, divorce, separated, or widowed. [c] Marital status was the only demographic factor showed significantly difference between screening participants vs. non-participants (p<.05).

Seventy percent of the women (88/125) reported they had had a Pap smear test before. The mean number of prior Pap smear tests was 2.42 among these women. Only fifty-eight percent of the women (73/125) had received a recent Pap smear test (within the past three years). A higher proportion of screening participants (89%) reported an intention to have a Pap smear test in the coming year, as compared with screening non-participants (57%) (p=0.000).

Screening related Psychosocial and Knowledge Scales

Perceived pros, perceived norms, and perceived risk scale

Item discrimination analysis showed that perceived pros (α=0.8751; 11 items) and perceived norms (α=0.7158; 4 items) had good internal consistencies. Therefore, no revisions were made on these two scales. Two items included in the perceived risk (susceptibility) scales were "I might get cervical cancer at some point during my life," and "I feel that my chance of getting cervical cancer is high." Although perceived risk (susceptibility) scale had a Cronbach alpha of 0.6849, it was considered acceptable with only two items in the scale.

Perceived cons scale

Two items from the perceived cons scale, "cancer treatment is worse than the cancer itself" and "I would rather not know if I had cancer," were dropped from the scale analysis. Data also showed both items had low correlation with other cons items (CITC less than 0.2). It was determined that although these two items may represent barriers to screening, they were not specific "costs" or "cons" of a Pap smear test itself. The revised cons scale included 9 items with Chronbach alpha as 0.6817.

Knowledge scale

In the knowledge scale (17 items), the item "Cervical cancer can be detected early with Pap smear tests" was removed because almost all women (99%) answered this item correctly. The remaining items showed sufficient correlation with other items in the knowledge scale (CITC greater than 0.2). Therefore, the final revision of the knowledge scale consisted of 16 items (α=0.7010). In item difficulty analysis for knowledge scales, 11 (70%) had an item mean greater than 0.7, indicating that over 70% of the women in the sample answered these questions correctly. The remaining 5 items showed moderate difficulty (item mean ranged 0.3-0.7). Data showed that the knowledge scale was relatively easy for the study participants because it mixed 70% easy and 30% moderately difficult items (Table 1.2).

Multiple Logistic Regression Analysis

Marital status was included in the multiple logistic regression models as a co-variable since it revealed a significant association with cervical cancer screening participation in the demographic analysis. Data showed significant associations between all the scales and women's screening behavior ($p<.05$), controlled for marital status. The adjusted odds ratios (ORs) were 1.08, 0.87, 1.25, and 1.14 for perceived pros (benefits), cons (barriers), norms, and knowledge, respectively (Table 1.3).

Table 1.2. Item Difficulty Analysis of the Knowledge Scale in the Needs Assessment Survey.

Item	Percent correct	SD
Q42. Cervical cancer is the most common cancer among women in Taiwan. (T)	0.90	0.30
Q43. People having sex without condoms have higher risk of getting cervical cancer. (T)	0.50	0.50
Q44. Pap smear test is done through drawing your blood sample. (F)	0.89	0.32
Q45. Women who are post-menopausal do not need Pap smear tests. (F)	0.88	0.33
Q47. If you have early stage cervical cancer, you will feel pain. (F)	0.54	0.50
Q48. Women who do not have regular cervical cancer screenings are more likely to have advanced cervical cancer when they were diagnosed. (T)	0.62	0.49
Q49. After women stop having children, they do not need Pap smear tests. (F)	0.94	0.25
Q50. A Pap smear test is most effective when you have one every year or two. (T)	0.94	0.25
Q51. Healthy adult women should have a Pap test smear every year. (T)	0.94	0.23
Q52. A Pap smear test is not important for women like me. (F)	0.94	0.25
Q53. Only women who have had many sex partners need to get a Pap smear test. (F)	0.93	0.26
Q54. A Pap smear test only finds problems when they are too far along to be treated. (F)	0.41	0.49
Q55. A Pap smear test is necessary even if there is no family history of cancer. (T)	0.92	0.27
Q56. Once I have a negative Pap smear test, I do not need to have any more. (F)	0.95	0.21
Q57. I need a Pap smear test only when I experience vaginal bleeding other than menstruation. (F)	0.92	0.27
Q58. A Pap smear test is the same thing as a cervix biopsy. (F)	0.59	0.49

Note: (T) – true statement; (F) – false statement.
Internal consistency of the knowledge scale (Cronbach alpha) = 0.7010 (16-items).

Table 1.3. Multiple Logistic Regression: Effect of each factor on screening adherence, adjusting for marital status

	Adjusted for marital status	
Scales	Odds Ratio	95% Confidence Interval
Pros	1.08*	(1.01, 1.16)
Cons	0.87*	(0.80, 0.95)
Norm	1.25*	(1.04, 1.50)
Knowledge	1.15*	(1.01, 1.30)

Note: Dependent variable: having a cervical cancer screening in the past three years.
* P values (Wald F test) <.05.

Discussion and Lessons Learned

All the scales used in this needs assessment revealed acceptable reliabilities with Cronbach alphas ranged 0.68 – 0.88. The cons scale had lower internal consistency (α=0.68). Developing or rewording existing items may strengthen the cons scale in the future. In addition, the survey only contained two items that measured women's perceived risk of getting cervical cancer. According to Nunnally & Bernstein (1994), a reliable measure of a construct should consist of at least 3 items. Additional items will need to be developed to make perceived susceptibility into a reliable scale.

This study revealed that 30% of the women had never had a Pap smear test. Wang and Lin (1996) surveyed women in Taipei in 1993, and found that 40% of the sampled women had never had a Pap smear test. The prior study was conducted 6 years before this needs assessment. The difference in findings may be due to the increases in accessibility of the screening through universal coverage of health insurance in Taiwan since 1996. Still, 30% represents a large proportion of women who had not been screened regularly. The needs assessment data indicated that recent cervical cancer screening rate was 58%. Other studies have found lower rates (Lee & Chou, 1997). A larger study is recommended to determine the true rate of screening among a representative sample of women in Taiwan.

Our results indicated that women's intention to have a Pap smear test was strongly associated with their screening status. This association is consistent with the Theory of Reasoned Action (Ajzen & Fishbein, 1980), which emphasizes the role of intention in health behavior. Although the direction of the relationship between intention and screening behavior was not explained, preliminary results indicated that future interventions designed to influence women's intention to have a Pap smear test could have an impact on screening behavior.

Marital status was the only demographic factor significantly associated with women's participation in cervical cancer screening. Similar findings were reported in Yi's (1998) study. Women who had never been married were less likely than currently and previously married women to have had a cervical cancer screening. It is possible that Chinese women, regardless of their age, believe that Pap smear test is necessary or appropriate only if they are or have been married. A comment from one of the participants in the focus group illustrated this perception well, "... age was not an issue. If I got married, I would have had a Pap".

Some never-been-married women from the focus group expressed the feeling as follows: "I want to keep my body as a whole. Especially in Chinese culture, we tend to view this as a very important thing." Several women even brought up the issue that doctors might be unwilling to perform a Pap smear test for girls who were not sexually active because they were afraid of being sued by girls' parents. Within the Asian culture, virginity is highly valued and can influence a woman's social status as well as her own self-esteem. The results of this study underscored the importance of considering cultural beliefs when designing interventions for cervical cancer screening.

Data from this needs assessment indicated that knowledge, perceived screening benefits, barriers, and screening norms were all significantly associated with prior screening participation. These significant associations were consistent with existing empirical evidence or theories (Lee & Chou, 1997; Ajzen & Fishbein, 1980; Gotay, 1998). Women who had a recent Pap smear test tended to have higher knowledge, perceived benefits (pros) and lower perceived barriers (cons), and higher screening norms. Such results suggest that effective intervention efforts should address these perceptions to increase perceived benefits as well as decrease perceived barriers (such as embarrassment, discomfort, nervousness, culture belief of sexuality, gender of physician, and lack of doctor's recommendation or reminder) of the cervical cancer screening. In addition, intervention development should also consider addressing women's perceptions on how other women behave in order to improve screening participation.

Limitations

One of the limitations in the study involves sample recruitment as well as the small sample size. Since all of the women voluntarily agreed to participate in the study, volunteer bias may exist. Study participants were recruited from female family members of inpatients who were admitted to the hospital during the data collection period. Since women were obtained from a hospital setting, it is possible that these women were more familiar with the health care system than women in the general population. These women may be different in that they were more open to health related information or they may be more likely to have ever been screened.

Similar to many other studies, this study relies on self-reported screening and might not reflect actual behavior. Since women could receive care from a wide variety of health care facilities in Taiwan, validation of their self-reported screening through medical record was not feasible. Still, evidence suggests that self-report for Pap smear test is valid (Suarez, Goldman, & Weiss, 1995). It is possible that social desirability bias could exist in self-reported screening behavior (Hancock, Sanson-Fisher, & Kentish, 1998). Self-report measurement might result in classifying some screening non-participants incorrectly thus over estimating the numbers of women had a recent Pap smear tests. On the other hand, the probability of classifying screening participants into non-participant group was low. A previous research has shown that when women reported screening non-participation, the majority were correct (95%) (Walter *et al.*, 1988). Therefore, since the screening participants group consisted of some non-participants, the actual difference between the two-group comparisons should be larger than what was shown by the study results.

In summary, in addition to identifying various screening-associated factors, this needs assessment study provides an important foundation for measuring these constructs in scales developed for Chinese women. Although some items were specifically created for Chinese culture, the results suggested that theory-based psychosocial constructs could be universally relevant. Larger studies are recommended to provide further confirmation of these relationships. Intervention efforts which address perceived pros, cons, norms, and knowledge related to cervical cancer screening could potentially impact women's screening participation in the future.

PHASE II: INTERVENTION DEVELOPMENT USING INTERVENTION MAPPING (IM), AN INNOVATIVE PROCESS OF DESIGNING EFFECTIVE INTERVENTION

Overview

This article describes the development of a program to increase cervical cancer screening behavior among Chinese women. Intervention mapping, an innovative process of intervention design, guided the development of this program. The development process integrated important factors influencing cervical cancer screening behavior relevant to Chinese women identified in the needs assessment in phase I. This phase specifically focused on the theoretical and empirical underpinning of the program and how qualitative and quantitative findings informed the intervention development. IM helped ensure that theory and evidence guided (a) the identification of psychosocial and environmental determinants relevant to cancer screening behavior, and (b) the selection of the most appropriate methods and strategies to address the identified determinants. The program used direct-mail communication as the main delivery channel. Methods used included information transmission, modeling, persuasion, and facilitation. Strategies used included role model stories and testimonials, and a telephone-counseling component. The delineation of specific plans for implementation and evaluation are also described in this phase. Details of the evaluation of program effectiveness are described in Phase III.

Significance

There are a few studies that have applied constructs from various social and behavioral science theories to guide the needs assessment and development of interventions to increase cervical cancer screening (Dignan, 1994; Earp, Altpeter, & Mayne, 1995). However, details were lacking pertaining to how the programs were designed and developed. There was also a lack of information regarding program linkage to specific intermediate outcomes that influence health behavior. Programs labeled *culturally sensitive*, for example, usually do not specify whether any formative research preceded program development or how the program addressed cultural needs. There is often no description of how the intervention methods were selected and why. A review conducted by Marcus & Crane (1998) among 65 cancer education programs for adult women across the United States showed that the target audience, the message being delivered, and the action being urged were often not clear in many materials they reviewed.

This phase of the chapter describes the development of a program called "*Love yourself before you take care of your family.*" It was designed to increase cervical cancer screening behavior specifically for Chinese women living in Taiwan. It was developed using Intervention Mapping, an innovative process of program intervention design (Bartholomew, Parcel, Kok, & Gottlieb, 2006). Intervention Mapping is a detailed process that provides explicit step-by-step guidance for planning and designing theory- and evidence-based health education programs. It intends to integrate theory, empirical findings from literature, and new data collected from study participants in the design of an intervention. IM has been used to develop intervention programs for a variety of health behaviors, including asthma management (Bartholomew et al., 2000), nutrition (Cullen, Bartholomew, Parcel, & Kok, 1998), sun protection (Tripp, Herrmann, Parcel, Chamberlain, & Gritz, 2000), and HIV and pregnancy prevention (van Empelen, Kok, Schaalma, & Bartholomew, 2003). This was the first program that used IM to develop a theory and evidence-informed program to increase cervical cancer screening.

Methods

Intervention Mapping (IM)

All of the six IM steps are described in this chapter: needs assessment, preparation of change objective matrices, selection of theoretic methods and practical strategies, program design, implementation planning, and evaluation (Bartholomew et al., 2006). This phase specifically focused on the theoretical and empirical underpinning of the program and how qualitative and quantitative findings informed intervention development. IM helped ensure that theory and evidence guided (a) the identification of psychosocial and environmental determinants related to cancer screening behavior, and (b) the selection of the most appropriate methods and strategies to address the identified determinants. Details of the evaluation of program are described in Phase III.

Step 1 - Conducting Needs Assessment

Intervention mapping depends on a thoroughly conducted needs assessment that specifies the problem of interest. To better design the program, we conducted a needs assessment to assess factors that influence cervical cancer screening behavior among Taiwanese women. The needs assessment consisted of both quantitative and qualitative assessment: a quantitative survey and qualitative focus group interviews exploring and assessing factors important to cancer screening behaviors. Details of the quantitative needs assessment survey is described in Phase I of the study. The needs assessment provided information on salient factors influencing screening behavior, such as knowledge, perceived pros and cons, and perceived norms. The information was used to guide the development of the current intervention. The purpose of the qualitative focus group interviews was to provide direction for the design of the program intervention approaches, concepts, messages, as well as explore potential factors influencing screening behaviors. Three focus groups were conducted during the pilot study (*N*= 24). Women were recruited from churches and community centers in Taiwan, through local community key informants. A semi-structured protocol with open-ended and probing questions was used to explore potential behavioral and environmental factors that might influence women's screening behavior in this particular population. Possible intervention ideas and strategies were also collected. The program theme "*Love yourself before you take care of your family*" was identified through the focus group discussions.

Step 2 - Creating Matrices of Change Objectives

This step provides the foundation for the program intervention by specifying who and what would change as a result of the intervention. The program change objectives are specific statements of what individuals need to learn or what must be changed in the environment related to the determinants in order for the performance objectives to be met. A series of matrices of change objectives, which combine performance objectives for cervical cancer screening behavior with selected personal and external determinants, are created to guide the intervention development.

Performance Objectives

In this program, our goal was to increase the cervical cancer screening adherence among women in Taiwan. The performance objectives are objectives that break down the behavior objectives to smaller steps. For example, in this case, they described what a woman needs to do in order to obtain a Pap smear test. Two behavioral performance objectives were delineated in this program (Table 2.1):

Behavioral Performance Objective 1: Screening non-adherent women (women who have not had a screening in the previous 12 months) will schedule a Pap smear test within 3 months.

Behavioral Performance Objective 2: Screening non-adherent women will obtain a Pap smear test within 3 months.

The environment could have an impact on individuals' behavior as well. The needs assessment phase indicated that common environmental factors influencing cervical cancer screening included cost, access (i.e., lack of physician referral), transportation, lack of child care, and gender of the physician (Centers for Disease Control and Prevention, 1998; Seow, Wong, Smith, & Lee, 1995; Yi, 1994). Issues regarding cost and access to screenings were not brought up by the focus group, probably because for women aged 30 and older in Taiwan, an annual Pap smear test is covered by the nation-wide universal insurance. One of the major environmental factors influencing screening brought up by women from the focus group were their preference to have a female provider perform the exam as most gynecologists are males in Taiwan. Environmental performance objectives describe what would change in the environment as a result of the program, and who would effect the change. To address the issues of availability of female providers for screening, the program included the following two environmental performance objectives (Table 2.1):

Environmental Performance Objective 1: Hospital administrators will approve the provision of Pap smear tests by female physicians in the community.

Environmental Performance Objective 2: Female physicians will commit to providing Pap smear tests in the community.

Determinants of Behavioral and Environmental Factors

The analysis from our needs assessment revealed several significant factors associated with cervical cancer screening participation. These included knowledge, perceived pros and cons to screening, and perceived norms about screening as demonstrated in Phase I study (Hou, Fernandez, Parcel, & Chen, 2003). These results were consistent with previous research findings (Gotay & Wilson, 1998; Neilson & Jones, 1998; Rakowski, Dube, Marcus,

& Abrams, 1992). Compared with screening non-participants, women received a recent Pap smear test tended to perceive higher benefits for screening and lower barriers to obtaining regular Pap smear tests. They were also more knowledgeable about cervical cancer and Pap smear tests and tended to perceive that other women obtain annual Pap smear tests. Some of the reasons women gave for non-participation at cervical screening included the beliefs that the test was unnecessary and that they were not at risk (low perceived susceptibility). In our focus group discussions, some women said that screening reminders could also help them to take action (cues to action).

During the focus group discussion, many women expressed that they did not have the intention to obtain Pap smear tests. They expressed they did not think that cervical cancer screening was necessary or relevant to their health. This data implied that intention as well as perceptions that cancer screening is necessary and relevant for their health could be important factors influencing women's decision to be screened.

The final list of determinants of the behavioral and environmental factors was compiled from previous studies, existing social and behavioral theories, and additional factors identified through the needs assessment. To prioritize the hypothesized determinants, an expert panel was consulted on the degree to which determinants were more important and changeable. The identified determinants included knowledge, perceived pros and cons from the Transtheoretical Model (Prochaska, Norcross, & DiClemente, 1994), perceived norms and intention from the Theory of Planned Behavior (Ajzen & Fishbein, 1980), and perceived susceptibility and cues to action from the Health Belief Model (Rosenstock & Krischt, 1974). Similarly, we identified factors influencing the Environmental Performance Objectives 1 and 2. These factors included knowledge, outcome expectations, and rewards and/or compensation.

Matrix of Change Objectives

To ensure that the supporting theoretical and empirical findings were appropriately applied in the intervention, we constructed an intervention matrix of change objectives for the program (see Table 2.1). This matrix was created by crossing the performance objectives with the selected determinants. The first row of the matrix listed critical behavioral determinants such as intention, knowledge, perceived susceptibility, perceived benefits and/or barriers (pros and cons), perceived norms, and cues to action. The performance objectives were presented in the left-hand column. Each cell in the matrix described the change objectives for the cancer-screening program. For example, for the performance objective of "schedule a screening," one of the change objectives regarding knowledge was that women could identify locations and schedules where a Pap smear test screening was offered. A change objective regarding "cues to action" was that women would receive screening reminders from the project staffs. The matrix of the change objectives served as a blue print to guide the program intervention development.

Table 2.1. Matrix of Change Objectives

Behavioral Objective: Screening non-adherent women will obtain a Pap smear test after 3 months of the intervention.							
	Personal Determinants						*External Determinants*
Performance Objectives (POs)	**Intention**	**Knowledge**	**Perceived benefits (pros)**	**Perceived barriers (cons)**	**Perceived norms**	**Perceived susceptibility**	**Cue to action**
PO1: Schedule a Pap smear test		1a) Identify locations and schedules that a Pap test screening is offered.	1b) State benefits of having an annual Pap. 1c) Point that scheduling an appointment is important to ensure that she will obtain a Pap.	1d) Set time aside to schedule a Pap. 1e) Obtain clinic's phone number.	1f) Express that other women like her call to schedule a Pap.	1g) Identify themselves at risk of getting cervical cancer.	1h) Women receive screening reminder from the program staffs.
PO2: Obtain a Pap smear test	2a) Express intention to obtain a Pap.	2b) Describe the Pap test procedure. 2c) List the "don'ts" before obtaining a Pap exam.	2d) Identify a Pap test can detect cell changes before they become cancerous. 2e) Define that regular Pap screening can help women find cancer early.	2f) Predict less embarrassment about having a Pap screening. 2g) Recognize her right to ask for a female nurse to be present during the procedure.	2I) Indicate that other women like her obtain their annual Pap. 2j) Review Pap screening as a routine medical procedure.		
Environmental Objective: Increased availability of alternative service by female doctors.							
	Personal Determinants			*External Determinants*			
Performance Objectives	**Knowledge**	**Outcome expectations**		**Reward/Compensation**			
PO1: Hospital administrators approve	1a) Hospital administrators recognize the importance of providing the alternative service.	1b) Hospital will receive good reputation in providing the outreach service. 1c) More community people will visit the hospital.		1d) Hospital will receive positive feedback from the community.			
PO2: Female doctor sign up the duty	2a) Relate that women prefer female doctor to perform the Pap exam.	2b) Women will show up in the outreach screening service. 2c) Community will appraise her and more women/patients would choose her at the hospital.		2d) Doctors will get compensation by signing up for the duty.			

Step 3 – Selecting Theory-based Methods and Practical Strategies

In this step, we created an inventory of theory-based intervention methods to address the program change objectives, developed in the previous step. Methods and strategies for the cervical cancer screening program were selected based on findings of the needs assessment, the objectives for the program, theory or findings from other studies, and the resources available. Methods selected for the program included information transmission, modeling, persuasion, and facilitation. Intervention strategies planned included direct mail communication, role-model stories and testimonies, and phone counseling. The following section describes how these methods were chosen and how they were translated into practical strategies arranged by the following three major categories of change objectives: (a) knowledge-related change objectives, (b) belief-related change objectives (i.e., intention, perceived pros and cons, norms, and susceptibility), and (c) environment related change objectives (i.e., cues to action and availability). See Table 2.2 for more details.

Table 2.2. Methods and Strategies

Change Objectives (COs)	Methods (Theory)	Strategies	Program Component	Descriptions/Messages
Knowledge determinate COs	1. Chunking & advance organizers (Theories of Information Processing) 2. Persuasive communication (PCM)	1. Use direct mail as a communication channel ; - Use question and answer format to guide what is to be learned and to aid memory. 2. Ensure attention, relevance & comprehension of the messages	1. Theory and evidence based cervical cancer brochure. 2. "Do you know" fact sheet.	1. See brochure (Fig. 2.1a & Fig. 2.1b). 2. Fact sheet about cervical cancer & Pap screening.
Intention, perceived pros/cons, susceptibility, and perceived norms determinate COs	1. Modeling (SCT) 2. Persuasive communication (PCM)	1..Modeling and persuasion through role model stories and reinforcement of the model 2. Persuasive communication (use stories, testimonials, and quotes from women in the target group to increase credibility and relevance)	1. Role model stories 2. Testimonials 3. "Do you know" factsheet 4. Women's quotes from Focus groups	1. See role model stories & testimonials (Fig. 2.2 ~ 2.4). 2. See fact sheet. 3. See women's sharing regards their Pap experience. (Fig. 2.5)
Cue to action & availability of alternative screening service	1. Facilitation (SCT)	1. Providing cues and enabling services. 2. Increase service accessibility 3. Increase availability of the screening.	1. Screening invitation letter 2. Doctor's schedule 3. Phone intervention 4. Community screening service provided by female doctor	1. Screening invitation letter 2. Telephone intervention to remind & schedule a Pap test

Notes: SCT: Social Cognitive Theory (Bandura, 1986)
PCM: Persuasion Communicaiton Matrix (McGuire, 1985)

Methods and Strategies Addressing Knowledge-Related Change Objectives

To influence knowledge-related change objectives, the primary method used was information transmission, which aimed at gaining attention as well as comprehension of factual messages (McGuire, 1984). The direct-mail educational communication was chosen as the primary intervention strategy because it could reach all of the target women and allowed them to read the information at their leisure. Compared with other kinds of intervention strategies, the direct-mail newsletter campaign is relatively inexpensive both in production and in delivery. The direct-mail newsletter campaign is also typically more effective in recruiting high-risk women than are mass media campaigns and is less expensive than personal contact (Dignan, Michielutte, Jones-Lighty, & Bahnson, 1994).

Components included in the direct-mail campaign were newsletters, cancer fact sheets, educational brochures, and pamphlets. These components contained information on the benefits of cervical cancer screening, a description of the Pap smear test procedure, and recommendations about the frequency of screening. The prevalence, risk factors, and signs and/or symptoms of cervical cancer were also provided. All of the educational materials used plain language and were printed in colors with an attractive layout. In addition, question and answer format were used to guide what was to be learned and to aid memorization (Fig. 2.1a & Fig. 2.1b).

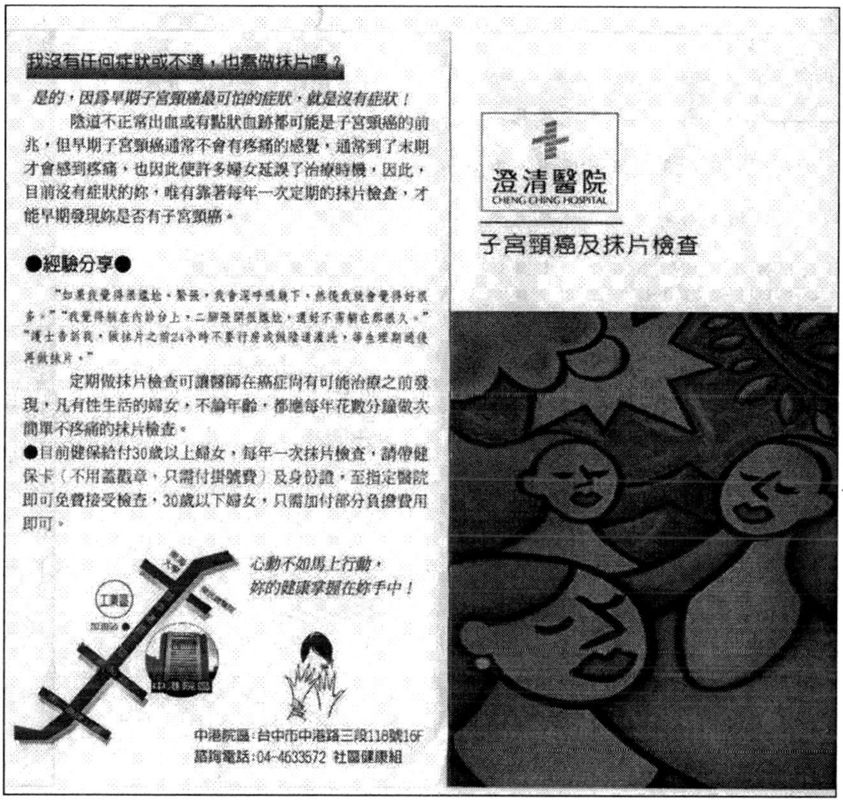
我沒有任何症狀或不適，也需做抹片嗎？
是的，因為早期子宮頸癌最可怕的症狀，就是沒有症狀！
陰道不正常出血或有點狀血跡都可能是子宮頸癌的前兆，但早期子宮頸癌通常不會有疼痛的感覺，通常到了末期才會感到疼痛，也因此使許多婦女延誤了治療時機，因此，目前沒有症狀的妳，唯有靠著每年一次定期的抹片檢查，才能早期發現妳是否有子宮頸癌。
●經驗分享●
定期做抹片檢查可讓醫師在癌症尚有可能治療之前發現，凡有性生活的婦女，不論年齡，都應每年花數分鐘做次簡單不疼痛的抹片檢查。
●目前健保給付30歲以上婦女，每年一次抹片檢查，請帶健保卡（不用蓋戳章，只需付掛號費）及身份證，至指定醫院即可免費接受檢查，30歲以下婦女，只需加付部分負擔費用即可。
心動不如馬上行動，
妳的健康掌握在妳手中！
中港院區:台中市中港路三段118號16F
諮詢電話:04-4633572 社區健康組
澄清醫院
CHENG CHING HOSPITAL
子宮頸癌及抹片檢查

Fig. 2.1a. Cervical cancer and screening brochure (outside - front and back).

Methods and Strategies Addressing Belief-Related Change Objectives

Modeling and persuasion were chosen to influence women's intention, perceived susceptibility, perceived pros and cons, and perceived norms about cervical cancer screenings. According to Bandura (1986), modeling is one of the most powerful ways to transmit values and beliefs. Because modeling is most effective if the target women can identify with the models (Bandura, 1986; McAlister, 1995), models were selected from the same demographic group as the target women in order to increase familiarity and similarity. Models that are similar to the target population may communicate their message more effectively than those who are not. Using the matrix of the change objectives as a guide (Table 2.1), we searched focus group data for appropriate stories and themes.

Persuasion was another method used to influence women's beliefs about cervical cancer screening. Persuasive communication is a very powerful way of influencing people and bringing about behavior change and can be defined as a non-coercive influence on the perceived value of particular behaviors (McGuire, 1984). According to Bandura (1986), a very important part of persuasive communication is changing perceptions about how behaviors are viewed.

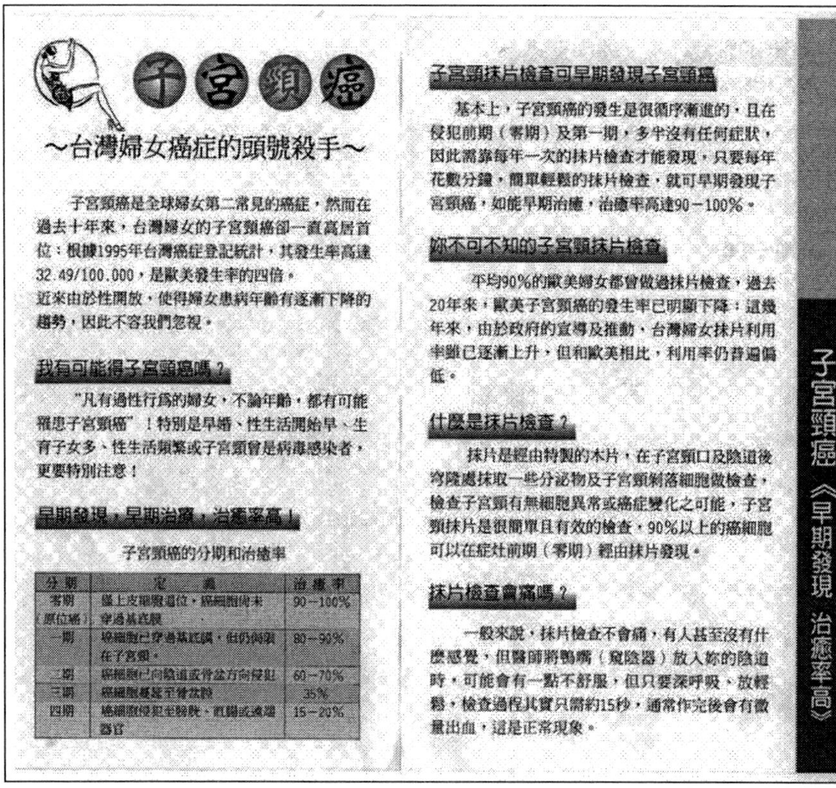
子宮頸癌

~台灣婦女癌症的頭號殺手~

子宮頸癌是全球婦女第二常見的癌症，然而在過去十年來，台灣婦女的子宮頸癌卻一直高居首位：根據1995年台灣癌症登記統計，其發生率高達32.49/100.000，是歐美發生率的四倍。
近來由於性開放，使得婦女患病年齡有逐漸下降的趨勢，因此不容我們忽視。

我有可能得子宮頸癌嗎？

"凡有過性行爲的婦女，不論年齡，都有可能罹患子宮頸癌"！特別是早婚、性生活開始早、生育子女多、性生活頻繁或子宮頸曾是病毒感染者，更要特別注意！

早期發現，早期治療，治癒率高！

子宮頸癌的分期和治癒率

分期	定義	治癒率
零期（原位癌）	鱗上皮細胞還位，癌細胞尚未穿過基底膜	90－100%
一期	癌細胞已穿過基底膜，但仍侷限在子宮頸。	80－90%
二期	癌細胞已向陰道或骨盆方向侵犯	60－70%
三期	癌細胞擴展至骨盆壁	35%
四期	癌細胞侵犯至膀胱、直腸或遠端器官	15－20%

子宮頸抹片檢查可早期發現子宮頸癌

基本上，子宮頸癌的發生是很循序漸進的，且在侵犯前期（零期）及第一期，多半沒有任何症狀，因此需靠每年一次的抹片檢查才能發現，只要每年花數分鐘，簡單輕鬆的抹片檢查，就可早期發現子宮頸癌，如能早期治療，治癒率高達90－100%。

妳不可不知的子宮頸抹片檢查

平均90%的歐美婦女都曾做過抹片檢查，過去20年來，歐美子宮頸癌的發生率已明顯下降；這幾年來，由於政府的宣導及推動，台灣婦女抹片利用率雖已逐漸上升，但和歐美相比，利用率仍普遍偏低。

什麼是抹片檢查？

抹片是經由特製的木片，在子宮頸口及陰道後穹窿處抹取一些分泌物及子宮頸剝落細胞做檢查，檢查子宮頸有無細胞異常或癌症變化之可能，子宮頸抹片是很簡單且有效的檢查，90%以上的癌細胞可以在症狀前期（零期）經由抹片發現。

抹片檢查會痛嗎？

一般來說，抹片檢查不會痛，有人甚至沒有什麼感覺，但醫師將鴨嘴（窺陰器）放入妳的陰道時，可能會有一點不舒服，但只要深呼吸、放輕鬆，檢查過程其實只需約15秒，通常作完後會有微量出血，這是正常現象。

子宮頸癌《早期發現 治癒率高》

Fig. 2.1b. Cervical cancer and screening brochure (Inside).

The program used role-model stories to convey positive values and persuasive messages related to annual Pap smear test. For example, in one story, Ms. Liu (28 years old) expressed that she now realized how important and beneficial a Pap smear test was for her health. She said that she felt confident that she could set time aside for a Pap smear test every year. Ms. Liu was a young working woman with two children. Although she was very busy with work, family, and kids, she made getting an annual Pap smear test her priority. Ms. Liu understood the perceived benefits and of setting time aside for a Pap smear test, and overcame her perceived lack of time to have a regular Pap smear test. [Figure 2.2]

Another woman, Ms. Chuang (36 years old), shared her experience of changing the way she thought about a Pap smear test:

> I was shocked when one of my close friends told me that she got cervical cancer. Her experience made me feel that I could get cervical cancer too [note from the author: perceived susceptibility]. I used to use laziness, no time for a Pap smear test, or "I won't be the one getting cancer" as excuses from obtaining a screening, but now I get a Pap smear test every year. I need to take care of myself so that I can take care of my family.

Everyone has time to stay healthy. Cervical cancer is not a disease that is far away. You could get it as well. [Figure 2.3]

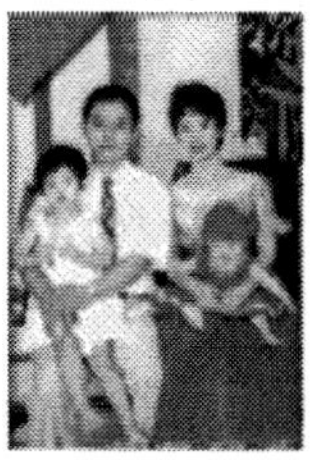

即使未滿30歲…

已婚或有性生活的的妳
也需要抹片檢查

劉太太

南屯區，28 歲，目前是全職職業婦女

我24歲結婚，我第一次做抹片是產後檢查，我想多了解自己的身體狀況，所以每年都定期檢查，至今已4年了。抹片檢查不會痛，雖然我還很年輕，但我不會覺得不好意思，不過每次檢查前還是會有點緊張，還好做抹片的過程很快，只需幾秒鐘就好了。

抹片檢查是很簡單的子宮頸癌症篩檢，可以在癌症早期還有可能治癒的時候就偵測出來，定期做抹片可讓我對我的健康放心，我的丈夫也很贊成我做抹片。他覺得我每年做抹片是我關心照顧自己健康及對家庭負責的一種表現。現在抹片篩檢已是非常例行的醫療檢查，我認識的人也認為子宮頸抹片檢查很重要，即使醫生沒有提醒，即使沒有陰道不適，我覺得抹片檢查也是必要的。

子宮頸癌是目前台灣婦女最常見的癌症，雖然我家族中沒有癌症的病史，但我覺得我在一生中仍有可能得到子宮頸癌。

預防勝於治療，
不要讓擔心害怕或不好意思造成你一生的遺憾！

社區健康諮詢電話：042-4633572
澄清醫院社區健康室 採訪製作 ©版權所有©

Figure 2.2 – (Ms. Lui, 28 years old) Even If You Are Under 30 Years Old, A Pap Smear Test Is Still Needed If You Are Married or Sexually Active.

抹片檢查 大家一起來!

莊媽媽

西屯區 *36*歲

我第一次做抹片是生完小孩，後來停了好長一段時間都沒有再檢查，因為抱著"反正我也不會得子宮頸癌"的心態，雖然我自己是護理人員，但我仍是覺得在別人面前脱褲子很不好意思，生產時是不得已，沒辦法。

三年前，我的學妹告訴我她得了子宮頸癌，我聽了很震驚，因為這就是真實在我身邊的人！她這麼年輕，才30歲出頭。印象中的她很乖、很認真、很聰明，我們唸書時她成績一直都是前幾名，我實在無法相信她會得子宮頸癌，她那陣子情緒一直很低落，我完全可以體會，要換成是我，我也很想去死。可是我很佩服她，她很勇敢的走過來，也調適的很好，我覺得假如我是她，我可能會受不了。

她的例子影響我很大，我開始每年定期做抹片，而且我也鼓勵我的朋友去做；我的孩子還這麼小，還有先生要我照顧，假如我得了子宮頸癌，那真是太可怕了，我可能不會考慮我自己，但我的孩子怎麼辦？我太在乎我的孩子了！

我的先生也很支持我做抹片，他和我説"醫生就是醫生，妳就去檢查，他們一天到晚都在看，為了健康，不要不好意思了，子宮頸癌的機率這麼高，電視常在講，只要有性生活，都有可能得到，妳可千萬別得到，妳要是怎麼樣，那我們家怎麼辦？"

子宮頸癌初期沒有什麼症狀，但子宮頸抹片檢查可以早期發現是否有子宮頸癌，早期治療治癒率可高達95%以上，檢查時會有一點點不舒服，不過一年只有一次，又不是時常做，總比死還好。所以為了健康，也為了那些關心妳的人，不要忘了你一年一次的抹片檢查，若是妳不想一個人去醫院，可以找個伴一起去做。

我的朋友聽了我學妹的例子，現在也都和我一樣每年定期做檢查。

妳也可以加入我們定期做抹片的行列！

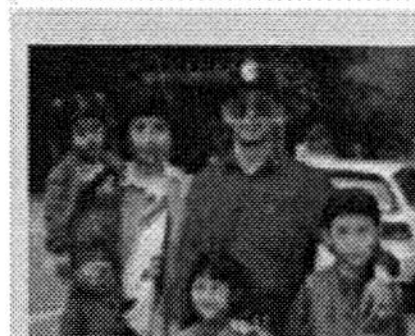

莊媽媽全家福

社區健康諮詢電話：042-4633572

澄清醫院社區健康室 採訪製作 ©版權所有©

Figure 2.3. (Ms. Chuang, 36 years old) Let's All Get a Pap Smear Test!

Testimonials were also used as a strategy for both modeling and persuasion. One example was Ms. Chao (65 years old), a cervical cancer survivor whose story included the following statements:

> Pap smear test could detect cervical cancer in the early stage. I had cervical cancer and had a surgery about one year ago. Now I am cured. I think all women should obtain regular Pap smear tests. Anyone can get cancer, and cervical cancer can be cured if you find it early [Figure 2.4].

By focusing on specific determinants, the theoretically derived role-model stories and testimonials served as a powerful communication channel to influence women's cancer screening decisions.

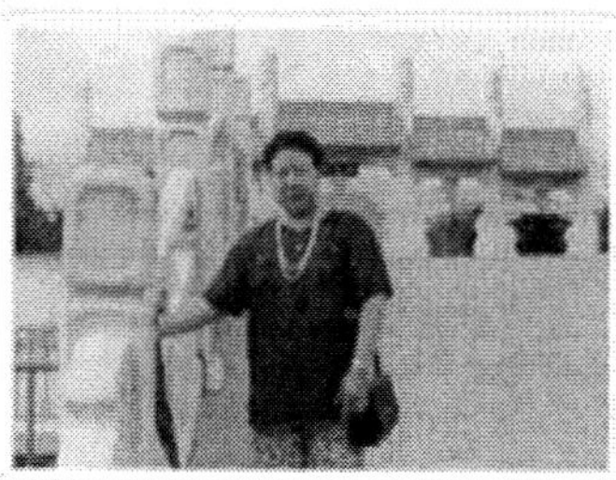

年紀大了，
更需要做抹片！

社區健康諮詢電話：042-4633572
澄清醫院社區健康室 採訪製作 ©版權所有©

趙媽媽 / 西屯區 · 65歲

我今年65歲。去年我和朋友一起去做健康檢查，結果醫師說子宮頸抹片結果好像有點問題，我半信半疑，我覺得我人很好，也沒什麼不舒服，本來我不想理它，但後來想想還是不放心，於是我又去另一家醫院檢查，那時我已比較有心理準備了（可能需要接受開刀）。醫師說還好只是癌症早期，去年5月，我做了子宮切除手術。

開刀到現在已一年多了，我沒有感覺任何不適，也不覺得自己是病人，也沒有怨天尤人，我覺得每個婦女都應去做抹片，沒有什麼不好意思。若生病了就更不得了。也不要以為老了就不用檢查，老了身體才要緊，所以不要緊張，也不要害怕，定期做抹片檢查，早期發現，早期治療，健康掌握在妳手中。

Figure 2.4. (Ms. Chao, 65 years old) A Pap Smear Test Is Even More Important When You Get Older.

Methods and Strategies Addressing Environment-Related Change Objectives

The results of the needs assessment indicated that environmental factors also influenced screening. Facilitation was used as a method to change the environment condition. The program increased access to screening services by providing a screening day with a female doctor at one of the community churches. To inform women about this service, a personalized screening invitation letter was mailed out along with directions to the church. Consistent with the Health Belief Model, the program provided "cues to action" (Rosenstock & Krischt, 1974). Women in the program also received a phone call to remind them to schedule screenings. Evening time slots were arranged for the screening to increase the accessibility for women.

Step 4 – Designing and Organizing Program

Designing Program Materials

The theme of the program was "Love yourself before you take care of your family." This theme addressed the importance of women's health. In Chinese culture, women are usually the caregivers for the whole family. Chinese women tend to sacrifice or ignore their health to take care of other family members. The theme emphasized and stressed the need for women to take care of themselves so that they can take care of their families. Sample intervention materials can be found in Figure 2.1~2.5.

個案#2
35歲／每年定期做，已四年了

關心家人，請先關心自己

每年定期抹片檢查很重要，我希望關心自己並關心另一半，我會特地安排時間做抹片，把它當成一件重要的事。

個案#3
34歲／過去1.2年，共做過2次

勇於愛自己—給婦女同胞多點勇氣

我有一位好友每年皆做抹片篩檢，結果在一次檢查中診斷為子宮頸癌前期而及早治療。我最需克服的是"懶"的去做這個因素，有朋友的例子後，馬上就克服了。我覺得子宮頸癌是身邊的事。不是電視上的事。

個案#4
39歲／四年前做第一次

妳的健康，是全家人的幸福

早期發現，早期治療，治癒率高；抹片檢查內容不複雜，有性生活及結婚的婦女都應定期檢查。

個案#13
31歲／每年一次

預防勝於治療『6分鐘護一生』

第一次是因產後40天，去婦產科回診，醫師順便幫我做抹片檢查。抹片檢查不痛，只是要尷尬一下下而已，我都告訴自己，反正醫師已經看膩了。

生孩子過後，比較不會害怕去婦產科內診，所以這是我敢去做的最主要因素，現在年齡漸大，越需要去做抹片，因生理機能、免疫力降低。

個案#14
31歲／去年第一次

愛自己就是愛你所愛的人，
保護自己，就是保護你所愛的人

去年做了第一次的抹片檢查，因為想了解自己的健康狀況，這是一種保護自己也保護自己所愛的人的方式，抹片檢查很簡單，很快就可檢查完畢。

Fig 2.5. Sample quotes from other women regarding their screening experience.

Pretest with the Target Group

One very important part of providing new information is to make sure that participants can understand the information given. The information provided in the brochure and the fact sheets was designed to simplify complex issues. The material was pre-tested with a group of women to make sure they understood the messages. Pre-testing print materials with the target audience is essential to receive feedback on attraction, comprehension, acceptability, self-involvement, and persuasion (Rice, 1991). The pretest result showed that most women were satisfied with the intervention content as well as with the layouts. Some women expressed their lack of knowledge regarding the screening procedure so that information was added to the material.

Program Theme:

"Love yourself before you take care of your family"

Scope and Sequence of the program:

1st month -
- personalized welcome letter
- cervical cancer/Pap brochure
- quotes of other women's experience
- screening schedule w/ doctors information

2nd month -
- personalized screening invitation letter
- screening service provided by female doctor
- role model stories
- knowledge-based fact sheet
- updated screening schedule

3rd month -
- phone intervention (reminder calls)
- reminding letters

Fig. 2.6. Scope and sequence of the cervical cancer screening program.

Scope and Sequence of the Program

The intervention lasted for 3 months. Female family members of inpatients admitted into one of the major teaching hospitals in Taichung, Taiwan, during fall of 1999 were interviewed about their screening status. Women who had not had a Pap smear test in the past 12 months were identified as screening non-adherent and were thus eligible to be recruited into the program. In the first month of the intervention program, women received a personalized welcome letter to the study, a theory- and evidence-based educational brochure, 14 quotes regarding other women's screening experiences, and a screening schedule with information about the doctors. In the second month, they received a personalized screening invitation letter with screening services provided by a female doctor in one of the community churches. Other materials included four role-model stories from adherent women and cervical cancer survivors, fact sheets regarding cervical cancer and Pap smear tests, and an updated screening schedule. In the third month, the program provided a phone consultation to remind women about the Pap smear tests and to help them schedule screening appointments (see Fig. 2.6).

Table 2.3. Adoption and Implementation Matrix

Adoption Matrix			
Adoption Performance Objectives	Determinants	Methods	Strategies
1. Hospital superintendent will review the propose program.	Knowledge and awareness Outcome Expectations	Attention Comprehension Persuasive Communication	Submission of the proposed program and expected outcomes
2. Hospital superintendent and the research review committee will consider the potential benefits of the program would worth investment.	Perceived benefits Perceived barriers	Persuasive Communication Goal setting Facilitation	Statistics on effectiveness of screening List of potential benefits both to the community and the hospital Identify existing resources and propose realistic budget
3. Hospital superintendent and the research review committee will approve funding of the program.	Outcome Expectations Expectancies	Shifting Perspective Previous Experience Contracting	Proposal submission Approval form
Implementation Performance Objectives	Determinants	Methods	Strategies
1. Program staffs will obtaining a group of non-adherent women	Knowledge Skills Self-efficacy	Information Modeling Cues to participate in training	Staff training on participant recruitment and identifying non-adherent women
2. Program staffs will schedule and mail the program intervention materials.	Knowledge Skills Self-efficacy	Demonstration Implementation guides Technical assistance	Staff training on protocols of scheduling and sending program materials
3. Program staffs will coordinate community screening services with female doctors.	Attitudes Team functioning Outcome expectations	Persuasive communication Skills training Advocacy	Information, persuasion, and negotiation with hospital superintendent. Provide incentives for female physicians agreed to provide services
4. Program staffs will conduct screening reminding calls to women in the program.	Self-efficacy Expectancies Logistics	Skill building with guided practice Reinforcement Persuasive communication	Providing phone call record sheets Staff training on protocols of conducting phone consultation.
5. Program staffs will mail the post-intervention surveys.	Self-efficacy Outcome expectations Reinforcement	Demonstration Feedback Reinforcement	Staff training on protocols of conducting post intervention mailed survey.

Step 5 – Program Implementation

This step aims to ensure an acceptable level of completeness and fidelity with program delivery. Planning can help identify dissemination strategies. In order to reach the aims, the intervention mapping suggests the need to develop an implementation plan, which includes adoption and implementation objectives, methods, strategies, and a training program to help create the workflow and documentation plans. Intervention mapping steps again serve as a guide to the development of the program implementation (Table 2.3).

Program delivery tasks would include obtaining a group of non-adherent women, scheduling and mailing the program intervention materials, coordinating community screening services with female doctors, and conducting screening reminding calls to women in the program. The program would provide training sessions on how to recruit and identify non-adherent women.

Program staffs would also be trained on how to schedule and send program materials, as well as how to conduct a telephone consultation.

Step 6 – Program Evaluation

Intervention mapping helps not only the design of an intervention program but also the specification of the evaluation measures. The purpose of this step was to determine whether decisions made about changing objectives, methods, strategies, and implementation were correct at each mapping step through program monitoring and evaluation. This intervention program was evaluated through a controlled randomized intervention trial.

Through referring to the matrices of change objectives, we developed several effect evaluation questions to measure the effectiveness of screening adoption and changes on cervical cancer screening related psychosocial beliefs and knowledge. Previous steps of intervention mapping and needs assessment also helped us in identifying process evaluation items to assess the completeness and fidelity of program delivery. For example, as part of the process evaluation, women in the intervention group were asked about program reach or exposures, reaction towards intervention materials, and questions related to methods and strategies assumptions. In addition, questions related to program implementation were asked among program staffs (see Table 2.4). Information about any cervical cancer screening–related community activities or media events was gathered to better explain possible threats to the internal validity of the study. Detailed program evaluation results of the controlled randomized trial are described in Phase III.

Discussion and Lessons Learned

By using the process of intervention mapping, the program developer was able to ensure systematical incorporation of empirical and new data and theories to guide the intervention design. The needs assessment provided an important foundation for this program by specifically identifying factors that influence cervical cancer screening behavior and environment conditions relevant for the Chinese women. Incorporating input from the target population throughout the process was essential. The process also helped the development of an evaluation plan, including the identification of specific research questions and the development of measures. The effectiveness of the intervention demonstrated that developing a program using a systematic process leads to the development of an effective program. Programs targeting other health-related behavior and using other methods or strategies can also be developed with this intervention mapping process.

Table 2.4. Effect and process evaluation questions

Effect evaluation questions (assessed among all screening non-adherent women at the post intervention) - Did you women schedule a Pap test during the past 3 months? If yes, where did you go? - What were your reasons to obtain a Pap test? - Did knowledge, perceived susceptibility, perceived pros and cons, and perceived norms changed after the intervention? (measured by various scales, see Appendix: Research instrument)
Process evaluation questions (assessed among women in the intervention group at the post intervention) - Did you receive our mailing information about cervical cancer and Pap screening in the past 3 months? - Did you read the information? - What did you think of the role model stories in the newsletters? - How often can you relate those role-model stories to yourself? - Has a program staff member contacted you for a Pap test arrangement in the past month? - Which program components were most effective in influencing your decision to have a Pap test? - Other open-ended questions included: (a) How do you feel about using direct mail to provide health information? (b) How can direct mail communication influence your health behavior? (c) How do you think other women's experience can influence your Pap decision? (d) How do you think a screening invitation letter or a reminding call can influence your Pap decision?
Program delivery evaluation questions (assessed among program staffs during the program implementation) - How many screening non-adherent women were you able to identify? - Did you schedule and mail program intervention material to women? - Did you organize a community screening service with a female doctor for women? - Did you offer a screening consultation call to women? - How were women's responses to the program service? - How many women were you not able to contact?

PHASE III: PROGRAM EVALUATION USING A CONTROLLED-RANDOMIZED INTERVENTION TRIAL

Overview

This phase of the study describes the effectiveness of a theory-based direct mail campaign to encourage screening non-adherent women, aged 30 and older, or younger if married, to obtain a Pap smear test. Participants were female family members of inpatients admitted to one of the major teaching hospitals in Taiwan during August - September 1999. A total of 424 women were recruited in the randomized intervention trial. Three months following implementation of the intervention, women in the intervention group reported a higher rate of cervical cancer screening than women in the comparison group (50% versus 32%) (p=0.002). Women in the intervention group also showed higher perceived pros of a Pap smear test at follow-up (p=0.031). Although women in both groups showed an increased knowledge and intention to obtain a screening, only the intervention group had significantly higher follow-up scores on perceived pros and susceptibility. The results showed that the intervention was effective in increasing cervical cancer screening among Chinese women within three months. The results also supported the use of Intervention Mapping, a systematic program development framework for planning effective interventions.

Significance

Although there are many educational interventions designed to increase Pap smear test utilization, few have targeted Chinese women. Intervention studies designed to increase screening have provided some information about methods and strategies that have been shown to be effective in other populations. For example, several studies have shown increased screening in response to written invitations (Byles, Redman, Sanson-Fisher, & Boyle, 1995; Bowman, Sanson-Fisher, Boyle, & Pope, 1995). However, another study found the invitation letter alone was not sufficient to encourage women to have a Pap smear test (Buehler & Parsons, 1997). Some study showed that mailed reminders combined with barrier counseling could significantly increase cervical cancer screening adherence (Lantz, Stencil, Lippert, Beversdorf, Jaros, & Remington, 1995; Taylor, et al, 2002). In a review article of cervical cancer screening intervention research, the authors suggested that direct mail may be especially effective in promoting screening when personalized letters or combined strategies were used (Marcus & Crane, 1998). The effectiveness of such strategies to increase screening compliance in Taiwan had not been studied. In addition, another gap in the literature is the lack of information describing the process regarding how information from behavioral studies examining the determinants of screening behavior can be translated into actual intervention methods and strategies.

As described earlier, the National Health Insurance Plan (1996) in Taiwan provides free health care coverage of annual Pap smear tests for women aged 30 and over. Married women under 30 are also entitled to this benefit with a small co-payment. Removing the cost barrier alone, however, does not ensure screening. It is clear that in Taiwan, although all women have access to free or low cost Pap smear test screening services, many do not utilize them. This paper describes a study to assess the effectiveness of an innovative intervention that addressed psychosocial factors influencing screening among women in Taiwan. The intervention was built on existing theories, empirical evidence, as well as findings from both qualitative and quantitative research with the target population (described in Phase I & II). The primary objective of this intervention trial was to assess the effectiveness of the intervention in encouraging non-adherent women (who had not had a Pap smear test within the preceding 12 months) to obtain a Pap smear test within 3 months. The secondary objectives are to assess the impact of the intervention on intermediate factors that might influence cervical cancer screening behavior, including perceived pros/cons of the Pap smear test, perceived norms, perceived susceptibility, and knowledge of cervical cancer and early detection.

Methods

Sample Selections

This study was conducted at one of the major teaching hospitals in Taichung, Taiwan. Female family members of inpatients admitted to the hospital during August and September 1999 were approached by program staff. A brief enrollment survey was conducted to determine women's screening status and eligibility. Women who had not had a Pap smear test in the previous 12 months and were aged 30 and older (or younger if married) were eligible for the study. Women were excluded from the study if they had undergone a hysterectomy or had been diagnosed with cervical cancer.

A total of 990 women were approached during the study period. Among these, 21 women (0.02%) had a previous hysterectomy. Among the remaining women, sixty-eight percent (656/969) reported they had not had a Pap smear test in the previous 12 months. Sixty-five percent (424/656) of these non-adherent women agreed to participate in the study. Those who declined participation (N=232) said that they were not interested or had low literacy level (Figure 3.1).

Study Design

This evaluation study used a true control group, pretest-posttest experiment design (Fig. 3.2). Women were randomly assigned to either intervention or control groups. Women with even research ID numbers were assigned to the intervention group, while women with odd numbers were assigned to the comparison group.

A total of 424 women participated in the study, with 212 women in each group at baseline. A follow-up survey was mailed to these women three months after the baseline survey. The overall response rate to the mailed follow-up survey was fifty-eight percent (N=247). Although about forty percent of the women were lost to follow-up, the drop out rate was the same in both intervention and comparison groups. Additionally, there were no significant differences found in demographics between women who dropped-out and those who completed follow-up.

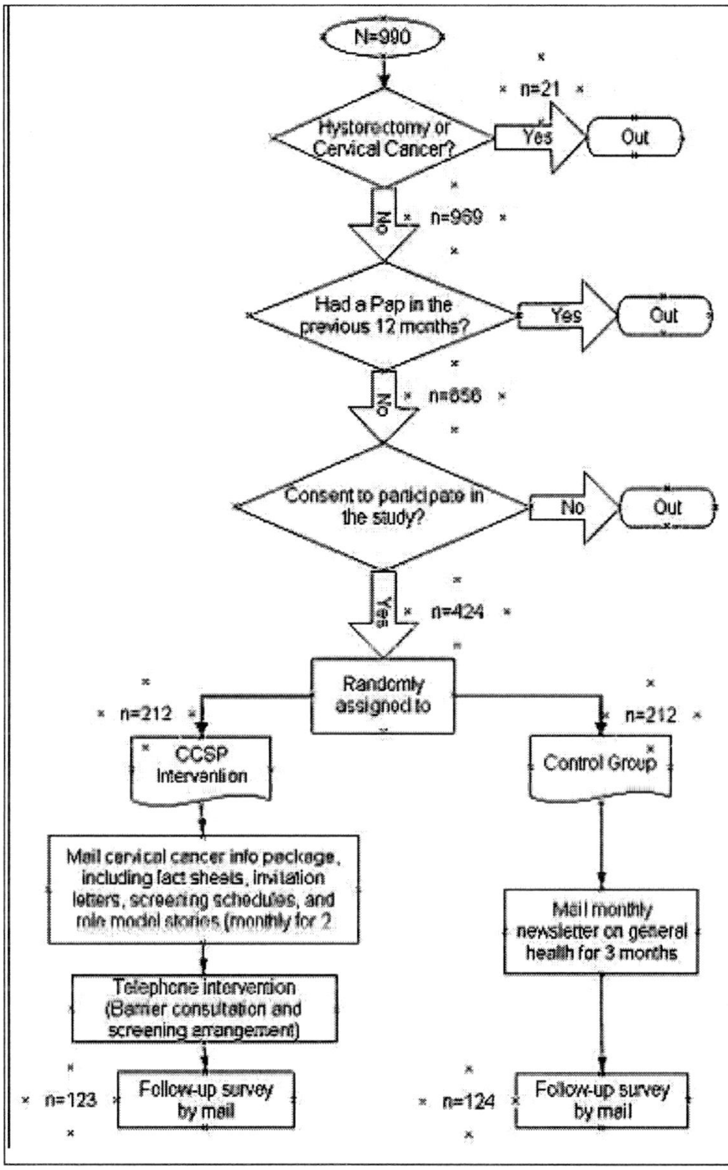

Figure 3.1. Flow chart of the controlled randomized trial.

Measurement

The measurement of the primary outcomes in the survey included items assessing women's screening behavior and screening intention in the coming year. Other variables of interests included constructs such as perceived pros/cons, perceived norms, perceived susceptibility, and knowledge related to cervical cancer and its screening. Demographic information was also obtained. The items making up the perceived pros, perceived cons, perceived norms, and susceptibility scales used 5-point Likert scale with response categories that ranged from strongly disagree (1) to strongly agree (5). The mean score calculated for each scale was the sum of the item scores divided by total number of items in that scale. The knowledge scale consisted of a sum of correct responses. Comments from the open-ended questions in the needs assessment survey were used to refine the measurement instrument. The final survey used in the evaluation study consisted of thirteen pros items (Chronbach α=.87), thirteen cons items (Chronbach α=.79), four norms items (Chronbach α=.63), three susceptibility items (Chronbach α=.81), and sixteen knowledge items (Chronbach α=.80).

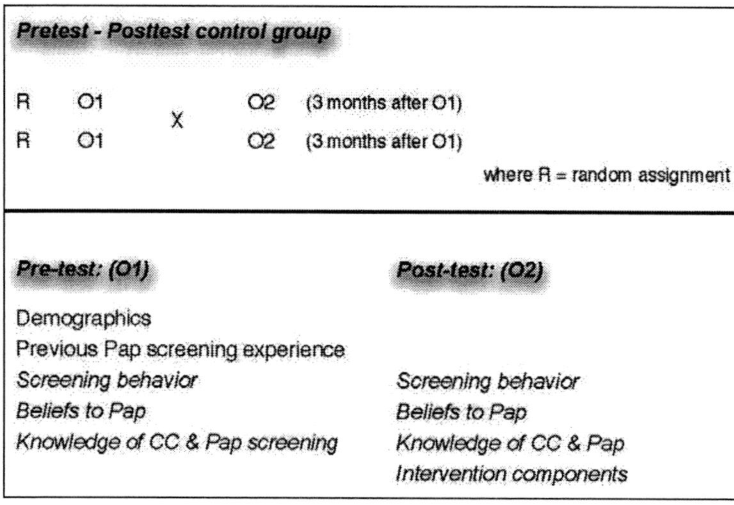

Figure 3.2. Evaluation design.

Data Analysis

Chi-square and t-test were used to assess group equivalency at baseline. There were no statistically significant differences found between groups at baseline. Chi-square tests were used to assess differences between groups on screening completion rates and to assess changes in screening intention among women in the intervention and comparison groups at follow-up. Paired t-tests were used to compare scale differences between pre-test and post-test within each group. Linear regression, including the pre-test scores and group effect as covariates, was used to compare the scale scores between groups at follow-up.

Results

Sample Characteristics and Group Comparisons at Baseline

Comparisons of the demographics and prior screening between intervention and comparison groups at baseline

The mean age of the women in the study was 33.87 (SD=8.61). Most women in the sample were married (90%). Forty percent of the women worked full time and twenty-eight percent of the women had a college education or higher. Prior screening behavior was similar between these two groups. About forty percent of the sample had never had a Pap smear test. The overall intention to have a Pap smear test in the coming year was sixty-three percent at baseline and did not differ significantly between groups. There were no significant differences in age, marital status, employment status, or education between women in the intervention and comparison groups. There were no statistically significant differences between groups at baseline in prior screening or intention to have a Pap smear test in the coming year (Figure 3.3).

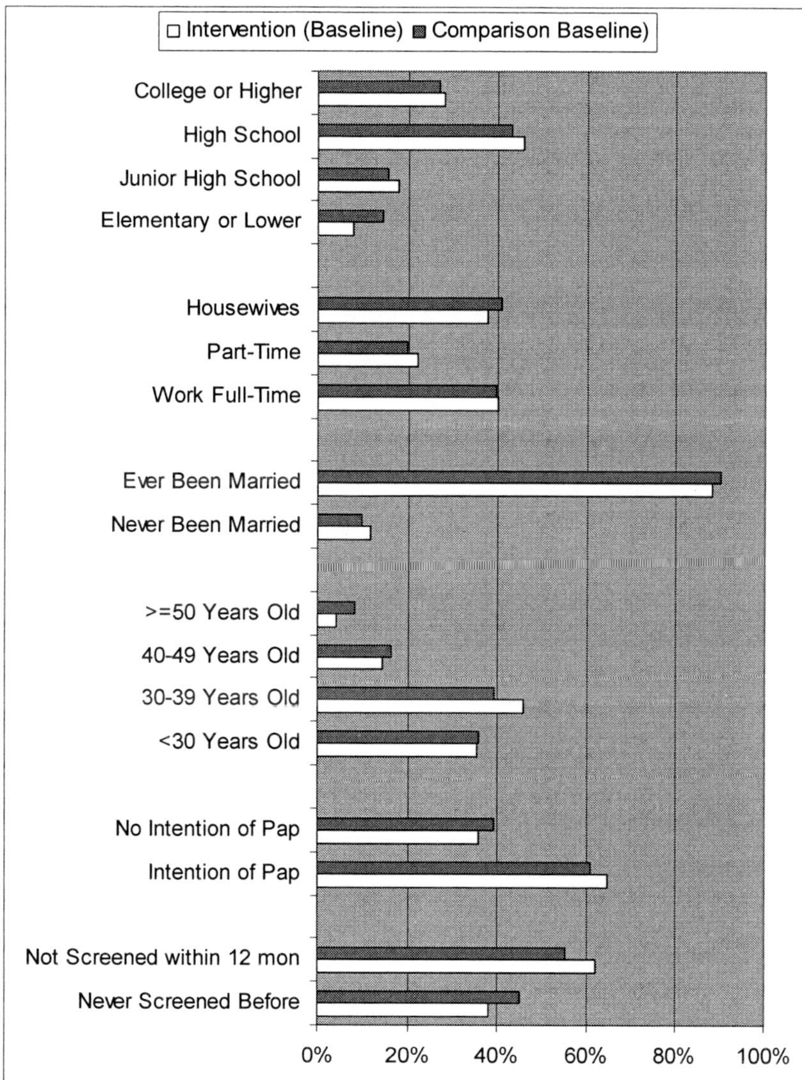

Fig. 3.3. Background information of the women in the intervention trail (N=424). Notes: No significant differences were found on any of the background factors between intervention vs. comparison groups at baseline.

Scales comparisons between groups at baseline

Knowledge, perceived pros, perceived cons, perceived norms, and perceived susceptibility were also assessed using the scales described above. There were no significant differences on these scales between women in the intervention and comparison groups at baseline. Women in both groups answered about 76% of the knowledge items correctly at baseline. The overall mean scores on the 5-point Likert scale for the perceived pros and cons were 4.17 (SD 0.41) and 2.78 (SD 0.54), respectively. The overall means and standard deviations for the perceived norms and susceptibility scales were 3.92 (0.49) and 2.83 (0.70), respectively (Figure 3.4).

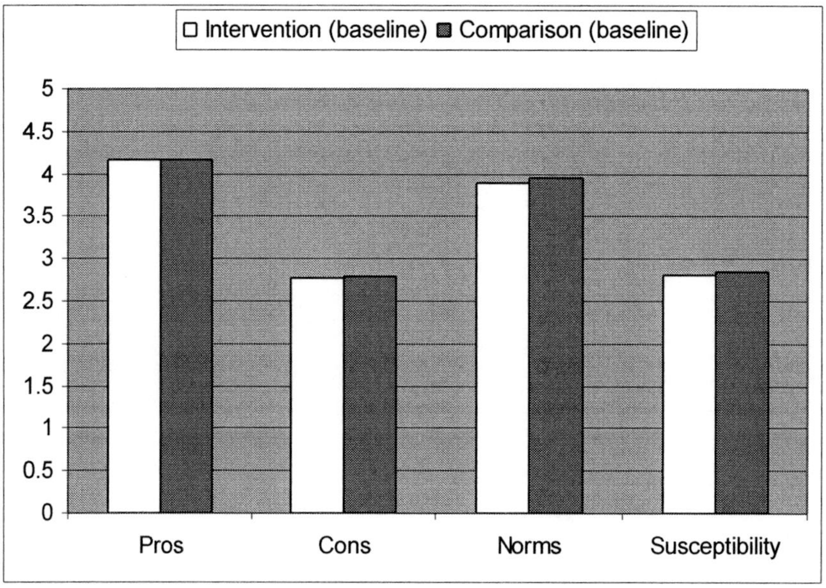

Figure 3.4. Summary of scale means between women in intervention and comparison groups (Baseline). Notes: No significant differences were found on any the beliefs scales between intervention vs. comparison groups at baseline.

Group Comparisons at Post-test on Screening Completion Rates, Intentions, and Factors Associated with Screening

The follow-up survey was conducted after three months of program implementation. At follow-up, women in the intervention group reported significantly higher rates of Pap smear test completion than women in the comparison group. Fifty-one percent of previously non-compliant women in the intervention group reported having had a screening within three months following recruitment, while only thirty-two percent of the women in the comparison group reported receiving a Pap smear test ($p=0.002$).

According to the Transtheoretical Model, women who reported no intention of a screening at baseline were classified as pre-contemplators, whereas women who reported an intention to obtain a Pap smear test at baseline were classified as contemplators in this study. Changes on intention to obtain a screening between groups among pre-contemplators and the screening completion rate between groups among contemplators were examined. Among pre-contemplators, the result showed no significant difference in intention change between women in the intervention and comparison groups at follow up ($p=0.310$). However, among contemplators, there was a significant difference in screening completion rate between groups at follow-up. A higher proportion of the contemplators in the intervention group (62%)

reported completing a Pap smear test at follow-up than women in the comparison group (38%), p=0.008. (Figure 3.5)

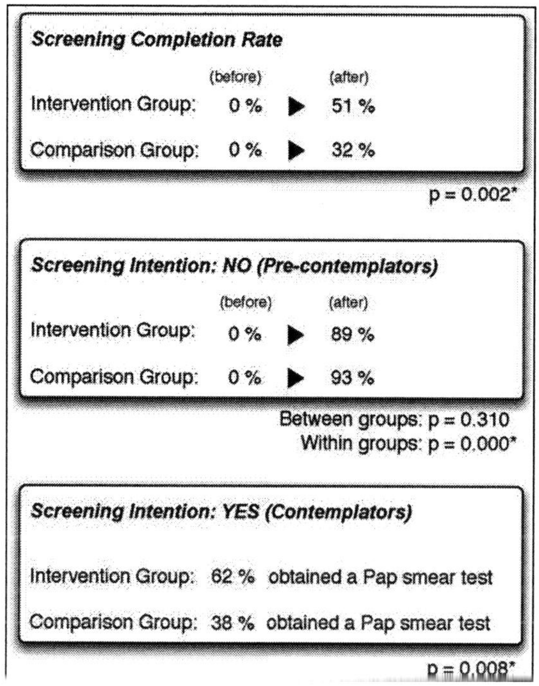

Figure 3.5. Cervical cancer screening (Pap smear test) completion rates.

Linear regression models were used to assess differences on the mean scores of various scales at post-test between women in the intervention and comparison groups. The analysis included pre-test scale scores and intervention condition as covariates. After adjusted for pre-test scale scores, no significant differences were found at post-test between groups on the scales measuring knowledge, perceived norms, or perceived susceptibility. Among women in both groups at follow-up, the overall means for knowledge, perceived norms, and perceived susceptibility scales were 0.81, 3.90, and 2.94, respectively (Table 3.1).

Table 3.1. Summary of scale means between women in intervention and comparison groups (post-test)

Scales	Intervention (N=123) Mean SD	Comparison (N=124) Mean SD	All (N=247) Mean SD	Standardized Coefficient β	P-value Adjusted	95% CI for Coefficients β
Knowledge	0.82 (0.16)	0.79 (0.17)	0.81 (0.17)	0.055	0.305	(-0.017, 0.054)
Pros	4.26 (0.45)	4.16 (0.42)	4.21 (0.43)	0.110	0.031*	(0.009, 0.181)
Cons	2.65 (0.60)	2.75 (0.53)	2.70 (0.57)	-0.088	0.059	(-0.204, 0.004)
Norms	3.88 (0.47)	3.90 (0.48)	3.90 (0.47)	0.008	0.880	(-0.096, 0.112)
Susceptibility	2.96 (0.59)	2.92 (0.71)	2.94 (0.65)	0.048	0.447	(-0.076, 0.173)

Linear regressions were used for the follow-up group comparisons to adjust the pre-test scale and intervention effects.

At follow-up, women in the intervention group perceived higher benefits to cervical cancer screening compared to women in the comparison group (p=0.031). The scale means at post-test was 4.26 for the intervention group and 4.16 for the comparison group. The intervention coefficient β was 0.110 (95% CI [0.009, 0.181]) for the pros scale. Women in the intervention group perceived lower cons (scale mean=2.65) of the Pap smear test than women in the comparison group (scale mean=2.75). The difference was not that significant, however, the p-value indicated that the difference approaches significance (p=0.059).

To further examine the relationships between perceived pros and screening behavior, logistic regression analysis was used. The results indicated that perceived pros significantly predicted women's screening behavior. Women who perceived higher benefits (pros) of a Pap smear test at follow-up were 2.45 times more likely to have received a screening (OR=2.45; 95% CI [1.330, 4.503]; p=0.004), as compared with women who perceived lower benefits of a Pap smear test screening.

Changes of scales scores within groups over time

We conducted further analysis of scales scores to assess changes over time within each group. Although there were no significant differences between intervention and comparison groups on women's knowledge, perceived norms, and perceived susceptibility, there were significant differences between pre- and post-test times among women within the intervention group on these variables. There were statistically significant differences between pre-test and post-test on knowledge 0.04 (p=0.016*), perceived pros 0.09 (p=0.008*), and perceived susceptibility 0.13 (p=0.011*) among women in the intervention group. For women in the comparison group, knowledge was the only factor that showed significant changes over time. The mean difference was 0.03 (p=0.02*) (Figure 3.6).

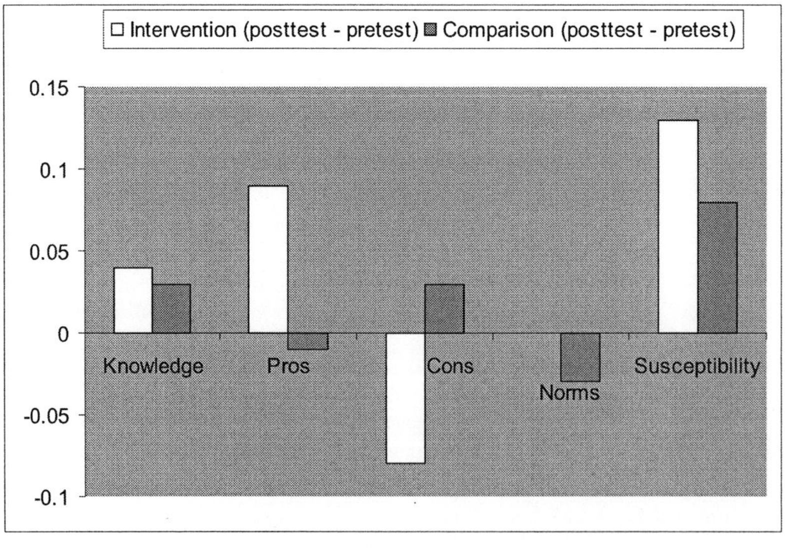

Figure 3.6. Within group comparison of scales between pre-test and post-test. Notes: Paired t-tests were used to compare the changes of scale means within intervention and comparison groups. [b] Significant changes of scale means within intervention groups: knowledge, pros, and susceptibility (p<.05). [c] Significant changes of scale means within comparison groups: knowledge (p<.05).

Discussion and Lessons Learned

The current study demonstrated that the intervention was successful to increase women's cervical cancer screening behavior. Results from this study also indicated that the intervention had successfully influenced women's perceived pros of screening. The perceived pros were found to be a predictor of women's cervical cancer screening behavior (OR=2.45). This was consistent with existing behavioral theory. In an article where the Transtheoretical Model was applied to the prevention of cancer, Ruggiero underlined one important construct included in the model: decisional balance, which involves the balance between the pros and cons of changing the behavior (Ruggiero, 1998). Decisional balance is critical, especially in the early stage of a behavior change. This model suggests that an individual must increase perceived pros or benefits of changing a behavior in order to move forward from pre-contemplation or contemplation to become ready to take action (Prochaska, 1994). The question may be raised as to why we observed a difference in pros scale but not the cons scale. The reason for the lack of significance found in the cons scale may be due to a larger variance observed in the responses of the cons scale compared with the pros scale. Although the *mean difference* between intervention and comparison groups at post-test was the same for these two scales, the post hoc power analysis for the cons scale indicated a power of only twenty-eight percent to detect a statistically significant difference between groups.

For the within group comparison, perceived norms was the only factor that did not change over time for either group. This indicates that perceived norms (women's perception about what other women do and think) about the Pap smear test might not be a salient factor, or might be more difficult to influence through the mailed educational packages and phone intervention than the other factors examined.

Because the study population was made up of mostly younger women (age mean=34), we cannot assume that the intervention would be the same level of effectiveness with older women. This study should be interpreted with the understanding that all the women agreed voluntarily to participate, and that thirty-five percent of the eligible women refused to participate, therefore, self-selection bias may be functioning. Although we may have expected that these women could have higher screening rates than the general population, similar rates of screening were observed. Data showed about sixty-eight percent (656/969) of the women we approached had not had a cervical cancer screening in the past year. In Lee and Chou's study conducted among a similar sample size of women in Taiwan (n=990), their finding revealed a comparable percentage of screening non-adherent women (72%).

It is possible that some women were concealing their non-attendance for screening by not responding to the follow-up survey (Bowman, et al., 1995). Although forty percent of the women responding to the baseline survey were lost to follow-up at post-test, the results did not show differential drop-out rates between women in two groups. Additionally, there was no evidence of demographic differences (age, marital status, employment status, or education level) between women who dropped out and women who remained in the study. Women who were lost to follow-up did have lower levels of knowledge and higher perceived cons compared with women who completed the follow-up. Still, among the women who were lost to follow-up, there were no significant differences found between women in the intervention and comparison groups on any demographics, prior screening behavior, intentions, as well as any factors associated with cervical cancer screening. Post hoc power calculation revealed the follow-up sample provided a power of eighty-nine percent to detect a difference of twenty percent magnitude in the screening completion rate (assuming $\alpha = 0.05$).

Although there was some evidence of inaccuracy in the self-reported screening behavior in previous research, the inaccuracy was usually in the direction of over-reporting screening (Bowman, et al., 1995). The chance that women who reported not being screened but had in fact been screened was minimal. The self-reported negative predictive value estimates were ninety-five to ninety-four percent (Suarez, Goldman, & Weiss, 1995; Walter, Clarke, Hatcher, & Stitt, 1988). Therefore, women in this study at baseline were likely to be a true sample of "under-screened" women. Questions about "when and where" women obtained a Pap smear test during the study period were asked in order to minimize the possibility of the over-reporting at post-test. If it occurred, it was assumed that the over-reporting rate was non-differential in intervention and comparison groups. Thus, the between group comparisons of screening behavior would not be affected.

The study results suggest that a theory and evidence-based direct mail intervention can increase cervical cancer screening behavior among Chinese women who were non-adherent to recommended screening guidelines. The direct mail intervention is a cost-effective way to change screening behavior and has the advantage of allowing women to read the information at their leisure. It is also relatively easy to disseminate. Future studies should investigate the role of perceived pros/cons on influencing cancer-screening behavior, especially for intervention programs that focus on populations in the early stages of a behavior change. Similar strategies with tailored messages to promote screening behavior can also be adopted to reach at-risk populations.

APPENDIX A: RESEARCH MEASUREMENT FOR THE CONTROLLED RANDOMIZED TRIAL

Appendix A: Research Instrument for the Cervical Cancer Screening Program for Chinese Women

台灣婦女子宮頸抹片篩檢研究調查

Cervical Smear Test Research Project among Women in Taiwan

研究單位: 美國德州大學公共衛生研究院 暨 澄清醫院社區健康室

Research Organizations: The University of Texas – School of Public Health, Houston, TX, U.S.A.

& Department of Community Health, Cheng-Ching Hospital, Taichung, Taiwan

研究計畫主持人 侯書逸

Principle Investigator: Su-I Hou

以下是有關子宮頸抹片檢查的敘述，請告訴我們您對每一個敘述的同意程度，分為—
[非常同意，同意，不確定，不同意，或非常不同意]五個等級

Following are statements related to cervical smear test. Please tell us whether you strongly agree (SA), agree (A), unsure (U), disagree (D), or strongly disagree (SD). 例如:
For example:

		非常同意	同意	不確定	不同意	非常不同意
	我覺得我的社區治安很好 I feel my neighborhood is very safe	SA	A	U	D	SD

		非常同意	同意	不確定	不同意	非常不同意
Q-1	我覺得做子宮頸抹片檢查很痛. I feel cervical smear test hurts.	SA	A	U	D	SD
Q-2	子宮頸抹片檢查可以在癌症發生之前查出問題. A cervical smear can find a problem before it develops into cancer.	SA	A	U	D	SD
Q-3	做子宮頸抹片檢查讓我覺得很困窘 / 不好意思. I feel embarrassed to have a cervical smear.	SA	A	U	D	SD
Q-4	子宮頸抹片檢查可以在癌症還有可能治癒的時候發現. A cervical smear can find cancer at a point when it is likely to be cured.	SA	A	U	D	SD
Q-5	做抹片檢查讓我很緊張. A cervical smear test makes me nervous.	SA	A	U	D	SD
Q-6	子宮頸抹片檢查是非常簡單而且快的過程. The cervical smear procedure is very simple and quick.	SA	A	U	D	SD
Q-7	定期做子宮頸抹片檢查可讓我對我的健康放心/安心. Regular cervical smear test gives me peace of mind about my health.	SA	A	U	D	SD
Q-8	每年定期做子宮頸抹片檢查讓我覺得我照顧自己的健康. Having a cervical smear every year gives me a feeling of control over my health.	SA	A	U	D	SD
Q-9	我的男朋友/丈夫不願意我去做子宮頸抹片檢查. My partner / husband would not want me to have a cervical smear.	SA	A	U	D	SD
Q-10	如果我每年定期做抹片，我的家人會覺得我很關心照顧我的健康. My family will think that I take care of myself if I have annual cervical smears.	SA	A	U	D	SD
Q-11	如果我做抹片，我的男朋友/先生會支持我. My partner / husband will support me if I want to have a cervical smear.	SA	A	U	D	SD
Q-12	我願意為了我的健康做抹片. I am willing to obtain a cervical smear for health reason.	SA	A	U	D	SD
Q-13	我可以鼓勵我的朋友去做抹片假如我自己也定期檢查. I can encourage my friends to have a cervical smear if I do it myself.	SA	A	U	D	SD
Q-14	我覺得定期做抹片是我對我的家庭負責的一種表現. I feel having annual cervical smear is a way to show I take care of my family.	SA	A	U	D	SD
Q-15	我會為了我的先生/小孩做抹片. I want to have a cervical smear because I need to take care of my family.	SA	A	U	D	SD

Q-16	早期子宮頸癌的治癒率很高. Cervical cancer in the early stage has high chance to be cured.	非常同意 同意 不確定 不同意 非常不同意 SA A U D SD
Q-17	我覺得我沒有時間作抹片. I do not have time for a cervical smear test.	非常同意 同意 不確定 不同意 非常不同意 SA A U D SD
Q-18	我覺得做抹片檢查很麻煩. It is too much trouble for me to obtain a cervical smear test.	非常同意 同意 不確定 不同意 非常不同意 SA A U D SD
Q-19r	做子宮頸抹片對我來說不重要. Getting a cervical smear is not an important thing for me (reverse coded).	非常同意 同意 不確定 不同意 非常不同意 SA A U D SD
Q-20	讓男醫師做抹片會使我覺得很尷尬 / 不舒服. I feel uncomfortable if a male doctor exam me.	非常同意 同意 不確定 不同意 非常不同意 SA A U D SD
Q-21	越早發現子宮頸癌,治癒率越高. The early a cervical cancer is detected, the higher chance of a cure.	非常同意 同意 不確定 不同意 非常不同意 SA A U D SD
Q-22	如果女醫師來做子宮頸抹片我會感覺更加願意. I would feel more comfortable to have a smear if a female doctor performs the procedure.	非常同意 同意 不確定 不同意 非常不同意 SA A U D SD
Q-23	我只有在醫師提醒之下才有可能做抹片. I would only have cervical smears if I got reminders from my doctor.	非常同意 同意 不確定 不同意 非常不同意 SA A U D SD
Q-24	我如果沒有陰道不適我是不會去做子宮頸抹片. I would not have a smear unless I had some vagina symptoms or discomfort.	非常同意 同意 不確定 不同意 非常不同意 SA A U D SD
Q-25	假如我還沒有性行為，我是不會去做抹片的. I will not have a cervical smear if I am not sexually active.	非常同意 同意 不確定 不同意 非常不同意 SA A U D SD
Q-26	假如我未婚，我不會去做抹片. I will not have a cervical smear if I am not married.	非常同意 同意 不確定 不同意 非常不同意 SA A U D SD
Q-27	子宮頸抹片已是非常例行的醫療檢查. Cervical smear is now a very routine medical test.	非常同意 同意 不確定 不同意 非常不同意 SA A U D SD
Q-28	我覺得我得到子宮頸癌的機率很高. I feel my chance of getting cervical cancer is high.	非常同意 同意 不確定 不同意 非常不同意 SA A U D SD
Q-29	我覺得其他婦女都定期做抹片. Other women in my age obtain a cervical smear regularly.	非常同意 同意 不確定 不同意 非常不同意 SA A U D SD
Q-30	所有的婦女都應該做定期的子宮頸抹片檢查. All women should have regular cervical smears.	非常同意 同意 不確定 不同意 非常不同意 SA A U D SD
Q-31	我在一生中有可能得到子宮頸癌. I might get cervical cancer at some point during my life.	非常同意 同意 不確定 不同意 非常不同意 SA A U D SD
Q-32	我認識的人認為抹片檢查很重要. People I know think cervical smear is very important.	非常同意 同意 不確定 不同意 非常不同意 SA A U D SD
Q-33	和其他婦女相比我有可能得到子宮頸癌. Comparing with other women, my chance of getting cervical cancer is high.	非常同意 同意 不確定 不同意 非常不同意 SA A U D SD

Appendix A-1: Rotated Factor Structure for the Cervical Smear Belief Inventory (CSBI) scale items (N=424).

Scale	Item #	Factor I	Factor II	Factor III	Factor IV
Pros	Q2	0.37			
	Q4	0.36			
	Q6	0.52			
	Q7	0.60			
	Q8	0.66			
	Q10	0.67			
	Q11	0.51			
	Q12	0.67	-0.31		
	Q13	0.67			
	Q14	0.67			
	Q15	0.58			
	Q16	0.44			
	Q19r	0.49			
	Q21	0.67			
Norms	Q27	0.43			
	Q29	0.37			
	Q30	0.67			
	Q32	0.38			
Cons	Q1		0.46		
	Q3		0.67		
	Q5		0.66		
	Q17	-0.38	0.41		
	Q18	-0.41	0.63		
	Q20		0.62		
	Q23		0.51		
	Q24	-0.30	0.47		
(Cultural belief)	Q25				0.76
	Q26				0.82
Susceptibility	Q28			0.72	
	Q31			0.68	
	Q33			0.88	
Eigenvalues		6.03	3.18	1.83	1.6
Variance explained (%)		19.44%	10.26%	5.9%	5.2%

Note: The loadings less than 0.30 were not shown in the table.

Brief Summary of the Research Instrument

This appendix contains measurement items of Cervical Smear Belief Inventory (CSBI) for Chinese Women. The baseline data, collected from the controlled randomized trial (n=424) described in Phase III, were used to examine the psychometrics of the research instrument. Reliabilities showed good internal consistency for the perceived Pros, Cons, and Susceptibility scales (α ranged .78 ~ .87). Factor analysis showed good construct validity of the scores of CSBI which revealed concordant patterns with existing social and behavioral theories, except that the Norms scale was loaded with the Pros scale (Appendix A-1). Moreover, in the Cons scale there appeared to be a "cultural belief toward virginity." Item-discrimination analysis showed that all items in the CSBI successfully discriminated women with favorable cervical smear beliefs from those with unfavorable beliefs ($p<.001$). In summary, many psychometric properties of the CSBI showed that the scores of the inventory were reliable and valid to assess belief towards cervical smear among Chinese women (Hou & Luh, 2005).

Acknowledgement

This study was supported by Cheng-Ching Hospital in Taichung, Taiwan. Special thanks to Pai-Ho Chen, director of the Department of Nursing, and staff at the Department of Community Health for their assistance with the coordination and implementation of the program. This research was approved by The Committee for the Protection of Human Subjects (CPHS) at The University of Texas – Houston Health Science Center, School of Public Health (HSC-SPH-99-013).

References

Ajzen I. & Fishbein M. (1980). Understanding attitudes and predicting social behavior. Englewood Cliffs, NJ: Prentice-Hall.

Ajzen, I. (1988). *Attitudes, personality and behavior.* Chicago: Dorsey Press.

American Cancer Society. (2006a). Cancer facts & figures 2006. Retrieved April 25, 2006, from http://www.cancer.org/downloads/STT/CAFF2006PWSecured.pdf

American Cancer Society. (2006b). Cancer prevention & early detection: Facts & figures 2006. Retrieved April 25, 2006, from *http://www.cancer.org/downloads/STT/CAFF2006PWSecured.pdf*

Bandura, A. (1986). *Social foundations of thought and action: A social cognitive theory.* Englewood Cliffs, NJ: Prentice Hall.

Bartholomew, Parcel, Kok, and Gottlieb. (2006). *Health Promotion Planning: An Intervention Mapping Approach.* 2nd Ed. San Francisco, CA: Jossey-Bass, 2006.

Bowman J, Sanson-Fisher RW, Boyle C, Pope S. (1995). A randomized controlled trial of strategies to prompt attendance for a Pap smear. *Journal of Medical Screening, 2*, 211-218.

Buehler SK, Parsons WL. (1997). Effectiveness of a call/recall system in improving compliance with cervical cancer screening: a randomized controlled trial. *Canadian Medical Association Journal, 157*, 521-526.

Buller D, Modiano MR, & Zapien JG, et al. (1998). Predictors of cervical cancer screening in Mexican American women of reproductive age. *Journal of Health Care for the Poor and Underserved, 9*(1), 76-95.

Burnett CB, Steakly CS, & Tefft MC. (1995). Barriers to breast and cervical cancer screening in underserved women of the District of Columbia. *Oncology Nursing Forum, 22*, 1551-1557.

Byles JE, Redman S, Sanson-Fisher RW, Boyle C. Effectiveness of two direct-mail strategies to encourage women to have cervical (Pap) smears. *Health Promotion, 10*, 5-16.

Centers for Disease Control and Prevention. (1998). The National Breast and cervical cancer early detection program; At-A-Glance, 1998. *US Department of Health and Human Services*, 1-6.

Cullen, K. W., Bartholomew, L. K., Parcel, G. S., & Kok, G. (1998). Intervention mapping: Use of theory and data in the development of a fruit and vegetable nutrition program for Girl Scouts. *Journal of Nutrition Education, 30*, 188-195.

Dignan, M.B. (1994). Development of a Cervical Cancer Education Program for Native American Women in North Carolina. *Journal of Cancer Education. 9*, 235-242.

Dignan, M.B., Michielutte, R., Jones-Lighty, D.D., & Bahnson, J. (1994). Factors influencing the return rate in a direct mail campaign to inform minority women about prevention of cervical cancer. *Public Health Report. 109*, 507-511.

Earp, J.L., Altpeter, M., & Mayne, L. (1995). The North Carolina Breast Cancer Screening Program: Foundations and Design of a Model for Reaching Older, Minority, Rural Women. *Breast Cancer Research & Treatment. 35*, 7-22.

Gotay, C.C., & Wilson, M.E. (1998). Social support and cancer screening in African American, Hispanic, and Native American women. *Cancer Practice. 6(1)*, 31-37.

Guidry JJ, Greisinger A, & Ada LA et al. (1996). Barriers to cancer treatment: a review of published research.

Hancock L., Sanson-Fisher R., & Kentish L. (1998). Cervical cancer screening in rural NSW: health insurance commission data compared to self-report. *Australian & New Zealand Journal of Public Health, 22(3)*, 307-312 (suppl).

Hou S, Fernandez M, Baumler E, & Parcel GS. (2002). Effectiveness of an intervention to increase Pap test screening among Chinese women in Taiwan. *Journal of Community Health, 27*(4), 277-290.

Hou, S., Fernandez, M., Baumler, E., Parcel, G & Chen, P. (2003). Correlates of cervical cancer screening among women in Taiwan. *Health Care for Women International, 24*(5), 384-398.

Hou, S., Fernandez, M., & Parcel, G. (2004). Development of a cervical cancer educational program for Chinese women using Intervention Mapping. *Health Promotion Practice, 5*(1), 80-87.

Hou, S. & Lessick, M. (2002). Cervical cancer screening among Chinese women: Exploring the benefits and barriers of providing care. *AWHONN Lifelines, 6*(4), 349-354.

Hou, S. & Luh, W. (2005). Psychometric properties of the Cervical Smear Belief Inventory (CSBI) for Chinese women. *International Journal of Behavior Medicine, 12*(3), 180-191.

Huang X.L. & Zhang M. (1994). Effects of two teaching programs on women's cervical cancer screening knowledge, health belief and behavior. [Chinese]. *Unpublished doctoral dissertation, National Taiwan University, School of Nursing, Taiwan.*

Jackson CC, Taylor VM, Chitnarong K, et al. (2000). Development of a cervical cancer control intervention program for Cambodian American women. *Journal of Community Health, 25*(5), 359-75.

Janz, N.K., Champion, V.L., & Strecher, V.J. (2002). The Health Belief Model. In K. Glanz, F.M. Lewis, & B.K. Rimer (Eds.), *Health behavior and health education: Theory, research and practice* (3rd ed., pp. 45-66). San Francisco: Kossey-Bass.

Kelly, AW, Fores CM, Wolan PC, Trapp MA, Weaver AL, Barrier PA, Granz WB, & Kottke TE (1996). A program to increase breast and cervical cancer screening for Cambodian women in a midwestern community. *Mayo Clinic Proceedings, 71*(5), 437-44.

Lee-Lin, F., & Menon, U. (2005). Breast and cervical cancer screening practices and interventions among Chinese, Japanese, and Vietnamese Americans. *Oncology Nursing Forum, 32*(5), 995-1003.

Lee T.F., Kuo H.S., & Chou B.S. et al (1997). Factors of Pap screening behavior among women in King-Men, Taiwan. *Public Health of Republic of China. 16 (3),*198-209.

Mandelblatt J, Traxler M, Lakin P, Thomas L, Chauhan P, Matseoane S, & Kanetsky P. (1993). A nurse practitioner intervention to increase breast and cervical cancer screening for poor, elderly black women. The Harlem Study Team. *Journal of General Internal Medicine, 8*(4), 173-8.

Marcus, A.C., & Crane, L.A. (1998). A review of cervical cancer screening intervention research: Implications for public health programs and future research. *Preventive Medicine. 27*, 13-31.

McAlister, A.L. (1995). Behavioral journalism: beyond the marketing model for health communication. *American Journal of Health Promotion. 9*, 417-420.

McGuire, W.J. (1984). Public communication as a strategy for inducing health promoting behavioral change. *Preventive Medicine. 13*, 299-313.

McGuire, W.J. (1985). Attitudes and attitude change. In G. Lindzey& E. Aronson (Eds.), *The handbook of social psychology: Vol. 2. Special fields and applications* (3rd ed., pp. 233-346). New York: Knopf.

Mickey RM, Duraski J, Worden JK, & Dangelis NL. (1995). Breast cancer screening and associated factors for low-income African-American women. *Preventive Medicine, 24*, 467-476.

National Health Insurance Plan. (1996). Department of Health, R.O.C. (Taiwan).

Neilson, A., & Jones, R.K. (1998). Women's lay knowledge of cervical cancer/cervical screening: accounting for non-attendance at cervical screening clinics. *Journal of Advanced Nursing. 28(3),* 571-575.

Nunnally J.C, & Bernstein I.H. (1994). Psychometric Theory. (3rd ed.). New York: McGraw-Hill, Inc.

Pearlman D.N., Rakowski W., Clark M.A., Ehrich B., Rimer B.K., Goldstein M.G., Woolverton H. III, & Dube C.E. (1997) Why do women's attitudes toward mammography change over time? Implications for physician-patient communication. *Cancer Epidemiology, Biomarkers & Prevention, 6*, 451-457.

Pham C.T. & McPhee S.J. (1992). Knowledge, attitudes, and practices of breast and cervical cancer screening among Vietnamese women. *Journal of Cancer Education, 7(4)*, 305-310.

Prochaska J.O., Norcross J.C., & DiClemente C.C. (1994). Changing for good (3rd ed.). New York: William Morrow and Company, Inc.

Rakowski W., Dube C.E., Marcus B.H., & Abrams D.B. (1992) Assessing elements of women's decisions about mammography. *Health Psychology. 11(2)*, 111-118.

Rakowski W., Fulton J.P., & Feldam J.P. (1993) Women's decision making about mammography: A replication of the relationship between stages of adoption and decisional balance. *Health Psychology. 12*(3), 209-214.

Rakowski W., Clark M.A., Pearlman D.N., Ehrich B., Rimer B.K., Goldstein M.G., Dube C.E., & Woolverton H. III. (1997) Integrating pros and cons for mammography and pap testing: Extending the construct of decisional balance to two behaviors. *Preventive Medicine, 26*, 664-673.

Rice, M.V.L. (1991). A simple guide for design, use and evaluation of educational materials. *Health Education Quandary, 18*, 79-85.

Ries, L.A., Wingo, P.A., Miller, D.S., et al. (2000). The annual report to the nation on the status of cancer, 1973 – 1997, with a special section on colorectal cancer. *Cancer, 88*(10),2398-2424.

Rosenstock I.M. & Krischt J.P. (1974). The Health Belief Model and personal health behavior. *Health Education Monographs, 2*, 470-473.

Seow A., Wong M.L., Smith WCS, & Lee H.P. (1995). Beliefs and attitudes as determinants of cervical cancer screening: A community-based study in Singapore. *Preventive Medicine, 24*, 134-141.

Straton JA, Sutherland GJ, & Hyndman JC. (1995). Cervical cancer screening for hospital inpatients: report of an intervention study. *Australian Journal of Public Health, 19*(3), 288-93.

Suarez L., Goldman D.A., & Weiss N.S. (1995). Validity of Pap smear and mammogram self-reports in a low-income Hispanic population. *American Journal of Preventive Medicine, 11*, 94-98.

Suarez L, Loyd L, Weiss N, Rainbolt T, & Pulley LV. (1994). Effect of social networks on cancer-screening behavior of older Mexican-American women. *Journal of National Cancer Institute, 86*, 775-779.

Taylor VM, Hislop TG, Jackson JC, et al. (2002). A randomized controlled trial of interventions to promote cervical cancer screening among Chinese women in North America. *Journal of National Cancer Institutes, 94*(9), 670-77.

Tripp, M. K., Herrmann, N. B., Parcel, G. S., Chamberlain, R. M., & Gritz, E. R. (2000). Sun protection is fun! A skin cancer prevention program for preschools. *Journal of School Health, 70*, 395-401.

U.S. Census Bureau. (2003). The Asian Population: 2000. Census 2000 brief. Retrieved April 25, 2006, from http://www.census.gov/prod/2002pubs/c2kbr01-16.pdf

U.S. Census Bureau. (2005). American community survey: 2003 data profile. Retrieved April 25, 2006, from *http://www.census.gov/acs/www/Products/Profiles/Single/ 2003/ACS/Tabular/010/01000US1.htm*

van Empelen, P., Kok, G., Schaalma, H. P., & Bartholomew, L. K. (2003). An AIDS risk reduction program targeting Dutch drug users: An intervention mapping approach to program planning. *Health Promotion Practice, 4*(4), 402-412.

Yi J.K. (1994). Factors associated with cervical cancer screening behavior among Vietnamese women. *Journal of Community Health, 19*(3), 189-200.

Yi J.K. (1998). Acculturation and Pap screening practices among college-aged Vietnamese women in the United States. *Cancer Nursing, 21*(5), 335-341.

Yu EH, Kim KK, Chen EH, et al. (2001). Breast and Cervical Cancer Screening Among Chinese American Women. *Cancer Practice, 9*(2),81-91.

Walter S.D., Clarke E.A., Hatcher J., & Stitt L.W. (1988). A comparison of physician and patient reports of Pap smear histories. *Journal of Clinic Epidemiology, 41*, 401-410.

Wang P.D. & Lin R.S. (1996). Socio-demographic factors of Pap smear screening in Taiwan. *Public Health, 110*(2), 123-127.

In: New Research on Cervical Cancer
Editor: George Z. Rolland, pp. 47-61

ISBN 1-60021-300-6

Chapter 2

ALTERNATIVE APPROACHES TO CERVICAL CANCER PREVENTION: RISK-ADAPTED MULTIMODAL LABORATORY CERVICAL SCREENING

Reinhard Bollmann[1], Alinda Dalma Varnai[1], Agnes Bankfalvi[2,*] and Magdolna Bollmann[1]

[1]Institute of Pathology, Bonn-Duisdorf, D-53124 Bonn, Germany;
[2]International Medical College (IMC), University of Münster, D-48147 Münster, Germany.

ABSTRACT

Cervical screening is acknowledged as currently the most effective approach for cervical cancer control. To date, there is extensive and strong evidence that cytology-based screening programs have been effective in reducing the incidence of and mortality from the disease in developed countries. However, conventional Papanicolaou (Pap) smears have inherent methodological shortcomings. New developments in cytology, such as liquid-based techniques and automated reading, seem to effectively overcome some of these limitations and have the potential to improve sensitivity and specificity of cytology both in diagnosis of and screening for cervical pre-cancer and cancer.

The recognition that cervical cancer is a consequence of an acquired infection with a few types of oncogenic human papillomaviruses (HPV) has led to novel opportunities for screening based on the use of HPV-tests. Current HPV testing systems are able to detect the presence of viral DNA in exfoliated cervical epithelial cells in close to 100% of invasive cervical cancer and up to 90% of its precursors. Thus, in terms of public health

* Correspondence concerning this article should be addressed to Dr Agnes Bánkfalvi, International Medical College (IMC), Gartenstrasse 21, D-48147 Münster, Germany. Tel: +49(0)251 210-86-39; Fax: +49(0)251 210-86-40; E-mail: bankfal@online.de.

and also for practical purposes, all cervical cancer cases should be considered to be caused by HPV infection. A number of clinical studies have also demonstrated HPV testing to be more sensitive for the detection of clinically relevant pre-invasive cervical disease than cytology alone and the combination of HPV tests and cytology may achieve a negative predictive value of >97% in detecting high grade intraepithelial neoplasia and cervical cancer.

However, in most women, cervical HPV infections remain asymptomatic and are transient, becoming undetectable in 1-2 years even by the most sensitive genetic tests. This is also true for high-risk HPV (HR-HPV) types. It is the long term persistence of certain HR-HPV genotypes that is strongly associated with cervical carcinogenesis in permissive cases. Therefore, discrimination between transient and persistent infections with a certain HPV genotype is essential for risk-adapted screening protocols, which can only be defined by genotyping of two consecutive probes.

Nevertheless, even the highly sensitive test combination of cytology and HR-HPV genotyping cannot predict the biological potential of prevalent cervical pre-cancers towards progression or regression. This can only be assessed by using an adequate biomarker of neoplastic transformation, e.g. DNA aneuploidy, in combination with morphological and HPV tests.

This review focuses on the clinical utility of conventional, ancillary and experimental methods for cervical screening and possible future directions for enhanced screening accuracy and prognostication using risk-adapted multimodal protocols.

Keywords: cervical screening, cytology, HPV-genotyping, DNA-cytometry

Current Epidemiological Status of Cervical Cancer – the European Union Perspective

Carcinoma of the cervix uteri is the second most common cancer in women worldwide with approximately 500 000 new cases diagnosed and 230 000 deaths each year. Almost 80% of new cases occur in the developing world where it is the leading cause of cancer-related death among women [1]. In the former European Union (EU), cervical cancer was estimated to comprise about 3% of cancers in women ranking eighth in importance and it was the tenth most common cause of cancer-related deaths in women in the year 1998 [2]. The recent expansion of the EU in May 2004 will certainly cause significant changes in cervical cancer rates, because there is a substantial excess in female mortality for the disease in most central and eastern European accession countries [3].

Cervical Screening – Past and Present

The objective of screening for cervical cancer is to reduce mortality and incidence of the disease. To date, there is extensive and strong evidence that this can be achieved by cytology-based screening programs as it was observed after the implementation of such regular population-based cervical screening in most developed countries in the 1960s. This has been mainly attributed to early detection and treatment of precancerous lesions. Where screening quality and coverage has been high, these efforts have reduced invasive cervical cancer by up to 90 percent [4,5]. Also in Germany, the age-standardized rates for cervical cancer incidence and mortality declined by 73% and 74% from 1960 to 1997 after the introduction of the statutory opportunistic cancer-screening program in the Western part of the country in 1971 [6]. Despite significant efforts in population-based screening that makes a free annual Papanicolau (Pap) test available to all women 20 years of age and older covered by statutory health insurance (slightly above 90% of the adult female population) [7], the age-standardized annual incidence of 13.3 and mortality rate of 3.0 per 100000 women were among the highest in Europe in 2002 [8]. This can be partly explained by the generally poorer effectivity of an opportunistic screening program compared to an active invitation system [9].

In the meantime, accumulating data from organized screening programs indicate that the marked declines seen until the mid-1980s have been slowing and may even be increasing in certain countries [10]. This could reflect increased cancer detection by using new diagnostic techniques, such as human papillomavirus (HPV) testing and cervicography, or it might be the result of a cohort effect. Another factor with potential effect on incidence trends is the increase in rates of adenocarcinomas and adenosquamous carcinomas, which account for about 10% of all cervical cancers in Western populations [11]. These tumor types and especially their precursors are frequently missed by conventional Pap smears. These data suggest that the maximum effect of Pap smear-based screening could have been reached and further reduction in cervical cancer rates will require the introduction of new technologies and/or more efficient population screening strategies.

Cytology-Based Cervical Screening

Screening for cervical cancer and its precursors have been performed by the conventional Pap smear method over the last half-century [12] with well-published public health success and inherent methodological limitations. High-quality cytology is a highly specific screening test with estimates of 97% as the mean (range 86-100%). In contrast, sensitivity of a single smear may be between 30-87% (51% as the mean), although the sensitivity for high-grade disease alone is between 70% and 80% [13]. Put another way, although the specificity of the Pap test is generally very high, the sensitivity to detect cervical intraepithelial neoplasia (CIN) or invasive cancer is low with poor sample processing and interpretation errors being the major problems. Blood, mucus and drying artefacts contribute to the difficulty of identifying abnormal cells in the traditional Pap smear, and up to 10% of slides can prove unsuitable for interpretation, necessitating repeat visits and sampling [14]. Many of these problems can be overcome partially by improving methods of cell collection and presentation, but there remains a clear need to improve the traditional Pap test.

Newer technologies developed with the intention of improving cytological assessment include liquid-based cytology (LBC; ThinPrep, Autocyte), computerized re-screening (PAPNET), and algorithm-based computer re-screening (AutoPap). Several sub-optimal studies (split-sample or historical) have been performed to determine sensitivity, specificity and predictive values of these new methods; however lack of an adequate reference standard in most of the studies hampers proper assessment and comparison of test characteristics [15].

Nevertheless, the available evidence indicates that using liquid-based cytology, sensitivity is modestly higher for detecting any degree of cervical intraepithelial neoplasia (CIN), whereas specificity is modestly lower than with conventional Pap smears [13]. This supports the conclusion that liquid based cytology is an acceptable alternative to conventional cervical cytology smears, which is reflected by the Food and Drug Administration of the US (FDA) approval of two liquid-based Pap systems for routine use.

Even though several independent reviews on comparing liquid-based versus conventional cervical cytology came to the conclusion that there is no significant difference between the two methods [16,17], there are three major advantages of liquid based cytology over conventional Pap smears: i) numerous investigators agree that liquid based cytology markedly improves specimen adequacy [18-20], ii) the residual material can be used for ancillary testing (e.g. for HPV DNA), and iii) recent studies have shown an improvement in sensitivity and specificity for biopsy proven adenocarcinoma in situ (AIS) and adenocarcinoma [21,22].

Although LBC may improve the cytological identification of abnormal epithelial cells when they are present, the identification of such cells ultimately relies on the ability of the investigator to distinguish atypical cells from normal ones by conventional histochemical staining and microscopy, and to interpret their meaning for the patient. Thus, there is an inherent subjectivity in the traditional Pap-test. This led to the development of imaging systems that can enhance screening accuracy or even replace human investigators in the identification of aberrant cells [23]. Whether such systems should be used either in primary screening or to assist the cytologist in identifying abnormal cells is the subject of current debate.

Detection of HPV DNA as a Marker of Precursor Lesions

It is now well established that the vast majority of cervical carcinomas and its precursors worldwide are caused by persistent infections with certain high-risk types of human papillomaviruses (HR-HPV) [24-26]. Under optimal testing conditions, HR-HPV DNA can be identified in nearly all specimens of invasive cervical cancer (99.7%), in at least 70 % of CIN1, 80% of CIN2 and 96% of CIN3 precursor lesions. Using the Bethesda system nomenclature, HR-HPV DNA can be identified in some 50% of borderline cytology lesions (ASCUS), 80% of LSIL and 90-95% of HSIL and invasive cancer cases [27-28]. In terms of public health, these data indicate that the existence of HPV-negative cervical cancer cases is negligible and does not require any interventional targeting by screening.

However, epidemiologic studies have shown not only that women without HPV do not get cervical cancer but also that most women with HPV do not get cervical cancer. This is due to the fact that most HPV infections are transient in nature, especially in younger age groups, resulting either in no symptoms or minimal cellular changes, or low-grade intraepithelial lesions [29,30].

Research is ongoing to determine acceptable protocols for HPV testing for three main screening- or management-related purposes: 1) as primary screening in asymptomatic women with cytology results being negative for intraepithelial neoplasia or malignancy for estimating prevalence and distribution of HPV in the normal screening population and to define baseline HPV status in these women for diagnostic follow-up [31], 2) reflex HPV DNA testing for triage of women with initial equivocal and abnormal Pap smear (≥ ASCUS) [32], and 3) follow-up for treated cases for improved surveillance of residual disease and/or recurrence [33].

Primary screening studies have demonstrated HPV testing to be more sensitive than cytology alone, whereas the specificity of HPV-tests is age dependent. In the younger age groups, specificity is lower than for cytology and, in age groups of 35 years and older (also country-dependent); the specificity of tests is similar [32,34,35]. One of the strongest gains of the combination of HPV tests and cytology lies in the very high negative predictive value of >99% for detecting CIN3 or cancer [31]. Such a testing combination could potentially allow screening intervals to be increased; e.g. from the minimum of 3 years up to 5 years or longer, depending on the population and risk profile [36]. Furthermore, HPV DNA detection can successfully be performed on self-collected samples as well, which may be advantageous in specific patient groups [37]. Additionally, unlike the Pap smear, which can determine only whether abnormal cells are presently detected, molecular HPV testing has predictive value for lesions that may develop in the future [27,38]. HPV DNA testing also appears to represent a significant enhancement for detection of endocervical adenocarcinomas, which are otherwise difficult to detect and prevent [39]. One of the main drawbacks of this approach is the loss in specificity with respect to either test in isolation due to the excessive number of patients who would need to be referred for colposcopy [40]. Nevertheless, results from large investigational trials, including the ASC-US/Low-grade Squamous Intraepithelial Lesion (LSIL) Triage Study (ALTS), provide an abundance of data to justify the use of HPV testing for triaging ASC-US cases and as a follow-up test [41].

At present there are two HPV testing systems in widespread clinical use. Current hybrid capture technology (HC2 test) detects the presence of 13 types of oncogenic HPVs and 5 low-risk types using respective probe cocktails. Results are group-specific and do not allow distinction between different HPV genotypes. For clinical purposes, only the high-risk probe cocktail is used, with a reported sensitivity for detecting high- grade cervical intraepithelial neoplasias (CIN 2-3) between 84% and 100% [28,42,43].

However, because only women with long-lasting latent HPV infections, even with low levels of oncogenic types, are at high risk for developing HSIL [44], discrimination between transient and persistent infection with high-risk HPV types is essential for risk-adapted screening protocols. Furthermore, the persistence of at least one oncogenic HPV type is necessary for the emergency of pre-cancer [45], which can only be defined by genotyping of two consecutive probes because of the possibility of a new infection with another high risk type during the follow up period. Since the median duration of transient infection is 6 – 11 months [29,35], a second type (variant)- specific HPV test about 12 months after the first positive genotype-test should identify persistent type specific infections.

Genotyping can be performed by using different established PCR techniques (PGMY09/11-Amplicor LBA, GP5+/6+-EIA, SPF10-LIPA, PPF1/CP5-Sequencing) [46,47]. Amplified HPV DNA is identified by either microplate hybridization for detection of PCR amplicons (GP5+/6+-EIA) or a reverse hybridization line blot assay (PGMY09/11-LBA, SPF10-LIPA) that provides information on the specific type(s) detected [48,49].

It is significant that with the development of PCR-based HPV tests, new HPV genotypes are permanently detected with yet undefined-risk for cervical cancer. Furthermore, there is now evidence, that the different HR-HPVs can differ by an order of magnitude in risk for cervical cancer and during different morphological phases of the multi-step carcinogenesis, different HPV types have different oncogenic potential [50,51]. Therefore, the identification of prevalent HPV type may aid in the stratification of women who are at greatest risk for cervical cancer.

Although, simultaneous reporting of cytology and HPV results seems to be ideal, it is not always feasible, e.g. due to reimbursement issues in several countries. However, stringent cytomorphological criteria for minor HPV-associated cellular changes could help in pre-selecting high-risk patients with borderline smear abnormalities for subsequent molecular HPV testing [20,52,53]. In our day-to-day diagnostic practice, the following non-classic features of HPV effect are assessed: i) *minor nuclear abnormalities* (mild hyperchromasia, mild nuclear variations and bi/multinucleation), ii) *disorders of keratinisation* (mild dyskeratosis and parakeratosis), iii) *measles cells and abortive koilocytes*, and iv) *degenerative changes* (macrocytes, cytoplasmic folding and keratohyalin-like granules). In a recent study we could show that all non-classic features were significantly associated with HPV in minimally abnormal cervical smears. Mild nuclear changes had 100% sensitivity and 100% negative predictive value for HPV infection [20]. Further, sensitivity and specificity of the combination of classical and non-classical HPV signs have nearly achieved 100% for PCR-based detection of HPV infection in women with squamous intraepithelial lesions (SIL) and high-grade intraepithelial lesions (HSIL), respectively [54,55]. Since >90% of HSIL is HPV infected, identification of even minor cytological changes suggestive of HPV infection could raise awareness of the screening cytologist more carefully to search for atypical cells. With complete lack of such minor abnormalities HPV infection and consequently the presence of HSIL is practically excluded and no further molecular HPV tests are needed.

Surrogate Biomarkers of Neoplastic Transformation

Theoretically, certain DNA, RNA or protein markers associated with neoplastic transformation of cervical epithelium subsequent to HPV infection could be applied in screening, diagnosis and prognosis. Because oncogenic HPVs are causative agents in cervical carcinogenesis and act via altering the cell cycle in infected epithelial cells, host genes interacting directly or indirectly with HPV oncoproteins have been extensively investigated in vitro [56,57]. The effect of the high-risk HPV early protein E7 on the function of the tumor suppressor pRB, which leads to over-expression of p16INK4A, a cyclin-dependent kinase inhibitor involved in cell cycle control has been investigated by several groups and a simple immunohistochemical assay has been developed for detecting p16 expression in both cell smears and tissue sections [58]. Diffuse, full thickness P16INK4A expression was found to discriminate low-grade from high-grade CIN and claimed to be a marker of high-risk HPV integration into DNA of infected squamous epithelial cells [59]. However, P16INK4A positivity in cervical glandular lesions was equivocal in different studies indicating limited utility of this biomarker in diagnosing suspicious glandular lesions, particularly in cytopathology [60].

Of markers of proliferative activity and differentiation, including Ki67, cell cycle regulators (Rb, p53, Cyclin A, E and D, p16, p21, p27, and telomerase), and cellular differentiation products (involucrin, CK13, CK14) combined quantitation of Ki67, Rb, CK13, and CK14 was found to predict progression risk of early CIN lesions [61].

From the above presentation of various putative molecular risk markers it is evident that no single marker reliably predicts the outcome of patients with abnormal cytology of any grade. A good candidate for a predictor of clinical outcome would be one that represents a wide range of significant genetic changes at early stages of carcinogenesis with a high positive and negative predictive value for abnormal and normal findings, respectively. Measurement of nuclear DNA content (DNA ploidy) is one approach that may fulfill these requirements. Normally, a non-dividing somatic cell contains 23 pairs or 46 chromosomes. This amount of DNA is called *diploid.* Just before cell division, the DNA is doubled and in mitosis, the 23 pairs of chromosomes are evenly distributed to two daughter cells. If no division follows the S-phase, the nucleus will then contain quadruples of DNA, making the cell *tetraploid.* Further doublings without cell division result in *polyploidy* that mean multiple copies of DNA in excess of diploidy. Polyploidisation often occurs in HPV infections, because the virus deranges the cell cycle. If the chromosomes are not uniformly distributed to the daughter cells or if parts of chromosomes become detached, the chromosomal segregation during mitosis is termed *unbalanced.* The unbalanced representation of chromosomes, i.e. gains or losses of chromosomal material, within nuclei is termed *aneuploidy,* which is a common feature in human cancers and pre-cancers [62].

Several lines of evidence indicate that aneuploidy is a cause rather than a consequence of malignant transformation and that it occurs early in carcinogenesis [63]. The development of genomic instability is an early and crucial event during HPV-associated cervical carcinogenesis, as well [64]. In line with others [65], we have recently reported that DNA ploidy measurement by image cytometry on cervical smears positive for HR-HPV help to detect women at high risk for developing high-grade cervical pre-cancer [66-68] This is supported by experimental results suggesting that increasingly deregulated expression of the E6-E7 oncogenes of HR-HPVs in epithelial stem cells first results in chromosomal instability and induces DNA aneuploidy followed either by subsequent integration of the HR-HPV genome into the affected cell clone [69] or alternative oncogene activation mechanisms [70]. Clinical studies support this concept in that cervical lesions with an aneuploid DNA profile are more likely to persist or progress than those with diploid or polyploid DNA content [71,72]. Thus, the assessment of DNA ploidy appears to have prognostic value in potentially malignant cervical lesions.

The method for measuring DNA ploidy uses automated image cytometry of nuclei from routinely processed cytology smears or separated nuclei from tissue samples, and needs little additional expertise over that currently available in most pathological laboratories.

Combination of Different Modalities

There is an increasingly large research literature on possible applications of new visual, microscopical and virological screening methods for prevention of cervical cancer [73]. Adding a second sensitive test to cytology, such as HR-HPV detection, yields a substantial increase in sensitivity and negative predictive value for high-grade CIN and cancer at the cost of concomitant decrease in specificity [35], which is of particular concern for large populations. A second test can be used sequentially as a triage method with the aim to restrict the number of screen-positives requiring referral. Among women with equivocal cytology results, HPV DNA testing is more accurate for detecting underlying CIN3 or cancer than repeat cytology. HPV DNA testing by virus group specific assays is not useful for triage of low-grade squamous intraepithelial lesions (LSIL in the Bethesda system) because of the very high HPV positivity [43]. Nevertheless, screening performance is largely influenced by population characteristics, especially the prevalence of underlying HPV infection. Therefore, all fundamental cervical screening statistics will vary greatly by region [73].

However, even the highly sensitive test combination of cytology and HR-HPV genotyping cannot assess the biological potential of prevalent cervical intraepithelial neoplasia towards progression or regression. An ideal test combination would indicate that an oncogenic HPV virus has already enhanced genetic instability and rendered cells susceptible to malignant transformation and consequent progression if left untreated. This can only be assessed by using adequate biomarkers in combination with morphological and/or HPV tests.

Sporadic published results of such preliminary approaches are available only from experimental and/or study settings up to date [61,65,67,69-71]. Our institution is the first in Germany, which introduced a multimodal, risk-adapted cervical screening protocol using the combination of cytology, HPV genotyping and DNA image cytometry in a pure clinical setting including a routine screening population of about 30000 women from the Bonn-region in Western Germany. Since January 1999, all cervical samples from women sent to our institute by referral gynaecologists from the region have been processed according to this screening profile (Fig.1). Our preliminary results from the year 2002 based on samples from 123 women with ≥ASCUS cytology and concomitant cervical biopsy showed that the combination of all three test modalities resulted in up to 6.9% increase in positive predictive value (PPV) for moderate to high-grade cervical dysplasias and carcinomas (≥CIN2) compared to single tests or double combinations [74]. This combined approach had the additional benefit of being able to predict the possible outcome of histologically proven CIN1 lesions detected as false positives by single tests. Positivity for HR-HPV and DNA aneuploidy in a CIN1 lesion signalise a high risk for progression, whereas HR-HPV positivity with diploid DNA content indicate a probable benign course. Accordingly, our multimodal cervical screening protocol might permit identification of those women with low-grade squamous intraepithelial lesions (LSIL/CIN1) likely to progress at earlier and curable stage of disease and distinguish them from transient minor lesions caused by productive HPV infection. Our multimpodal screening and surveillance protocol may also help to individually predict the clinical outcome of cervical diseases post-surgery [75]. Using a combination of methods, although more expensive per screening, might be cost effective if the increased sensitivity permits lengthening of the screening interval in women at low risk for cancer development and progression [76,77]; and the ability to distinguish between low-worry and high-worry individuals could potentially reduce unnecessary invasive diagnostics and therapy with beneficial socio-economical impact.

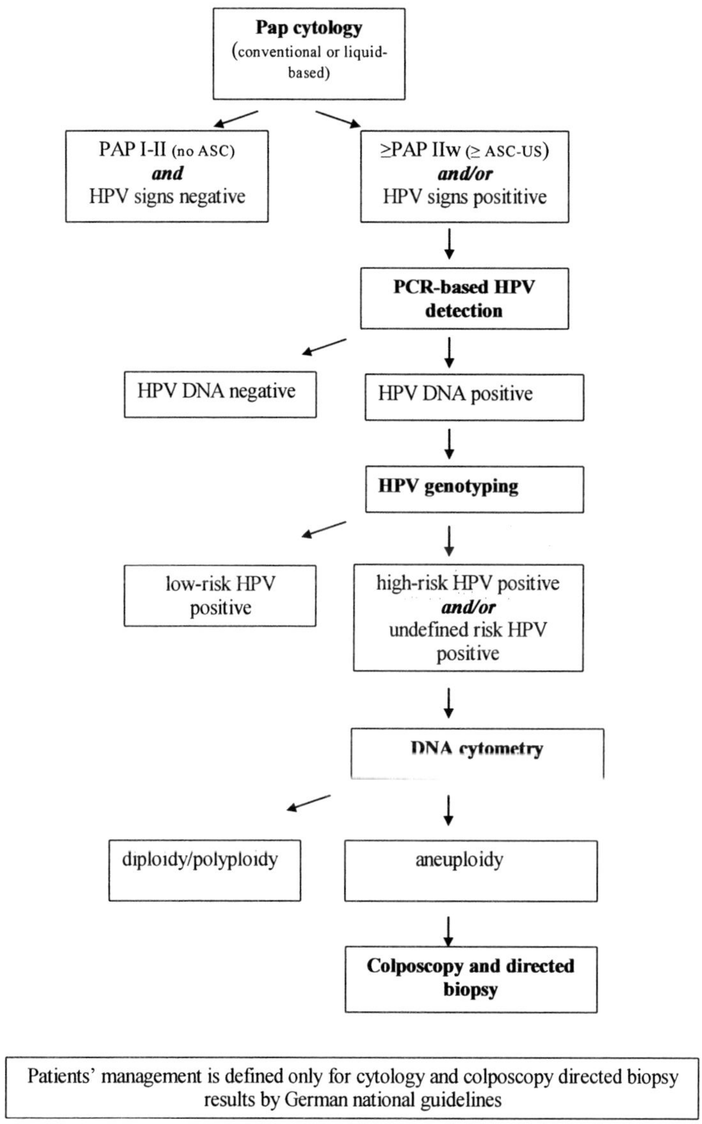

Figure 1. Risk-adapted, multimodal cervical screening program (the Bonn-scheme) using a combination of cytology and PCR-based HPV detection with adjuvant DNA-cytometry in the routine clinical setting. For the ideal case, the major steps include: 1) conventional Pap-test, or liquid-based cytology with special focus on assessing HPV-related cytomorphological changes (classic and non-classic HPV signs)(17), 2) cytology results of ≥PapIIw are managed by using reflex PCR-based HPV DNA testing, 3) in HPV DNA + cases, genotyping by sequencing, 4) in high-risk HPV+ cases, DNA cytometry for assessing gross chromosomal instability as progression marker (14), 5) only DNA aneuploid cases should be referred to immediate colposcopy and directed biopsy, 6) treatment is reserved for biopsy-confirmed ≥CIN3 cases 7) after ablation, Pap-smears are to be scheduled at 6-months with a repeated HPV DNA test.

Conclusion

To date, there are several good methods available for cervical screening. With appropriate screening programs and early diagnosis and treatment, cervical cancer may become a preventable public health issue in the foreseeable future. Based on good evidence, highly accurate screening for cervical cancer and high-grade intraepithelial neoplasias is now technically feasible. Given the abundant options for detecting its precursors, it is not a conceptual or technical challenge, but a matter of policy and financing which delays the elimination of this malignancy.

References

[1] Parkin, DM; Bray, FI; Deves, SS. Cancer burden in the year 2000. The global picture. *Eur J Cancer* 2001;37: 4-66.

[2] Ferlay, J; Bray, F; Sankila, R; Parkin, DM. *EUCAN: Cancer Incidence, Mortality and Prevalence in the European Union 1998.* version 5.0: IARC CancerBase No. 5. Lyon, IARC Press, 1999.

[3] Levi F; Lucchini, F; Negri, E; La Vecchia, C. Trends in mortality from major cancers in the European Union, including acceding countries, in 2004. *Cancer* 2004; 101:2843-50.

[4] Gustafsson, L; Ponten, J; Zack, M; Adami, HO. International incidence rates of invasive cervical cancer after introduction of cytological screening. *Cancer Causes Control* 1997; 8: 55-63.

[5] Nieminen, P; Kallio, M; Hakama, M. The effect of mass-screening on incidence and mortality of squamous and adenocarcinoma of cervix uteri. *Obstet Gynecol* 1995; 85:1017-21.

[6] Becker, N. Epidemiological aspects of cancer screening in Germany. *J Cancer Res Clin Oncol* 2003; 129:691-702.

[7] Schenck, U; Karsa von, L. Cervical cancer screening in Germany. *Eur J Cancer* 2000; 36:2221-26.

[8] Working group of population-based cancer registries in Germany: Krebs in Deutschland: Häufigkeiten und Trends. www.rki.de/KREBS; 2006.

[9] Nieminen, P; Kallio, M; Anttila, A; Hakama, M. Organised vs spontaneous PAP-smear screening for cervical cancer: a case-control study. *Int J Cancer* 1999; 83:55-58.

[10] Vizcaino, AP; Moreno, V; Bosch, FX; Munoz, N; Barros-Dios, XM; Parkin, DM. International trends in the incidence of cervical cancer: II Squamous cell carcinoma. *Int J Cancer* 2000;86:429-35.

[11] Vizcaino, AP; Moreno, V; Bosch, FX; Munoz, N; Barros-Dios, XM; Parkin, DM. International trends in the incidence of cervical cancer: I Adenocarcinoma and adenosquamous carcionomas. *Int J Cancer* 1998; 75:536-45.

[12] Papanicolau, GN. Survey on the actualities and potentialities of exfoliative cytology in cancer diagnosis. *Ann Int Med* 1949; 31:661-74.

[13] Nanda, K; McCrory, DC; Myers, ER; Bastian, LA; Hasselblad, V; Hickey, JD; Matchar, DB. Accuracy of the Papanicolaou test in screening for and follow-up of cervical cytologic abnormalities: a systematic review. *Ann Intern Med* 2000;132:810-19.

[14] Doorbar, J; & Cubie, H. Molecular basis for advances in cervical screening. *Mol Diagn* 2005;9:129-142.

[15] Hartmann, KE; Nanda, K; Hall, S; Myers, E. Technologic advances for evaluation of cervical cytology: is newer better? *Obstet Gynecol Surv* 2001;56:765-74.

[16] Davey, E; Barratt, A; Irwing, L; et al. Effect of study design and quality on unsatisfactory rates, cytology classifications, and accuracy in liquid-based versus conventional cervical cytology: a systematic review. *Lancet* 2006; 367: 122-32.

[17] Obwegeser, J; Schneider, V. Thin-layer cervical cytology:a new meta-analysis. *Lance*t 2006; 367:88-89.

[18] Diaz-Rosario, LA; Kabawat, SE. Performance of a fluid-based, thin-layer Papanicolaou smear method in the clinical setting of an independent laboratory and an outpatient screening population in New England. *Arch Pathol Lab Med* 1999;123:817-21.

[19] Saslow, D; Runowicz, CD; Solomon, D; et al. American Cancer Society Guideline for the early detection of cervical neoplasia and cancer. *CA Cancer J Clin* 2002;52:342-62.

[20] Bollmann, M; Bánkfalvi, A; Trosic, A; Speich, N; Schmitt, C; Bollmann, R. Can we detect cervical human papillomavirus (HPV)-infection by cytomorphology alone? Diagnostic value of non-classic cytological signs of HPV effect in minimally abnormal Pap tests. *Cytopathology* 2005;16: 13-21.

[21] Bai, H; Sung, CJ; Steinhoff, MM. ThinPrep Pap test promotes detection of glandular lesions of the endocervix. *Diagn Cytopathol* 2000;23:19-22.

[22] Ashfaq, R; Gibbons, D; Vela, C; Saboorian, MH; Iliya, F. ThinPrep Pap Test. Accuracy for glandular disease. *Acta Cytol* 1999;43:81-85.

[23] Wilbur, DC. Cervical cytology automation: an update for 2003. The end of the question nears? *Clin Lab Med* 2003; 23:755-74.

[24] Schiffman, MH; Bauer, HM; Hoover, RN; et al. Epidemiologic evidence showing that human papillomavirus infection causes most cervical intraepithelial neoplasia. *J Natl Cancer Inst* 1993;85:958-64.

[25] Bosch, FX; Manos, MM; Munoz, N; et al. Prevalence of human papillomavirus in cervical cancer: a worldwide perspective. International biological study on cervical cancer (IBSCC) Study Group. *J Natl Cancer Inst* 1995;87:796-802.

[26] Walboomers, JMM; Jacobs, MV; Manos, MM; et al. Human papillomavirus is a necessary cause of invasive cervical cancer worldwide. *J Pathol* 1999;189:1–3.

[27] Nobbenhuis, M; Walboomers, JM; Helmerhorst, TJ; et al. Relation of human papillomavirus status to cervical lesions and consequences for cervical-cancer screening: a prospective study. *Lancet* 1999; 354:20–25.

[28] Clavel, C; Masure, M; Bory, JP; et al. Human papillomavirus testing in primary screening for the detection of high-grade cervical lesions: a study of 7932 women. *Br J Cancer* 2001;84:1616-23.

[29] Ho, GY; Bierman, R; Beardsley, L; Chang, CJ; Burk, RD. Natural history of cervicovaginal papillomavirus infection in young women. *N Engl J Med* 1998; 338:423-8.

[30] Moscicki, AB; Shiboski, S; Hills, NK; et al. Regression of low-grade squamous intra-epithelial lesions in young women. *Lancet* 2004; 364:1678-83.

[31] Sherman, ME; Lörincz, AT; Scott, DR; Baseline cytology, human papillomavirus testing and risk for cervical neoplasia: a 10-year cohort analysis. *J Natl Cancer Inst* 2003; 95:46-52.

[32] Schiffman, M; Herrero, R; Hildesheim, A; et al. HPV DNA testing in cervical cancer screening: results from women in a high-risk province of Costa Rica. *JAMA* 2000;283:87-93.

[33] Wright, TC; Schiffman, M; Solomon, D; et al. Interim guidance for the use of human papillomavirus DNA testing as an adjunct to cervical cytology screening. *Obstet Gynecol* 2004; 103:304-9.

[34] Schneider, A; Hoyer, H; Lotz, B; et al. Screening for high-grade cervical intra-epithelial neoplasia and cancer by testing for high-risk HPV, routine cytology or colposcopy. *Int J Cancer* 2000; 89:529-34.

[35] Cuzick, J; Szarewski, A; Cubie, H; et al. Management of women who test positive for high-risk types of human papillomavirus: the HART study. *Lancet* 2003; 362:1871-6.

[36] Advisory Committee on Cancer Prevention. Recommendations on cancer screening in the European Union. *Eur J Cancer* 2000; 36:1473-78.

[37] Dannecker, C; Siebert, U; Thaler, CJ; Kiermeir, D; Hepp, H; Hillemanns, P. Primary cervical cancer screening by self-sampling of human papillomavirus DNA in internal medicine outpatient clinics. *Ann Oncol* 2004;15:863-9.

[38] Schlecht, NF; Platt, RW; Duarte-Franco, E; et al. Human papillomavirus infection and time to progression and regression of cervical intraepithelial neoplasia. *J Natl Cancer Inst* 2003; 95:1336-43.

[39] Davey D; & Zarbo, RJ. Human papillomavirus testing – Are you ready for a new era in cervical cancer screening? *Arch Pathol Lab Med* 2003; 127:927-29.

[40] Franco, EL.Chapter 13: Primary screening of cervical cancer with human papillomavirus tests. *J Natl Cancer Inst Monogr* 2003; 31:89-96.

[41] Schiffman, M; Solomon, D. Findings to date from the ASCUS-LSIL Triage study (ALTS). *Arch Pathol Lab Med* 2003; 127:946-49.

[42] Wright, TC; Denn, L; Kuhn, L; Pollack, A; Lorincz, A. HPV DNA testing of self-collected vaginal samples compared with cytologic screening to detect cervical cancer. *JAMA* 2000; 283: 81-86.

[43] Arbyn, M; Buntinx, F; Van Ranst, M; et al. Virologic versus cytologic trial of women with equivocal Pap smears: a metaanalysis of the accuracy to detect high-grade intraepithelial neoplasia. *J Natl Cancer Inst* 2004; 96:280-93.

[44] Ho, GY; Burk, RD; Klein, S; et al. Persistent genital human papillomavirus infection as a risk factor for persistent cervical dysplasia. *J Natl Cancer Inst* 1995; 87:1365-71.

[45] Kjaer, SK; van den Brule, AJ; Paul, G; et al: Type specific persistence of high risk human papillomavirus (HPV) as indicator of high grade cervical squamous

intraepithelial lesions in young women: population based prospective follow up study. *BMJ* 2002; 325:1-7.

[46] Coutlee, F; Gravitt, P; Kornegay, J; et al. Use of PGMY primers in L1 consensus PCR improves detection of human papillomavirus DNA in genital samples. *J Clin Microbiol* 2002; 40:902-7.

[47] Poljak, M; Marin, IJ; Seme, K; Vince, A. Hybrid Capture II HPV Test detects at least 15 human papillomavirus genotypes not included in its current high-risk probe cocktail. *J Clin Virol* 2002; 25 Suppl 3: S89-97.

[48] Kay, P; Meehan, K; Williamson, AL. The use of nested polymerase chain reaction and restriction fragment length polymorphism for the detection and typing of mucosal human papillomaviruses in samples containing low copy numbers of viral DNA. *J Virol Methods* 2002; 105:159-70.

[49] Perrons, C; Kleter, B; Jelley, R; Jalal, H; Quint, W; Tedder, R. Detection and genotyping of human papillomavirus DNA by SPF10 and MY09/11 primers in cervical cells taken from women attending a colposcopy clinic. *J Med Virol* 2002; 67:246-52.

[50] Munoz, N; Bosch, FX; de Sanjose, S; et al. Epidemiologic classification of human papillomavirus types associated with cervical cancer. *N Engl J Med* 2003; 348:518-27.

[51] Bolkmans, NW; Bleeker, MC; Berkhof, J; Voohosrt, FJ; Snijders, PJ; Meijer, CP. Prevalence of types 16 and 33 is increased in high-risk human papillomavirus positive women with cervical intraepithelial neoplasia grade 2 or worse. *Int J Cancer* 2005; 117:177-181.

[52] Schneider, A; Meinhardt, G, de Villiers, EM, Gissmann, L. Sensitivity of the cytologic diagnosis of cervical condyloma in comparison with HPV DNA hybridization studies. *Diagn Cytopathol* 1987; 3:250-5.

[53] Checchini, S; Confortini, M; Bonardi, M;et al. "Nonclassic" cytologic signs of cervical condyloma. *Acta Cytol* 1990; 6:781-4.

[54] Bollmann, R; Mehes, G; Torka, R; Speich, N; Schmitt, C; Bollmann, M. Human Papillomavirus Typing and DNA Ploidy Determination of Squamous Intraepithelial Lesions in Liquid-Based Cytologic Samples. *Cancer Cytopathol* 2003; 99:57-62.

[55] Speich, N; Schmitt, C; Bollmann, R; Bollmann, M. Human papillomavirus (HPV) study of 2916 cytological samples by PCR and DNA sequencing: genotype spectrum of patients from the west German area. *J Med Microbiol* 2004; 53:1-4.

[56] Alazawi, W; Pett, M; Arch, B; Scott, L; Freeman, T; Stanley, MA; Coleman, N. Changes in cervical keratinocyte gene expression associated with integration of human papillomavirus 16. *Cancer Res* 2002; 62:6959-65.

[57] Al Moustafa, AE; Foulkes, WD; Wong, et al. Cyclin D1 is essential for neoplastic transformation induced by both E6/E7 and E6/E7/ErbB-2 cooperation in normal cells. *Oncogene* 2004; 23:5252-6.

[58] Klaes, R; Friedrich, T; Spitkovsky, D; et al. Overexpression of P16INK4a as specific marker for dysplastic and neoplastic epithelial cells of the cervix uteri. *Int J Cancer* 2001; 92: 276-84.

[59] Hu, L; Guo, M; He, Z; Thornton, J; McDaniel, LS; Hughson, MD. Human papillomavirus genotyping and p16(INK4a) expression in cervical intraepithelial neoplasia of adolescents. *Mod Pathol* 2005; 18:267-73.

[60] Murphy, N; Heffron, CC; King, B; et al. P16(INK4A) positivity in benign, premalignant and malignant cervical glandular lesions: a potential diagnostic problem *Virchows Arch* 2004;445:610-15.

[61] Kruse, AJ; Skaland, I; Janssen, EA; et al. Quantitative molecular parameters to identify low-risk and high-risk early CIN lesions: role of markers of proliferative activity and differentiation and Rb availability. *Int J Gynecol Pathol* 2004; 23:100-9.

[62] Sen, S. Aneuploidy and cancer. *Curr Opin Oncol* 2000; 12:82-8.

[63] Duesberg, P; & Li, R. Multistep carcinogenesis. A chain reaction of aneuploidizations. *Cell Cycle* 2003; 2:202-210.

[64] zur Hausen H. Papillomavirus causing cancer: evasion from host cell control in early events in carcinogenesis. *J Natl Cancer Inst* 2000; 92:690-698.

[65] Lorenzato, M; Bory, JP; Cucherousset, J; et al. Usefulness of DNA ploidy measurement on liquid-based smears showing conflicting results between cytology and high-risk human papillomavirus typing. *Am J Clin Pathol* 2002; 118:708-13.

[66] Bollmann, R; Bollmann, M; Henson, DE; Bodo; M. DNA cytometry confirms the utility of the Bethesda system for the classification of Papanicolaou smears. *Cancer Cytopathol* 2001 93:222-8.

[67] Bollmann, R; Mehes, G; Torka, R; Speich, N; Schmitt, C; Bollmann M. Determination of features indicating progression in atypical squamous cells with undetermined significance: human papillomavirus typing and DNA ploidy analysis from liquid-based cytologic samples. *Cancer* 2003; 99:113-17.

[68] Bollmann, R; Mehes, G; Speich, N; Schmitt, C; Bollmann, M. Aberrant, highly hyperdiploid cells in human papillomavirus positive, abnormal cytologic samples are associated with progressive lesions of the uterine cervix. *Cancer Cytopathol* 2005; 105:96-100.

[69] Melsheimer, P; Vinokurova, S; Wentzensen, N; Bastert, G; von Knebel-Doeberitz, M. DNA aneuploidy and integration of human papillomavirus type 16 e6/e7 oncogenes in intraepithelial neoplasia and invasive squamous cell carcinoma of the cervix uteri. *Clin Cancer Res* 2004; 10:3059-63.

[70] Sathish, N; Abraham, P; Peedicayil, A; Sridharan, G; John, S; Chandy G. Human papillomavirus 16 E6/E7 transcript and E2 gene status in patients with cervical neoplasia. *Mol Diagn* 2004; 8:57-64.

[71] Bibbo, M; Dytch, HE; Alenghat, E; Bartels, PH; Wied, GL. DNA ploidy profiles as prognostic indicators in CIN lesions. *Am J Clin Pathol* 1989; 92:261-65.

[72] Bocking, A; Nguyen, VQ. Diagnostic and prognostic use of DNA image cytometry in cervical squamous intraepithelial lesions and invasive carcinoma. *Cancer Cytopathol* 2004;102:41-54.

[73] Ferreccio, C; Bratti, MC; Sherman, ME; et al. A comparison of single and combined visual, cytologic, and virologic tests as screening strategies in a region at high risk of cervical cancer. *Cancer Epidemiol Biomarkers Prev* 2003; 12:815-23.

[74] Bollmann, R; Bankfalvi, A; Griefingholt, H; et al. Validity of combined cytology and human papillomavirus (HPV) genotyping with adjuvant DNA-cytometry in routine cervical screening: results from 31031 women from the Bonn-region in West Germany. *Oncol Report* 2005; 13:915-922

[75] Bollmann, M; Varnai, AD; Griefingholt, H; et al. Predicting treatment outcome in cervical diseases using liquid-based cytology, dynamic HPV genotyping and DNA cytometry. *Anticancer Res* 2006; 26:1439-46.

[76] Maxwell, GL; Carlson, JW; Ochoa, M; Krivak, T; Rose, GS; Myers, ER. Costs and effectiveness of alternative strategies for cervical cancer screening in military beneficiaries. *Obstet Gynecol* 2002; 100: 740-748

[77] Goldie, SJ; Kim, JJ; Wright, TC. Cost effectiveness of human papillomavirus DNA testing for cervical cancer screening in women aged 30 years or more. *Obstet Gynecol* 2004; 103:619-631

In: New Research on Cervical Cancer
Editor: George Z. Rolland, pp.63-107
ISBN 1-60021-300-6

Chapter 3

UNDERLYING CERVICAL CANCER PORTRAY: FROM HPV/CO-INFECTIONS AND HOST GENETIC PROFILES TO GENE EXPRESSION SIGNATURES

Martín C. Abba[*] and Carlos D. Golijow
Basic and Applied Genetics Research Center, National University of La Plata (UNLP), La Plata, Argentina.

ABSTRACT

Over the past years, the knowledge on natural history and epidemiology of the *Human Papillomavirus* (HPV) infection has advanced tremendously. Besides numerous ongoing efforts to understand the biological basis of complex traits as cervical cancer, many questions concerning the interaction of the virus with its host remain unanswered. Worldwide, HPV is one of the most prevalent sexual transmitted agents and, at the same time, cervical cancer is the rare consequence of HPV infection. Despite the prominent role of HPV in genital cancer development, other genetic, epigenetic and environmental factors have also been involved. The aim of the present study was to evaluate in a multifactorial fashion the HPV (genotyping, viral load), *Herpes Simplex Virus* and *Chlamydia trachomatis* infections combined with *k-ras*, *c-myc* and *c-erbB-2* oncogene status, as co-factors in cervical carcinogenesis in a set of 304 preneoplastic and neoplastic cervical cancer tissue. Furthermore, genetic polymorphisms belonging to the HLA-DQA1 gene and the tumor suppressor gene p53 were also evaluated, in order to define their role in cervical cancer development. Principal component analysis (PCA) was employed to perform an integrative multifactorial analysis and to view the overall trend of the data. In addition, genome-wide expression profiling obtained by DNA

[*] Correspondence concerning this article should be addressed to: Dr. Martín C. Abba, Basic and Applied Genetics Research Center (CIGEBA), National University of La Plata (UNLP). Calle 60 y 118 s/n, B1900AVW, La Plata - Argentina. Tel/Fax: +54-221-421-1799. E-mail address: mabba777@hotmail.com

microarray platform was downloaded from public available databases. Our statistical analysis identified 167 transcript differentially expressed between normal cervical tissue and invasive carcinomas ($p<0.01$). Finally, *Single Nucleotide Polymorphisms* (SNPs) analysis in cervical cancer research were also discussed.

Keywords: HPV, HPV-cofactors, genetics polymorphisms, gene expression signature

INTRODUCTION

Human Papillomavirus (HPV): the Central Hypothesis in Cervical Cancer

Worldwide, carcinoma of the uterine cervix is one of the most common cancers affecting women, being responsible for a high prevalence of women death in several parts of the world. Cervical carcinoma is a sexually transmitted disease, positioning as the third most common malignancy among women worldwide, especially in developing countries [1,2].

Research in relation to the aetiology of cervical cancer has made substantial progress over the past three decades, both in scientific and practical terms. For many time, the epidemiological profile of women with cervical cancer was recognised as suggestive of a sexually transmitted infection [3], and several microorganisms were previously proposed over the past years as the possible aetiological agents, including syphilis, gonorrhea, *Chlamydia trachomatis* and type 2 herpes simplex virus (HSV-2) [4].

The major discovery in cervical cancer aetiology has been the recognition that this disease is the rare consequence of an infection by some types of *Human Papillomavirus* (HPV) [4]. Since the first works pointing out the possible role of HPV as the aetiological agent of squamous cervical cancer [5], a large body of evidence has been achieved concerning the central role of this virus in cervical disease. In the one hand, epidemiological studies allowed the identification of the tight relationship between the virus and the disease. In the other hand, the progresses made in the field of molecular biology let established many ways of the interaction between the HPV and the host cell [6,7]. Furthermore, the complete viral genome has been sequenced and the protein functions have been identified, indicating that the HPV genome code for at least six different early and two late proteins [8]. Moreover, almost all the viral gene functions have been established and the molecular targets of the infected cells have been mainly recognized [7]. However, many ways of action in HPV infection and cell transformation still not completely understood [9].

Human Papillomavirus comprise a heterogeneous group of viruses, revealing a significant diversity of genotypes. So far, 85 HPV types have been recognized and fully sequenced and more than 120 alleged novel types have been partially characterized. The different HPV genotypes have been classified according to their oncogenic potential in two main groups: i) high-risk HPV types (16, 18, 31, 33, 45, etc.) mainly related to high grade cervical lesions and squamous cervical cancer and ii) low-risk HPV types (6, 11, 34, 53, 54, etc.) related to low grade cervical intraepithelial lesions and genital warts.

Despite the necessary role of HPV in cervical cancer development, other genetic and epigenetic factors should been considered as additional and required steps in the process of cell transformation and cancer progression [7,10,11,12]. As mentioned previously, cervical cancer is the rare consequence of the persistent infection with oncogenic HPV types. In this sense, cervical tumors have been shown to harbor HPV-DNA sequences in as many as 99.7% of the samples studied, implying a need for the sustained presence of viral DNA during cervical carcinogenesis [13]. So that, additional factors should support over time the HPV infection in order to become persistent, favouring the cell transformation process with a dead end in the malignant phenotype.

Sexual Transmitted Infections (STIs) as Co-Factors in Cervical Cancer Development

Since the early 90', it is suspected that co-infections with certain microorganisms could predispose to cervical cancer development [14,15,16]. In this sense, any sexual transmitted infection could be acting as a co-factor in cervical carcinogenesis, either promoting genomic changes or simply bringing a permissive environment for HPV infection and viral persistence. Among the possible viral and bacterial infections, HSV-2 and *Chlamydia trachomatis* infections have been proposed as co-factors in cervical cancer development and progression [17,18,19].

The importance of sexually transmitted infections (STIs) in the development of invasive cervical carcinoma (ICC) and its associated precursor low and high-grade squamous intraepithelial lesions (LGSIL, HGSIL) has become increasing recognized over the last 20 years [20]. Taking into account that the presence of HPV infection alone is unlikely to be sufficient for cervical carcinogenesis, and other STIs may increase the risk of cervical neoplasia or ICC, in conjunction with HPV infection [21].

Chlamydia Trachomatis and Cervical Cancer Development

Chlamydia trachomatis is an obligate intracellular bacterium that infects human epithelial cells of the genital tract and ocular tissue. It is one of the most common STIs worldwide, with an estimated 89 million new cases per year [22]. Despite its generally asymptomatic course, genitourinary tract infections due to *C. trachomatis* are a major cause of morbidity in the sexually active individuals [23] and can cause severe sequelae, including pelvic inflammatory disease, ectopic pregnancy, and tubal infertility.

Chlamydial infections have also been associated with clinical cervical hypertrophy [24] and the induction of squamous metaplasia [25], providing supportive evidence for a possible role of *C. trachomatis* in the etiology of cervical disease. Recent epidemiological studies, based on the detection of type-specific *C. trachomatis* serum antibodies, have suggested that *C. trachomatis* infection may increase the risk of ICC among HPV DNA-positive women [17] and in prospective studies after controlling for HPV seropositivity [26]. Although *C. trachomatis* DNA has been found in ICC tissue using highly sensitive PCR-based methods, the prevalence has generally been low (3-22%) [27,28], suggesting that chlamydial infection does not persist in ICC tissue. Some recent studies addressed that *C. trachomatis* could participate in cervical carcinogenesis through an indirect effect, modulating epithelial gene expression mainly affecting some tumor suppressor genes [29].

Herpes Simplex Virus Type II: a Cofactor in Cervical Carcinogenesis?

The role of Herpes Simplex Virus infection in cervical neoplasia is subject of an active controversy. Firstly, HSV-2 infection was considered the major cause of cervical cancer, but the epidemiological data available in the 1980s, along with the lack of detection of HSV-2 DNA in cervical tissues, substantially weakened such hypothesis [30,31]. To date, serologic studies have reported conflicting results about the relationship of HSV-2 and cervical cancer. Whereas some authors detected a significant association of HSV and cervical cancer using HPV-adjusted models, no evidence of such link was found by others [17,32,33,34].

On the other hand, laboratory studies have demonstrated that DNA sequences of HSV-2 are capable to transform epithelial cells in conjunction with HPV, leading to mutations and/or rearrangements of cellular genes, which may have critical growth regulation functions [17]. However, the significance of HSV-2 in cervical cancer remained questioned because HSV-2 DNA sequences were not consistently detected in cervical tissues. To date, a few studies have explored the relationship between HSV-DNA and cervical cancer using highly sensitive techniques, such as the polymerase chain reaction (PCR) assay, with variable results [35,36]. Some *in vitro* studies suggested that HSV-2 infection induce the over-expression of E1, E2 and E6 genes up to 3-fold, increasing the risk of cervical cancer by over-expression of both HPV regulatory and oncogenic genes [37].

Alterations in the host Genome: Activation of Proto-Oncogenes

Alterations at the cellular genome level, affecting the function and expression of genes involved in the control of cell growth and cell differentiation are considered crucial events for the development and progression of cancer. A critical property of the malignant phenotype is the deregulation of cell signalling and cell proliferation, which commonly occurs through the over-expression or mutation of proto-oncogenes and the inactivation of tumor suppressor genes. An altered oncogenic activity is a characteristic mainly associated with many malignant and pre-malignant phenotypes [38,39,40], and the activation of several oncogenes has been found linked to many tumors, including squamous cervical carcinoma [41,42,43]. Proto-oncogenes activated in human tumors mainly belong to one of three families: *myc*, *erbB* and *ras* [10]. These proto-oncogenes have also been extensively studied in cervical cancer tissue [42,44,45,46,47] but the obtained results were sometimes not entirely conclusive [42,44,45,48,49,50].

The c-myc Proto-Oncogene

The *c-myc* proto-oncogene is the cellular homologous of the *v-myc* transforming gene [51], and encodes a helix–loop–helix leucin zipper domain transcription factor. Constitutive expression of *c-myc* enforces uncontrolled proliferation [52,53,54], avoids differentiation [55] or, in some cases, sensitizes cells to apoptosis, depending on the protein levels [56].

The *c-myc* proto-oncogene has been found amplified in many solid tumors and a variety of human cancer cell lines [57,58,59]. In epithelial solid tumors, activation of this proto-oncogene is frequently reached by gene amplification or deregulation of its expression as a consequence of mutations in *trans* [10,60].

As stated in several works, gene amplification appears to underlie most of *c-myc* over-expression in a high percentage of epithelial carcinomas [61,62,63,64,65,66], and protein over-expression is often associated with more aggressive tumors [61,65]. In this sense, *c-myc* over-expression is a common event in cervical carcinomas and correlate with the biologic behavior of the neoplasm [67,68,69]. The expression of c-myc protein appeared increased not only in cervical cancer specimens but also in the premalignant lesions. So that, increased c-myc protein expression in stromal cells could facilitate a suitable microenvironment which may support the growth and proliferation of transformed cells [70].

A recent study showed that several tumors have low-levels of oncogene amplification, with 3-7 copies of *c-myc* gene and also that this alteration was found more often in HPV related cases. This finding indicates that HPV-associated cervical carcinomas bear frequent alterations of this gene, which may has a critical biologic impact on the development and progression of carcinomas of the uterine cervix [71]. In addition, in HPV-18 positive cervical tumors, the region surrounding *c-myc* is indeed a hot spot of viral integration [72], suggesting a synergistic role for HPV and this proto-oncogene in the development of cervical carcinoma [67,72,73]. A recent study suggests that over-replication and breakage-fusion-bridge-type mechanisms are involved in the genomic instability associated with HPV cervical cancers [74]. Also, different amplification patterns seem to be correlated with disease outcome, providing new insights into HPV-related carcinogenesis and tumor progression [74]. Although high levels of *c-myc* oncogene are observed in many cases of cervical cancer, the actual meaning of *c-myc* in the process of HPV-mediated transformation is still unclear [75].

The c-erbB-2 Proto-Oncogene

The *c-erbB-2* proto-oncogene (also known as *her-2/neu*) encodes a transmembrane tyrosine kinase receptor, showing high sequence homology to the epidermal growth factor receptor gene (EGFR). The aberrant over-expression of the *neu* gene has been implicated in the induction of a malignant phenotype [76,77]. It has been postulated that overexpression of the oncoprotein leads to autoactivation of the tyrosine kinase domain and the activation of signal transduction pathways, cellular transformation, or cellular proliferation [78]. Since the 80's, *c-erbB-2* gene amplification and protein over-expression are known events that strongly correlate with node-positive breast carcinoma and the reduction in overall disease free survival [79,80]. *c-erbB-2* amplification also has been commonly found in ovarian cancer and grade 2 and 3 bladder carcinomas [81,82].

To date, several studies focusing on *c-erbB-2* gene amplification and protein over-expression have appeared either in cervical carcinoma or preneoplastic lesions [41,83,84,85,86], revealing that *c-erbB-2* amplification or protein over-expression are rare events in cervical carcinogenesis. Contrarily, the study performed by Soh et al. (2002) showed a statistically significant trend for increasing risk with higher quartiles for *c-erbB-2* [49]. Interestingly, two recent *in vitro* studies performed in normal oral epithelial cells and in a mammary cell line transduced with *c-erbB-2* showed that HER-2, E6, and E7 cooperate with endogenous EGFR to yield fully transformed cells [87,88].

At present, *c-erbB-2* gene amplification has been described in a wide variety of human cancers, but it has been poorly studied in noncancerous cytological samples from genital specimens positive for low-risk or high-risk HPV types. Little is known about *c-erbB-2* amplification in low-grade lesions of the uterine cervix, and the relationship between this genetic event and the presence of HPV.

The K-Ras Proto-Oncogene

The proto-oncogene *k-ras* encodes a 21-kDa protein (known as p21) involved in the transduction of the external cell signals, most likely growth factors. These proteins engage in guanine triphosphate (GTP) binding, and possess GTPase activity. Point mutations in codons 12, 13 or 61 appear to inactivate this GTPase activity, resulting in constitutive stimulation of autonomous growth and contributing to neoplastic development [89,90]. Point mutations at codon 12 are the most frequently found *ras* mutation in human malignancies [90] and today is widely recognized that the presence of mutant *ras* genes may identify tumors with poor prognosis [91].

However, the role of *k-ras* gene mutation in the carcinogenesis process of the uterine cervix remain obscure. Consequently, the question of whether spot mutations of the *k-ras* gene or an excessive protein expression level are an essential condition for the generation of the neoplastic phenotype of the cervical epithelial cells stays without an explicit answer [92]. The relationship of *ras* genes and HPV infection has been described in cervical carcinomas, but in the meantime the information concerning their implication in premalignant lesions of the uterine cervix stills quite restricted [93]. Meanwhile some authors described a tight association between HPV infection and *k-ras* gene mutations [41,93], other authors reported an absence of association between these two events [92,94]. So, the real meaning and effect of *ras* mutations in cervical carcinogenesis continue under investigation.

Single Nucleotide Polymorphisms (SNPs), Genetic Profile and Risk of Cervical Cancer

Human cancer is the result of many genetic and epigenetic changes in a determined group of cells, affecting also the surrounding stroma and producing new blood vessels. These genetic alterations produce a disruption in several cell's molecular pathways leading to a state of self-sufficiency concerning the growth signals [95]. At the same time, these genetic alterations induce insensitivity to growth-control signals and the evasion of programmed cell death, eliminating the replicative potential, and also sustaining the angiogenesis, invasion and metastasis processes [96,97]. Human cancer susceptibility is partially attributable to the presence of rare mutations in genes with major effects on tumor growth or survival. On the other hand, there is a lot of evidence pointing out that the combination of polymorphisms in low penetrance genes may account for a substantial part of cancer susceptibility [95]. An individual's susceptibility to develop cancer is mainly determined by the environment and the combination of inherited cancer susceptibility and resistance polymorphisms in a variety of high and low penetrance genes [98]. The impact of these polymorphisms on cancer risk and the efficacy of therapy are only now becoming unraveled [99].

Given the evidence that persistent HPV infection is a prerequisite for cervical carcinogenesis [100], it is suspectable that host genetic differences influencing the host response against viral infection may determine those people who are at highest risk for developing cervical lesions and progressing to invasive carcinoma. Genetic polymorphisms present in genes related to viral infection, immune response, DNA repair systems and tumor suppressor genes may influence and determine the excessive risk to develop cervical cancer [101,102].

Identifying those genes involved in cancer development is urgent to fully understand the biology of the disease, for developing new therapeutics and providing methods for cancer prevention and detection. The use of genetic markers, particularly SNPs, promises to provide a comprehensive tool for the analysis of the human genome in order to identify those genes or genomic regions tightly associated to the cancer phenotype [103].

TP53 Codon 72: The first Described SNP in Cervical Cancer

The frequent mutation of p53 gene in human cancers shows its critical participation in the carcinogenesis process [104]. Essentially, p53 exists in two main polymorphic forms at codon 72: i) arginine (72R) or ii) proline (72P) [105]. This polymorphism is balanced, although the selective pressure maintaining this situation is not known [106].

Storey and co-workers (1998) proposed that the polymorphism at codon 72 in the p53 gene could be associated with an increased risk for cervical cancer. Experimental studies have indicated that the protein containing an arginine residue at position 72 was more efficiently targeted for degradation by the HPV-16 E6 protein, suggesting that individuals homozygous for the Arg-encoding allele may have an increased susceptibility to HPV-related cervical cancer [107]. In this sense, the proportion of p53 Arg-homozygous genotype was significantly higher in cervical cancer patients than in the normal population [107,108,109]. Many epidemiological studies have so far failed to confirm such excess of p53 Arg-homozygous genotype [110,111]. In fact, the association of p53 codon 72 polymorphism with HPV-associated cervical squamous carcinoma risk has been studied by several groups obtaining inconsistent results. A recent meta-analysis performed by Koushik and co-workers [112] showed that the major failure in the published studies was the departure from Hardy-

Weinberg equilibrium in the control groups, diminishing the statistical power of the obtained results.

It has been reported that p53 arginine is only enriched in *in situ* cervical carcinoma, whereas the low grade and high grade CINs have a similar proportion to the control samples. This situation could be explained if p53 polymorphism plays a role only in the transformation of a high grade lesion into an invasive one [113].

Human Leukocyte Antigens (HLA) and Risk of HPV Infection and Cervical Disease Progression

As previously stated, a hereditary feature for cervical disease has been postulated and several studies indicate that the host genetic background is an important component in cervical cancer susceptibility. Among those genetic determinants that could contribute in susceptibility/resistance properties to disease outcome, certain polymorphic genes of the major histocompatibility complex (MHC) have been intensively studied [114].

The relationship of HLA Class II DRB1*13/DBQ1*0603 alleles and a protective effect for cervical cancer is the most consistent HLA finding in the published literature [115]. Opposite, carriers of other HLA class II alleles, *e.g.* DRB1*1501 and DQB1*0602, are at more risk to HPV-16 infection and the development of cervical carcinoma [116].

There are only a few studies focused in HLA-DQA alleles and risk of cervical carcinoma. Helland and co-workers (1998) reported that DQA1*0102-DQB1*0602 haplotype gives an increased risk of developing CIN for women infected with HPV-16. Other study, performed by Ferrera et al. (1999) suggests that the allele DQA1*03011 (in linkage desequilibrium with HLA-DR4 alleles), gives an increased risk for high grade cervical dysplasia and invasive cancer (RR=3.45), meanwhile the HLA allele DQA1*0501 (found in several DR52 haplotypes), confer a protective effect against cervical disease (RR=0.30) [117]. In fact, the whole region containing the HLA-DQ and HLA-DR genes appeared associated with the risk of developing squamous cell carcinoma [118].

Although many polymorphisms have been proposed as genetic markers for cervical cancer development and progression, further analyses studying larger samples are needed in order to describe the exact relations between these genes and susceptibility for CIN and cervical cancer with an adequate statistical power [119].

Gene Expression Profiling of Cervical Cancer

Transcriptomic alterations affecting key cellular processes such us cell proliferation, differentiation and genomic stability are considered essential for the development and progression of cancer. Large-scale gene expression profiling is allowing us to identify candidate proteins that may serve as diagnostic and/or prognostic markers. Tumor gene expression profiling is currently being explored as an additional tool to identify tumors with different clinical outcomes. Since cervical carcinomas develop through identifiable stages, the recognition of putative early markers that predict the progression from the pre-invasive stages to invasive carcinomas remains as an important task. A complete and simultaneous analysis of gene expression should therefore lead to important insights into the transcriptional mechanism. Two major systems have emerged for a compressive high-throughput gene expression profiling of the cancer transcriptome: i) DNA microarrays, and ii) *Serial Analysis of Gene Expression* (SAGE) platforms. These techniques are powerful instruments for understanding the complexity of gene interactions in carcinogenesis process, providing by far the most comprehensive view of active biological processes taking place in cells or tissues.

Very large amounts of expression profiling data are now available and the major main is to extract their biological meaning. A number of bioinformatic infrastructures have been established to collect and compile the data from high throughput analysis with the goal of molecular characterization of physiological and pathological processes. Among the most important are the *Cancer Genome Anatomy Projects* (CGAP, http://cgap.ncbi.nih.gov), the *Gene Expression Omnibus* (GEO, http://www.ncbi.nlm.nih.gov/geo/), and the *ONCOMINE* database (http://www.oncomine.org) [120,121,122]. Several bioinformatics tools are available in CGAP, GEO and *ONCOMINE* for data depositing, retrieving and mining. An upstanding resource in CGAP is SAGE Genie tools, which involve perhaps the *SAGE Anatomic Viewer* (digital northern among normal and malignant human tissues), *SAGE Digital Gene Expression Displayer* (provides significant differences in expression profiles between two SAGE libraries groups) and *SAGE Library Finder* (searches for tissue-specific libraries from the SAGE database). GEO is publicly available gene expression profiling resource, allowing data submission, search (*SAGEmap* and *Geo profiles*) and retrieval. *ONCOMINE* is a cancer microarray database and integrated data-mining platform, facilitating gene expression profiling comparison, annotation, and correlations across 118 microarrays studies involved 31 different cancer types.

A limited number of studies have been developed using functional genomics approaches in cervical cancer research. These studies were addressed to the identification of transcripts involved in cancer progression, radiotherapy response of SCC, molecular classification and HPV-host cell pathways interactions [123,124,125,126,127,128,129,130,131]. Global analysis of gene expression patterns identified functional groups of genes differentially modulated in early stages of cervical carcinogenesis, that may be involved in tumor progression.

MATERIALS AND METHODS

Samples

Three-hundred and four cervical specimens, previously studied for Pap and/or histopathological diagnosis, were collected from Caucasian women in gynaecological departments of hospitals from La Plata, Argentina. The mean age (±S.D.) of the samples was 32.4 (±11.2). Among these samples, 79 were classified as normal smears (Pap I/II used as controls), 190 pre-invasive specimens (36 condilomas, 79 LGSIL, 75 HGSIL) and 35 cervical carcinomas (SCC). Endo/Exocervical tissue scrapes were collected and suspended in 5 ml of 1x PBS, maintained at 4°C, and processed within 24 h. Paraffin embedded samples were processed by routine techniques for histological analysis. Four 10 μm paraffin embedded tissue from each biopsy were used for DNA extraction and analysis. Tissue scrapes and paraffin embedded biopsies were processed according to the methods previously described [132]. The obtained DNA was purified by phenol-chloroform-isoamylalcohol (25:24:1) extractions and collected by ethanol precipitation.

HPV-DNA Detection, Genotyping and Viral Load Determination

DNA samples were subjected to an ultra sensitive nested PCR for the detection of the HPV genome, according to the method previously described [133]. My09 and My11 were used as outer primers and GP05+/06+ were used as inner primers. HPV-DNA genotyping was performed by two well studied methods: i) PCR-LIS-SSCP (*Low Ionic Strength Single Strand Conformational Polymorphisms*) and ii) PCR-Reverse hybridization. PCR-LIS-SSCP was carried out according to the method described elsewhere [134]. Briefly, 4 μl of the nested PCR product was added to 10 μl of LIS solution (10% sucrose, 0.01% bromophenol blue, and 0.01% xylene cyanol FF). The mixture was incubated for 10 min at 97 °C, chilled on ice and applied on to a 10% polyacrylamide (39:1) minigel. The band pattern for each viral type was obtained by direct amplification from the plasmid-HPV clones comprising HPV-6, -11, -16, -18, -31, -33, -34 and -51 (Figure 1).

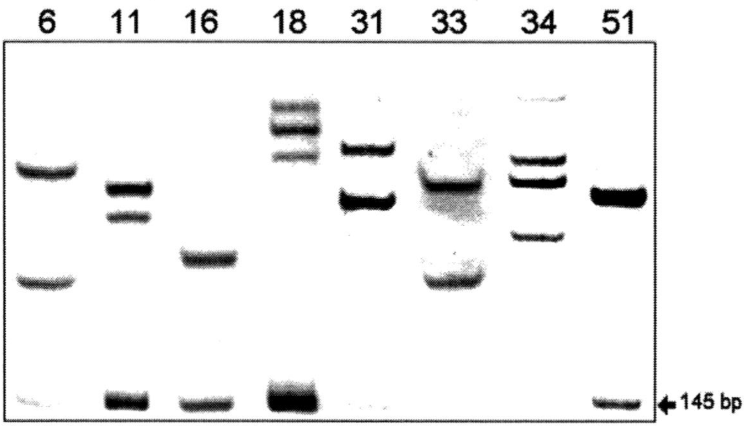

Figure 1. HPV-DNA genotyping by PCR-LIS-SSCP technique. DNA corresponding to HPV-6b, -11, -16, -18, -31, -33, -34 and -51 are shown. Electrophoresis was carried out on a 10% gel at 4°C during 4 hs (45 mA).

PCR-Reverse Hybridization was done with slight modifications according to previously described techniques [135,136]. In brief, GP06+ inner primer was modified by adding a biotin molecule in its 5' end. GP05+/06+Bio were then used for the second round of amplification as in the ultra sensitive nested PCR. The presence of an amplification product of the correct size was checked out on a 2% agarose gel and ethidium bromide staining. A neutral nylon membrane (Amersham Pharmacia, Sweden) was cut in strips (8 cm x 0.5 cm) and blotted with 13 different probes, comprising HPV-6b, -11, -16, -18, -31, -33, -34, -35, -

39, -45, -51, -52, and -58, according to the sequences provided by van den Brule et al. [126] and Lin et al. [127]. Optimal probe concentration was determined at 100 pmol each. Hybridization was carried out in hybridization solution containing 5X SSPE (0.9 M NaCl, 50mM NaH_2PO_4-H_2O, 5mM EDTA, pH=7.4) and 0.5% SDS at 33°C for 60 min. The strips were then incubated with streptavidin-HRP conjugated at 33°C for 20 min. One stringent wash was performed with 2.5X SSPE and 0.1% SDS at 33°C for 8 min. After the stringent wash the strips were left in citrate buffer (pH=5) for 5 min for pH stabilization. Colour development was accomplished with tetramethyl bencidine (TMB) and hydrogen peroxide for 20 min. Blue signals appeared on the strips when the amplified product hybridize with one or more of the spotted probes. HPV genotypes were read directly from the strips (Figure 2).

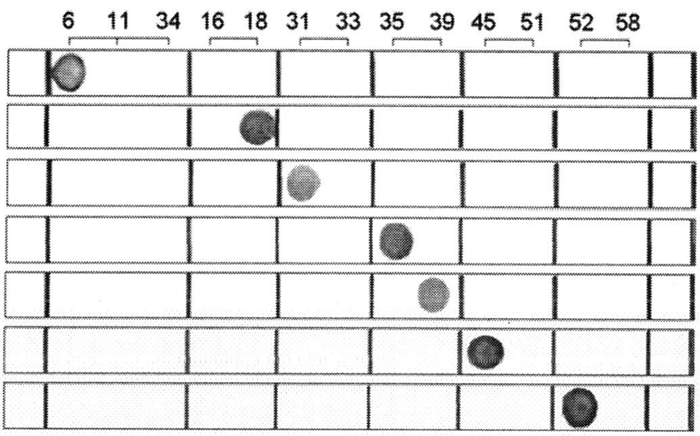

Figure 2. HPV-DNA genotyping by Reverse Hybridisation technique. Strips corresponding to HPV-6b, -18, -31, -35, -39, -45, -52 are shown. Neutral nylon membranes were blotted with 15 different probes and hybridised with biotinilated PCR amplicons at 33°C during 60 min.

Viral load determination was performed using low stringency PCR (LS-PCR) for DNA semiquantification [137]. PCR amplification was done in a final volume of 25 μl using 2.5 mM $MgCl_2$, 200 mM of each dNTP, 10 pmol of primers GP05/GP06, and 0.3 units of Taq DNA polymerase (Promega, Madison, USA), in PCR buffer (20 mM Tris-HCl, pH 8.4; 50 mM KCl). The reactions were cycled as follows: 1 cycle at 94°C for 4 min; 10 high-stringency cycles (30 sec at 92°C, 60 sec at 45°C, 60 sec at 72°C) followed by 30 low-stringency cycles (30 sec at 92°C, 60 sec at 40°C and 60 sec at 72°C). Detection of the amplified fragments was made by electrophoresis on an 8% polyacrilamide gel and SYBR-Green I DNA staining (Molecular Probes, Eugene, OR). Gel electrophoresis images were captured by means of a Kodak Digital Science camera and the bands net intensity were quantified using the *Kodak Digital Science 1D Image Analysis Software* (New Haven, CT, USA). To obtain the number of viral particles present in the infected cells, the ratio between the area and net intensity of the Gp and an arbitrary reference human band was compared with a calibration curve [138]. As described by other authors, 100 viral particles per cell was established in order to define a cut-off between low-viral load and high viral load for each sample [139].

HSV-DNA Detection and Genotyping

Primers flanking viral DNA polymerase gene were used to detect HSV-1/-2 as previously described [140]. PCR amplification was performed in a final volume of 25 μl, using 5 μl (1 ng/ml) of purified DNA, 2 mM $MgCl_2$, 200 mM of each dNTP, 25 pmol of each primer, and 1.25 U of Taq DNA polymerase in PCR buffer (20 mM Tris-HCl; pH 8.4 and 50 mM ClK). The reactions were cycled as follows: 1 cycle of 94°C for 2 minutes and 35 cycles of 1 minute at 94°C, 1 minute at 57°C, and 40 seconds at 72°C. Detection of the amplified fragments was made by electrophoresis onto a 2% agarose gel and ethidium bromide staining. HSV-DNA genotyping was performed by restriction fragment length polymorphisms (RFLP) using the obtained amplicon as described elsewhere (Figure 3) [140].

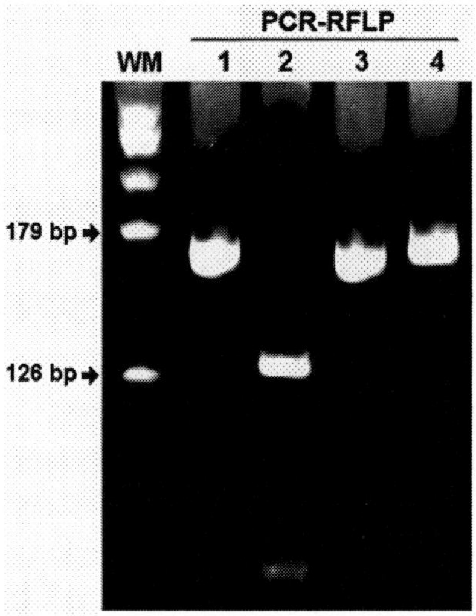

Figure 3. HSV-DNA genotyping by PCR-RFLP analysis of viral DNA polymerase gene. Lane 1 and 3: non-digested HSV-1 and HSV-2 amplicons respectively. Lane 2 and 4: HSV-1 and HSV-2 amplicons digested with *Bst*NI respectively. WM: molecular weight marker (pGEM® DNA marker, Promega).

Chamydia Trachomatis DNA Detection

C. trachomatis DNA was detected in cervical samples by PCR using PL6.1 and PL6.2 primers, as previously described [141]. These primers amplify a 155-bp fragment of the chlamydial multicopy bacterial plasmid. PCR amplification was performed in a final volume of 50 μl using 2.5 mM $MgCl_2$, 200 mM of each dNTP, 25 pmol of each primer, 0.3 units of Taq DNA polymerase, and PCR buffer (20 mM Tris–HCl, pH 8.4; 50 mM KCl). The reactions were cycled as follows: one cycle at 94°C for 2 min; and then 40 cycles without final extension (1 min at 94°C, 1 min at 56°C, 1 min at 72°C). Detection of the amplification products were made by electrophoresis onto 6% polyacrylamide/bis-acrylamide (19:1) minigels and then stained with ethidium bromide and exposed to UV 320 nm.

c-erbB-2 and c-myc Gene Amplification Analyses

Detection of *c-erbB-2* gene amplification was performed using the genomic differential PCR with the single-copy reference gene *thymidine kinase*, which represents the control gene located on the same chromosome. The multiplex PCR amplification was performed according to the method described elsewhere [44,81]. Detection of the amplified fragments was made by electrophoresis on a 8% polyacrylamide gel and SYBR Green I DNA staining (Molecular Probes, Eugene, OR). The *Kodak Digital Science 1D Image Analysis Software* (Kodak, Rochester, NY) was used to determine the ratio between net intensity bands of *c-erbB-2* and *thymidine kinase* (*TK*) (Figure 4A). Samples were considered to be *c-erbB-2* amplified when the ratio between net intensity bands was greater than ±2SD. All samples were examined in duplicate in order to confirm the obtained value.

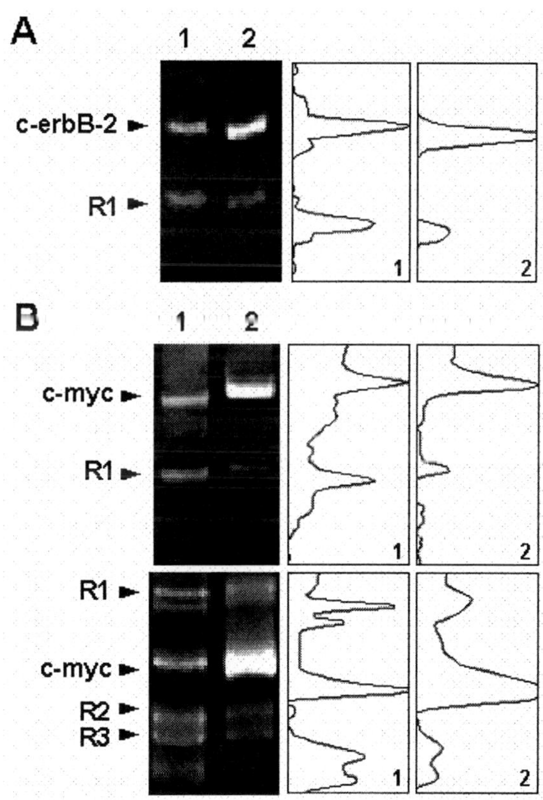

Figure 4. *c-erbB-2* and *c-myc* gene amplification analyses. A) Electrophoresis of RG-PCR products. Lane 1: normal sample; Lane 2: *c-erbB-2* amplified sample. B) Electrophoresis of RG-PCR (top) and LS-PCR (botton) products. Lane 1: normal sample; Lane 2: *c-myc* amplified sample. Arrows on the left hand of the figure indicate the target band (*c-erbB-2* or *c-myc*) and the reference bands (Rs). Boxes on the right hand of the figure indicate the net intensity/area bands digital pixels profiles.

The analysis of *c-myc* gene amplification was performed using the Low Stringency-PCR (LS-PCR) and the Reference Gene-PCR (RG-PCR) methodologies for DNA semiquantification. PCR amplification was done according to the method described elsewhere [142]. Detection of the amplified fragments was made by electrophoresis on an 8%

polyacrylamide gel and SYBR-Green I DNA staining (Molecular Probes, Eugene, OR, USA). Gel electrophoresis images were capture by means of a digital camera and the bands net intensity were quantified using the *Kodak Digital Science 1D Image Analysis Software*. To asses the degree of amplification, the net intensity from the c-*myc* band was divided by the sum of three arbitrary reference bands named as R1, R2 and R3 (Figure 4B). All the samples were analyzed in duplicates in order to confirm the obtained data and avoid false positive or negative results. Samples with *c-myc* amplification obtained by LS-PCR technique were further evaluated by RG-PCR method [142], confirming the obtained results (Figure 4B).

Detection of K-Ras Codon 12 Mutations

Mutations at the first and second bases at codon 12 of the *k-ras* gene were detected using the *Artificial Refractory Mutation System* (ARMS-PCR) [143,144]. This technique allows the selective amplification of mutant *k-ras* variants from cell suspensions through the creation of unique restriction enzyme sites. After elimination of the wild-type copies by restriction enzyme digestion, the assay allows for further mutant amplification, providing a sensitive approach to detecting *ras* gene mutations. The first round of PCR amplification was done using the primers 5BKIM and 3KiE [143]. An aliquot of 12 μl from the reaction was digested with *Bst*NI (New England Biolabs). The second round of amplification was performed using the entire digested product in a PCR reaction containing the primers 5BKIM and 3AKIL [143]. An aliquot of this second reaction was then removed and incubated with *Bst*NI. Detection of the amplification products were made by electrophoresis in 8% polyacrilamide gels and then stained with ethidium bromide and exposed to UV 320 nm (Figure 5A). Additionally, PCR-LIS-SSCP using 5BKIM and 3AKIL primers was employed to confirm *k-ras* codon 12 mutations (Figure 5B).

Analyses of p53 Codon 72 and HLA-DQA1 Polymorphisms

The p53 genotype was study by allele specific PCR using the primers and conditions previously described [107]. Briefly, PCR amplification was done in a final volume of 50 μl using 1.25 units of Taq DNA polymerase, 1.3 mM $MgCl_2$, 200 mM of each dNTP in PCR buffer (20 mM Tris–HCl, pH 8.4; 50 mM KCl), and 20 pmol of each primer. Reactions were cycled as follows: 1 cycle of 94°C for 2 min and 35 cycles of 40 sec at 94°C, 40 sec at 55°C (p53Pro) or 57°C (p53Arg), 40s at 72°C. Detection of the amplified fragments was made by electrophoresis on a 6% polyacrylamide minigel and ethidium bromide staining.

PCR amplification for HLA-DQA1 typing was done in a final volume of 50 μl using 1.25 units of Taq DNA polymerase (Promega, Madison, Wisconsin, USA), 2 mM $MgCl_2$, 200 μM of each dNTP in PCR buffer (20 mM Tris-HCl, pH 8.4; 50 mM KCl), and 25 pmol of each primers [145]. The amplicon covers the second exon of the HLA-DQA gene (242 bp). The reactions were cycled as follows: 1 cycle of 94°C for 2 min; 32 cycles of 30 sec at 94°C, 30 sec at 63°C, 30 sec at 72°C and finally, 1 cycle of 72°C for 5 min for chain elongation. Detection of the amplified fragments were made by electrophoresis on a 2% agarose gel and

SYBR-Green I® (Molecular Probes, Eugene, USA) DNA staining. HLA-DQA1 genotyping was performed using the commercial kit *Amplitype® HLA DQα PCR Amplification and Typing* (Perkin-Elmer, Branchburg, EEUU) according to the recommendations of the suppliers (Figure 6).

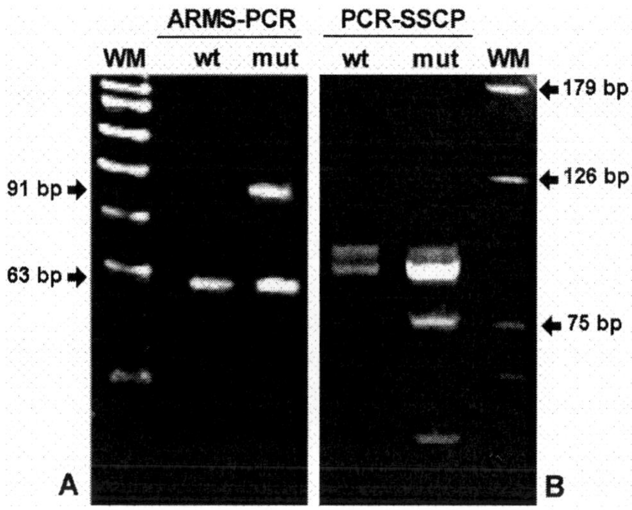

Figure 5. *K-ras* codon 12 mutation analysis using ARMS-PCR and PCR-LIS-SSCP techniques. A) Electrophoresis of wild type (wt) and mutated (mut) *k-ras* codon 12 samples on an 8% polyacrylamide gel. WM: molecular weight marker (φX174DNA/*Hinf*I). B) LIS-SSCP electrophoresis of wild type and mutated *k-ras* codon 12 samples on a 10% polyacrylamide gel. WM: molecular weight marker (pGEM® DNA marker, Promega).

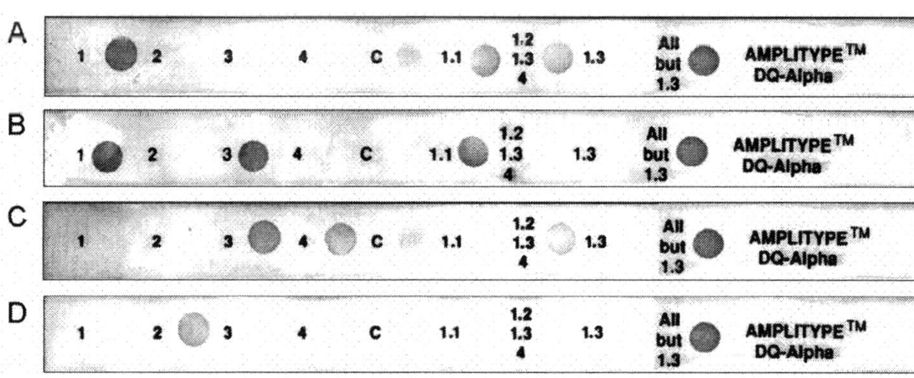

Figure 6. HLA-DQA1 genotyping by Reverse Hybridisation. Strip A: DQA1*0101-1*0102 genotype; Strip B: DQA1*0101-1*0301 genotype; Strip C: DQA1*0301-1*040 genotype; Strip D: DQA1*0201-1*0201 genotype.

Statistical Analysis

The associations between variables were assessed by chi-square test with Yates' correction. The odd ratios (OR) were computed as estimates of the relative risks, with 95% confidence interval (CI). Multivariate analysis was performed by Principal Component Analysis (PCA). In order to enable visualization of the factorial analysis, we employed a 3-D representation of component plot in rotated space. The basic significance level was fixed at $p < 0.05$ and all data was analyzed using SPSS® statistic software (SPSS Inc., Chicago, IL).

Processing and Statistical Analysis of DNA Microarray Data

GEO is an open access gene expression database (http://www.ncbi.nlm.nih.gov/projects/geo), that allow data browsing, query and retrieval. A previously published gene expression database of normal tissue and cervical carcinomas (GSE527) was download from GEO website and used for this study. This dataset was generated by Wong et al. 2003, using a custom-printed DNA arrays containing 11.000 DNA elements. Only the microarray experiments from 8 normal and 11 cervical carcinomas (FIGO stage IB) were selected.

To compare the normal and carcinoma groups, we utilized the *t* test statistical analysis application provided by the TIGR MultiExperiment Viewer (MeV 3.0) software [146]. This analysis allowed us to identify transcripts with significantly different expression levels ($p<0.01$). Furthermore, MeV software was employed for normalization and average clustering of the gene expression profiles. Briefly, the normalization included logarithmic transformation followed by median centering by samples and genes. We used standard average hierarchical clustering techniques to classify and illustrate further the differences found by *t* test, showing the clusters of differentially co-expressed genes between the normal and cervical invasive carcinoma groups.

For automated functional annotation and classification of genes of interest based on Gene Ontology terms, we used the *Expression Analysis Systematic Explorer* software (*EASE*) available at the *Database for Annotation, Visualization and Integrated Discovery* (*DAVID*) at http://david.niaid.nih.gov/david [147].

RESULTS AND DISCUSSION

Multivariate Analysis

Principal component analysis (PCA) is a multivariate and unsupervised strategy that allows the exploration of the data without any prior model revealing the natural grouping of variables. PCA of 304 cervical tissue samples (Figure 7, Table 1) identified statistical significant positive correlations between HPV (prevalence, viral load), HSV infections and cervical lesions ($p<0.001$). *c-myc* and *k-ras* activation were correlated with HPV (prevalence and viral load) and HPV/C. trachomatis infections respectively ($p<0.01$). It is interesting to note that p53 codon 72 polymorphism was not associated with HPV infection ($p=0.186$), HPV viral load ($p=0.484$) or cervical lesions ($p=0.219$) (Table 1).

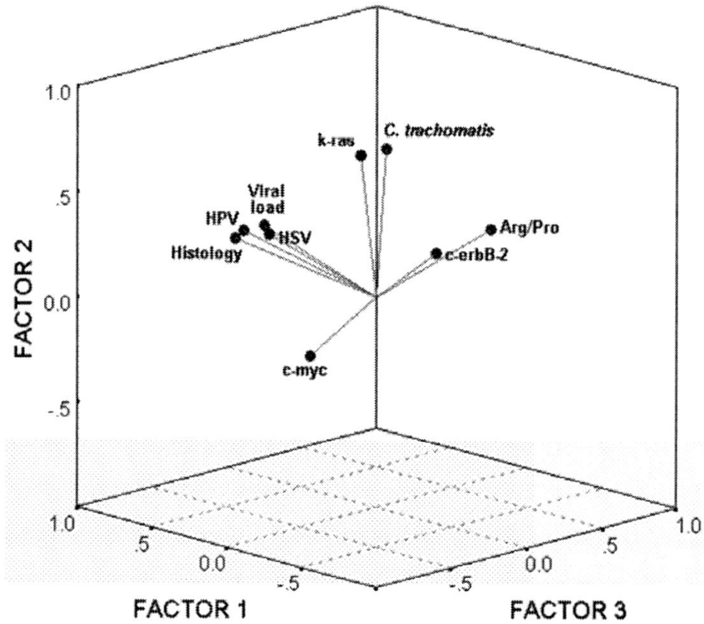

Figure 7. Principal component analysis of 304 cervical samples.

Table 1. PCA correlation matrix

	Variables	Histology	HPV	VL	CTM	HSV	*k-ras*	*c-erbB-2*	*c-myc*
Kendall's Tau-b	HPV	.670							
	Viral load	.577	.727						
	CTM	.137	.177	.192					
	HSV	.185	.114	.056	.046				
	k-ras	.161	.156	.122	.139	.088			
	c-erbB-2	.006	.087	.062	.079	-.004	.015		
	c-myc	.261	.256	.140	-.037	.033	.011	.023	
	p53	-.045	-.051	-.002	.073	-.099	.083	.075	-.006
p values	HPV	.000							
	Viral load	.000	.000						
	CTM	.008	.001	.000					
	HSV	.001	.023	.163	.211				
	k-ras	.002	.003	.017	.008	.063			
	c-erbB-2	.461	.065	.139	.086	.471	.395		
	c-myc	.000	.000	.007	.263	.282	.422	.343	
	p53	.219	.186	.484	.103	.042	.074	.096	.458

VL: HPV viral load; CTM: *C. trachomatis*

Sexual Transmitted Infections (STIs) as Co-FActors in Cervical Cancer

Human Papillomavirus DNA was found in 80.3% (244/304) of the studied samples. In the control group (Pap I/II), the prevalence of latent HPV infection was 30% (24/79). Among the abnormal specimens, 97.8% (220/225) appeared as HPV-DNA positive (Table 2). Whereas high-risk HPV-DNA was found in 69.3% (169/244) of the samples, the remaining infected samples were positive for low-risk HPV genotypes (Figure 8). The HPV-16 was found more frequently than other viral genotype, comprising 48% (117/244) of the analysed infected samples (Table 2) (Figure 8). Multiple infections were less frequent than single infection, comprising 18.4% (45/244) of the infected specimens studied.

Table 2. HPV, HSV and *C. trachomatis* infections among normal and cervical lesions groups

	Histology					
	Pap I/II	**Codilomas**	**LGSIL**	**HGSIL**	**SCC**	**Total**
HPV-DNA (-)	55 *(70%)*	- *(0%)*	4 *(5%)*	1 *(1,4%)*	- *(0%)*	60 *(19,7%)*
HPV-DNA (+)	24 *(30%)*	36 *(100%)*	75 *(95%)*	74 *(98,6%)*	35 *(100%)*	244 *(80,3%)*
High-risk	8 *(33,3%)*	20 *(56%)*	43 *(57,3%)*	64 *(86,5%)*	34 *(97%)*	169 *(69,3%)*
Low-risk	16 *(66,7%)*	16 *(44%)*	32 *(42,7%)*	10 *(13,5%)*	1 *(3%)*	75 *(30,7%)*
HPV-16	7 *(29,2%)*	15 *(41,7%)*	29 *(38,7%)*	42 *(56,7%)*	24 *(68,6%)*	117 *(48%)*
Low viral load	21 *(87,5%)*	23 *(64%)*	54 *(72%)*	39 *(53%)*	16 *(45,7%)*	153 *(62,3%)*
High viral load	3 *(12,5%)*	13 *(36%)*	21 *(28%)*	35 *(47%)*	19 *(54,3%)*	91 *(37,3%)*
HSV-DNA (-)	62 *(78,5%)*	27 *(75%)*	56 *(71%)*	49 *(65%)*	17 *(48,6%)*	211 *(69,4%)*
HSV-DNA (+)	17 *(21,5%)*	9 *(25%)*	23 *(29%)*	26 *(35%)*	18 *(51,4%)*	93 *(30,6%)*
***C. trachomatis* (-)**	70 *(88,6%)*	22 *(61%)*	46 *(58,2%)*	40 *(53,4%)*	28 *(80%)*	206 *(67,7%)*
***C. trachomatis* (+)**	9 *(11,4%)*	14 *(39%)*	33 *(41,8%)*	35 *(46,7%)*	7 *(20%)*	98 *(32,3%)*
Nº	79	36	79	75	35	304

When HPV-DNA positivity was evaluated, highly significant differences were observed between samples with normal and abnormal epithelia (χ^2=168.3, p<0.0001; OR=100.8, CI=36.8-276.2). Furthermore, high-risk viral types showed a strong association with the HGSIL/SSC groups with respect to the other histological stages (χ^2=212.3, p<0.0001; OR=68, CI=7.8-591).

Viral load was estimated for the 244 infected samples. A high-viral load (>100 HPV-DNA copies/cell) was found in 37.3% (91/244) of the analyzed samples following a non-parametric distribution (median=30 copies/cell, range 1-10500 copies/cell). HPV viral load analysis based on histopathologic group showed a strong correlation between high viral load infections and more advanced cervical lesions (Table 2), increasing the risk for condiloma

(χ^2=4.1, p=0.04; OR=3.9, CI=1-15.8), HGSIL (χ^2=9.2, p=0.002; OR=6.3, CI=1.7-22.9) and SCC (χ^2=10.6, p=0.001; OR=8.3, CI=2.1-33) development.

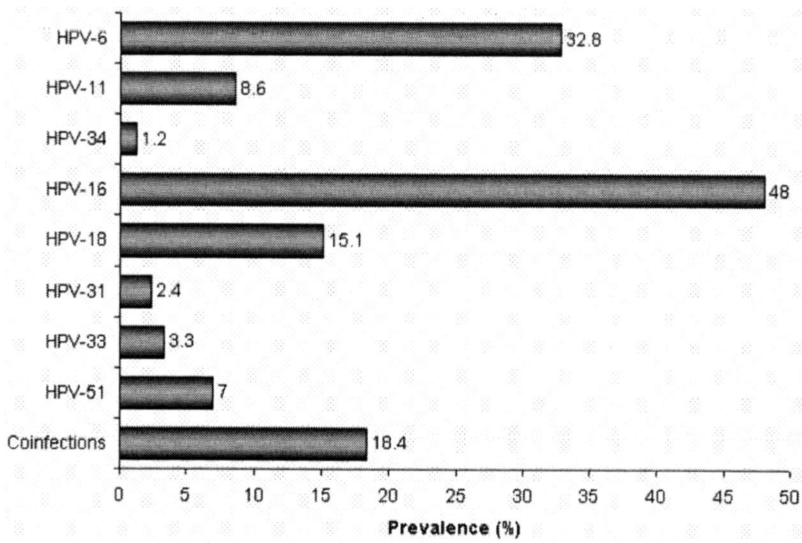

Figure 8. HPV genotypes distribution of the 244 positive cervical samples.

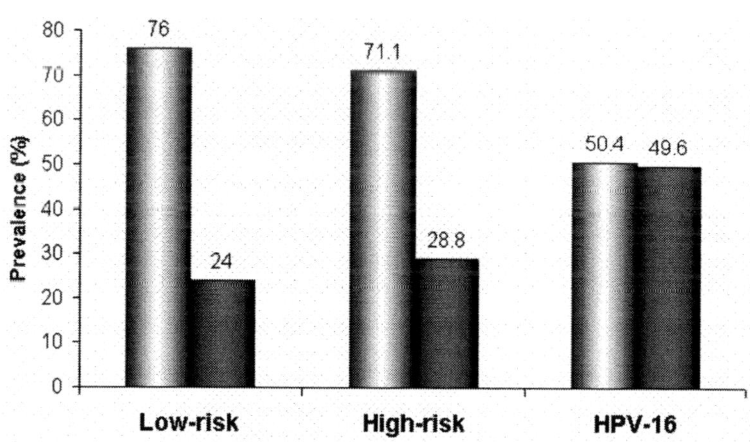

Figure 9. HPV viral load distribution among low-risk and high-risk viral types.

In the samples infected with high-risk viral types, 43.2% (73/169) presented a high-viral load, against 24% (18/75) found for the samples infected with low-risk types (χ^2=8.2, p=0.004). When only the samples harbouring the HPV-16 were considered, nearly 50% (58/117) showed a viral load above 100 particles per cell, a significantly higher value than 29% (15/52) obtained for other high-risk viral types (χ^2=12.5, p=0.0004) (Figure 9). Logistic regression analysis showed that HPV-16 and high-viral load association was independent of histopathological stage (χ^2=2.6, p=0.625).

The overall prevalence of HSV was 21.5% (17/79) in normal tissues compared with 35% (26/75) in HGSIL and 51.4% (18/35) among SCC (Table 2). In all the stages of cervical disease, HSV-2 was the prevalent type, with approximately 85% of the positive infections.

The prevalence of HSV in HPV-negative samples (21.8%) was approximately the same as that obtained in HPV-positive specimens (20.8%) ($p>0.05$). In addition, it is noteworthy that HPV and HSV-DNA positivity did not seem to be associated with a particular age's interval ($p>0.05$).

C. trachomatis DNA prevalence increased from low levels in women with normal cytology (11%) to those with HGSIL (47%) (χ^2=23.4, p=0.0001; OR=6.8, CI=3-15.6) (Table 2). However, *C. trachomatis* infection was not significantly higher in women with SCC than those with normal cytology (χ^2=1.5, p=0.22). In the age-adjusted model, the risk of HPV infection was not higher among *C. trachomatis* DNA positive than negative women ($p>0.05$). *C. trachomatis* DNA positivity did not appear associated with a particular age's interval (p=0.05).

For HSV-1 and -2, early *in vitro* experiments provided evidence about an effect modifier role. It was demonstrated that HPV-immortalized epithelial cells transfected with HSV-2 DNA became tumorigenic in nude mice, and several mechanisms of interaction were suggested [32]. However, loss of HSV-DNA in the transformed cell phenotype lead researchers to suggest a ''hit and run'' mechanism for cancer induction, suggesting that the expression of the HSV genes would be necessary for the initiation of the transformation process, but not for its progression [148]. Future *in vitro* studies are required to reveal the molecular mechanisms underlying the transformation abilities of HSV-2 DNA.

Our results, using highly sensitive PCR-based methods, found an association of *C. trachomatis* and both LGSIL and HGSIL lesions based on the direct identification of both pathogens. These results suggest that *C. trachomatis* acts as a cofactor to HPV in the earlier steps of cervical disease, possibly through chronic inflammatory responses produced in the cervical epithelia. In terms of biological plausibility, laboratory studies have shown that chlamydia has a cytotoxic activity through the mediators of the inflammatory response [149], possibly due to the overexpression of cytokines [150] or the alteration of cell-to-cell adhesion and cell differentiation patterns that predispose the cervical epithelia to HPV infection [151].

A limited number of studies have used highly sensitive polymerase chain reaction-based methods to examine the association between cervical cancer and HSV or *C. trachomatis* infections. In this study, the data indicated that neither HSV nor *C. trachomatis* infection were associated with HPV positivity among women with normal cytology. Furthermore, patients infected with HSV types 1/2 or with *C. trachomatis* were not at increased risk of cervical cancer.

The present study provides additional information concerning the presence of HSV and *C. trachomatis* DNA in normal and neoplastic cervical tissues. Patients with cervical cancer were not associated to HSV and *C. trachomatis* DNA, after controlling for age and HPV-DNA. However, there exists the possibility that other confounding sources, such as sexual behavior including woman's age at first intercourse or number of sexual partners, may have partially biased the obtained results. Indeed, this study has a relatively small sample size, although it has the advantage that the whole spectrum of cervical stages was examined. Nevertheless, the potential relationship between these pathogens and cervical disease awaits further evaluation in larger studies to clarify their true role in cervical carcinogenesis.

Proto-Oncogen Activation and Cervical Cancer

c-myc gene amplification was detected in 7.6% (6/79) of the normal specimens and 29.3% (66/225) of the cervical lesions showing high significant differences (χ^2=25.1, p<0.0001; τ-b=0.26, p<0.0001) (Table 3). When the frequency of *c-myc* activation was compared considering HPV infections, significant differences were detected between the HPV negative samples (5%) and those infected by HPV low-risk viral types (18.7%) (χ^2=5.6, p=0.017), as well as with the HPV high-risk infected group (25%) (χ^2=9.1, p=0.0002). Moreover, when only the samples harboring the HPV-16 were considered, near 36% (42/117) showed *c-myc* amplification (χ^2=20, p<0.0001). This fact indicates the strong association between the presence of this type of high-risk HPV and the activation of the *c-myc* oncogene.

Table 3. *k-ras, c-erbB-2* and *c-myc* proto-oncogene activations in normal and cervical lesions

	Histology					
	Pap I/II	**Codilomas**	**LGSIL**	**HGSIL**	**SCC**	**Total**
k-ras						
Wild-type	76 *(96,2%)*	30 *(83,3%)*	73 *(92,4%)*	59 *(78,7%)*	30 *(85,7%)*	268 *(88,2%)*
Mutated	3 *(3,8%)*	6 *(16,7%)*	6 *(7,6%)*	16 *(21,3%)*	5 *(14,3%)*	36 *(11,8%)*
c-erbB-2						
Normal	76 *(96,2%)*	31 *(86,1%)*	66 *(83,6%)*	67 *(89,3%)*	33 *(94,3%)*	273 *(89,8%)*
Amplified	3 *(3,8%)*	5 *(13,9%)*	13 *(16,4%)*	8 *(10,7%)*	2 *(5,7%)*	31 *(10,2%)*
c-myc						
Normal	73 *(92,4%)*	29 *(80,5%)*	62 *(78,5%)*	45 *(60%)*	23 *(65,7%)*	232 *(76,3%)*
Amplified	6 *(7,6%)*	7 *(19,5%)*	17 *(21,5%)*	30 *(40%)*	12 *(34,3%)*	72 *(23,7%)*
N°	79	36	79	75	35	304

c-erbB-2 gene amplification was found in 3.8% (3/79) of normal specimens and 12.4% (28/225) of the cervical lesions, showing the highest gene amplification frequency in LGSIL stage (χ^2=6.9, p=0.008) (Table 3). Non statistical significant differences were detected for *c-erbB-2* gene amplification in HGSIL (χ^2=2.7, p=0.1) and SCC (χ^2=0.21, p=0.64) groups. Furthermore, *c-erbB-2* amplification appeared correlated with low-risk viral types, particularly HPV-6 (χ^2=6.8, p=0.009).

k-ras codon 12 mutation was detected in 3.8% (3/79) of normal specimens and 14.7% (33/225) of the cervical lesions, showing the highest frequency in HGSIL group (χ^2=10.9, p<0.001) (Table 3). However, non statistical significant differences were detected between LGSIL and control groups (χ^2=1.06, p=0.3). When *k-ras* mutation was analysed considering

HPV infections, significant differences were detected between the HPV negative samples (5%) and those infected by HPV low-risk viral types (6.7%) (χ^2=4.35, p=0.036), as well as with the HPV high-risk infected group (16.6%) (χ^2=5.06, p=0.024). However, non statistical significant differences were detected in *k-ras* mutation frequency among different high-risk viral types (χ^2=0.52, p=0.47). Interestingly, principal component analysis showed a positive correlation between cervical samples infected with *C. trachomatis* and *k-ras* codon 12 mutation (τ-b=0.139, p=0.008). Further analyses should be conducted to corroborate this association.

Gene amplification is an important event in tumor induction and tumor progression. The *c-myc* oncogene has been implicated in the regulation of cellular proliferation, differentiation and apoptosis [54,55,152], and it was previously studied in cervical carcinogenesis as well as other malignant diseases, being proposed as a potential marker for cervical carcinoma development [67,153]. *c-myc* over-expression in conjunction with p53 inactivation in diploid cells markedly accelerates the spontaneous development of genomic instability [154]. In this sense, *c-myc* proto-oncogene is an important potential target because it is a critical point between the upstream *Ras* network of signalling pathways and the downstream Myc/Max/Mad matrix, affecting different aspects of cell behavior, including proliferation, differentiation and apoptosis by modulating distinct target genes [155,156]. Several works reported that different patterns of *myc* oncogene alterations could been associated with the integration of HPV-DNA in genital tumors, promoting the activation of the proto-oncogene via a mechanism of insertional mutagenesis and/or gene amplification [157]. Recently, it has been demonstrated a recurrent motif of amplification of HPV sequences upon DNA integration that suggest a common mechanism of gene amplification (perhaps *c-myc*/*c-erbB-2* amplification) based on homologous recombination as a result of over-replication [158]. Furthermore, we do not detect any statistical significant association between *c-myc* amplification events and *C. trachomatis* or HSV-2 infections (p>0.05). However, it has been recently shown that *C. trachomatis* mediate the up-regulation of *c-myc* expression in the transformation zone of non-neoplastic cervical tissue [159]. This study reveals a putative pathway by which *C. trachomatis* infection may contribute to neoplastic changes cooperating with HPV mediated transformation.

The obtained results showed that *c-myc* amplification appeared associated with the presence of HPV, particularly HPV-16, confirming the hypothesis of a correlation between the infection with high-risk HPV types and the activation of the *c-myc* oncogene through a gene amplification process. In addition, this work showed that *c-myc* amplification could be detected in a low percentage of pre-invasive lesions and a significantly high proportion of invasive ones, demonstrating that *c-myc* amplification takes place in the pre-malignant stage and could cooperate in the progression to more compromised lesions [158].

To date, *c-erbB-2* gene was shown to be amplified and over-expressed in a variety of human cancers [160,161,162,163,164], and both amplification and over-expression are associated with poor prognosis and overall reduction in disease-free survival [160,162,165]. We found an association between amplification of the *c-erbB-2* with HPV-6 infection. Also, *c-erbB-2* amplification was associated to the cytopathological stage LGSIL. This fact could reflect genetic changes happened for the acquisition of certain kind of low-grade lesions but not necessary for full neoplastic transformation. In the samples analysed, most of the LGSIL stage was characterized by the presence of koilocytes. So amplification of *c-erbB-2* could be related to the presence of this kind of cellular alteration. Since the cells could regress from these low-grade lesions to normal epithelia, amplification of the *cerbB-2* appears to be insufficient to achieve full cell transformation. These results are in agreement with other studies shown that amplification or overexpression of *c-erbB-2* plays a minor role in the oncogenesis of cervical carcinoma [161,166].

Several authors have examined the role of activated or over-expressed *ras* oncogenes in cervical carcinomas [167,168,169,170,171,172]. This study shows that *k-ras* codon 12 point mutations occur at relatively low rate in cervical premalignant lesions. Only 7.6% of the cases of LGSIL were found to carry mutation in *k-ras* codon 12 compared with 19% for HGSIL/SCC (21/110). The results of our analysis indicate that *k-ras* gene is possibly implicated by mutational activation in the development of a subset of cervical neoplasias. The fact that *k-ras* mutations were detectable in premalignant lesions indicates a possible role of *k-ras* at the initial stages of cervical carcinogenesis. Our findings are in accordance with previous studies, detecting *k-ras* mutations in association with high-risk viral types infection [170,171]. Interestingly, expression levels of *H-ras* and *N-ras* genes but not *k-ras* gene were found to be increased in cervical carcinomas compared with normal cervical epithelium [172].

In conclusion, *c-myc* amplification and *k-ras* activation, most likely triggered by high-risk HPV infection, may be an important step in the development and progression of premalignant cervical lesions. The detection of *c-myc* and *k-ras* mutations at initial stages of neoplastic cervical diseases underlines some of the crucial role in the multistep process of cervical carcinogenesis.

TP53 Codon 72 Polymorphism

p53 genotypes distribution among HPV infection and histological stages is presented in tables 1 and 2, respectively. Approximately 38% of the control group (Pap I/II) were found to be homozygous for the arginine allele (Arg/Arg); 50.6% were heterozygous (Arg/Pro); and 11.4% were homozygous for the proline allele (Pro/Pro). The frequency of proline (0.34) and arginine (0.66) alleles not deviated significantly from Hardy-Weinberg equilibrium (χ^2=0.63, p=0.427).

Non statistically significant differences were found for the frequencies of the different p53 genotypes in the different histological groups compared with normal counterpart (χ^2=4.7, p=0.79) (Table 4). Moreover, non statistical significant differences were detected for TP53 Arg/Pro polymorphism and HPV prevalence (χ^2=3.6, p=0,453), HPV-16 (χ^2=5.9, p=0,43) or high viral load infections (χ^2=0.48, p=0,975) (Table 5).

Many studies have attempted to repeat the results of Storey et al. [107], because it was assumed that the potential for increased degradation of p53 mediated by the E6 oncoprotein might contribute substantially to the risk of cervical cancer development. The results obtained in this study showed a lack of association between the Arg homozygous genotype and cervical disease progression, and thus they did not support the hypothesis that p53 polymorphism could be associated with an increased risk for cervical lesions development. In addition, these results showed non-significant differences for the frequency of the Arg/Arg genotypes between HPV-infected and non-infected samples. Moreover, no significant differences were found between the control group and those specimens with high-risk HPV, HPV-16 and high viral load infections. p53 codon 72 polymorphism meta-analysis based on 45 different studies clearly showed that there is not association between the Arg/Arg genotype and the increased risk for cervical cancer [112].

Table 4. p53 codon 72 polymorphism among normal and cervical lesions

				p53 codon 72 genotypes			
Histology	**Casos**	**Arg/Arg**		**Arg/Pro**		**Pro/Pro**	
Pap I/II	79	30	*(38%)*	40	*(50,6%)*	9	*(11,4%)*
Condilomas	36	16	*(44,4%)*	17	*(47,2%)*	3	*(8,4%)*
LGSIL	79	31	*(39,2%)*	38	*(48,1%)*	10	*(12,6%)*
HGSIL	75	36	*(48%)*	33	*(44%)*	6	*(8%)*
SCC	35	12	*(34,3%)*	21	*(60%)*	2	*(5,7%)*
TOTAL	304	125	*(41,1%)*	149	*(49%)*	30	*(9,9%)*

Table 5. p53 codon 72 polymorphism and HPV infection

				p53 codon 72 genotypes			
Characteristics	**Casos**	**Arg/Arg**		**Arg/Pro**		**Pro/Pro**	
HPV (-)	60	24	*(40%)*	29	*(48,3%)*	7	*(11,7%)*
HPV (+)	244	101	*(41,4%)*	120	*(49,2%)*	23	*(9,4%)*
Low-risk	75	30	*(40%)*	34	*(45,3%)*	11	*(14,7%)*
High-risk	52	25	*(48,1%)*	22	*(42,3%)*	5	*(9,6%)*
HPV-16	117	46	*(39,3%)*	64	*(54,7%)*	7	*(6%)*
Low viral load	153	65	*(42,5%)*	74	*(48,4%)*	14	*(9,1%)*
High viral load	91	36	*(39,6%)*	46	*(50,5%)*	9	*(9,9%)*

With the present evidence, it cannot be ruled out that p53 protein containing an arginine residue at position 72 could be more efficiently targeted for degradation by the HPV-16 E6 gene, although our results seems to indicate that polymorphism at codon 72 of TP53 gene is not associated with an increased susceptibility to cervical cancer development.

HLA-DQA1 Polymorphism

HLA-DQA1 genotyping was performed in 148 out of 304 cervical samples. Allele frequencies in each histopathological stage as well as in relation to HPV were detailed in tables 6 and 7. No departures from Hardy-Weinberg equilibrium were observed in HLA-DQA1 gene frequencies both in cases and control groups ($p>0.05$). The comparison of gene frequencies between cases and controls showed no significant differences ($p<0.05$). When the analysis was restricted to each histopathological stage, a significant increment of the allele DQA1*0101 was observed in the condiloma/LGSIL group (27.4%) whit respect to the control group (10.6%), with the concomitant increment in the estimated risk (OR=3.17, CI95%=1.40-7.14; χ^2=8.23, p=0 004) (Table 6). The other histopathological stages showed no deviations with respect to the control group (p>0.05). When dividing the cases in relation to the type of HPV present (high and low risk HPV types) the analysis of HLA-DQA1 allelic variants showed an absence of association with respect to the type of HPV present (p>0.05) (Table 7). No association was found between a specific HLA-DQA1 allele and the HPV viral load (χ^2=3.70, p=0.054) (Table 7).

Table 6. HLA-DQA1 allelic distribution in normal tissue and cervical lesions

Allelic variants	Control	Condilomas LGSIL	HGSIL	SCC	Cervical lesions	Total
1*0101	10 *(10,6%)*	23 *(27,4%)*	9 *(11%)*	7 *(18%)*	39 *(19,3%)*	49 *(16,5%)*
1*0102	12 *(12,7%)*	12 (14,3%)	15 *(19%)*	6 *(16%)*	33 *(16,3%)*	45 *(15,2%)*
1*0103	8 *(8,5%)*	3 *(3,6%)*	5 *(6%)*	1 *(3%)*	9 *(4,4%)*	17 (5,7%)
1*0201	16 *(17%)*	15 *(17,8%)*	11 *(14%)*	6 *(16%)*	32 *(15,8%)*	48 *(16,2%)*
1*0301	18 *(19,1%)*	10 *(11,9%)*	14 *(18%)*	6 *(16%)*	30 *(14,8%)*	48 *(16,2%)*
1*040	30 *(31,9%)*	21 *(25%)*	26 *(32%)*	12 *(31%)*	59 *(29,2%)*	89 *(30,1%)*

At present, only a limited amount of data concerning HLA-DQA1 and cervical cancer is available. Most of the published studies were focused in HLA Class I antigens or other HLA Class II genes and cervical cancer progression. Ferrera and co-workers [173] reported an increased risk for cervical cancer in women carrying the DQA1*0301 allele, which is in linkage desequilibrium with all the HLA-DR4 alleles. Other studies, such as the one performed by Maciag and co-workers [174], found that DQA1*0101/04 was inversely related to cancer development and progression. Contrarily, the results obtained in the present study indicated that DQA1*0101 was more frequent in the condiloma/LGSIL group than in controls, slightly raising the estimated relative risk. In general, all the studies between HLA genes and cervical diseases brought weak associations, with only small increments of relative risks [175]. Considering this situation, it is difficult to determine the true role of HLA antigens until larger series of patients and a higher number of MHC genes will be studied, so that more data became available.

Table 7. HLA-DQA1 allelic variants distributions and HPV infection

Allelic variants	HPV (-)	HPV (+)	Low-risk	High-risk	HPV-16	Low viral load	High viral load
1*0101	13 *(15,8%)*	36 *(16,8%)*	10 *(18,5%)*	26 *(16,5%)*	19 *(17,9%)*	21 *(16,9%)*	15 *(16,7%)*
1*0102	10 *(12,2%)*	35 *(16,3%)*	9 *(16,7%)*	26 *(16,5%)*	18 *(17%)*	20 *(16,1%)*	15 *(16,7%)*
1*0103	8 *(9,7%)*	9 *(4,2%)*	2 *(3,7%)*	7 *(4,3%)*	5 *(4,7%)*	8 *(6,4%)*	1 *(1,2%)*
1*0201	15 *(18,3%)*	33 *(15,4%)*	8 *(14,8%)*	25 *(15,6%)*	16 *(15,1%)*	19 *(15,3)*	14 *(15,6%)*
1*0301	13 *(15,8%)*	35 *(16,3%)*	8 *(14,8%)*	27 *(16,9%)*	15 *(14,1%)*	21 *(16,9%)*	14 *(15,6%)*
1*040	23 *(28%)*	66 *(30,8%)*	17 *(31,5%)*	49 *(30,6%)*	33 *(31,1%)*	35 *(28,2%)*	31 *(34,4%)*

Gene Expression Signature of Cervical Cancer

The primary goal was to identify the most commonly occurring transcriptome changes in the transition from normal cervical epithelium to invasive carcinoma. To this end, DNA microarray data publicly available obtained from 19 cervical samples were compared. Our statistically analysis revealed 167 transcripts commonly deregulated ($p< 0.01$) across the board when comparing normal tissue with cervical carcinoma. Among the 167 transcripts, 51 were down-regulated and 116 were up-regulated transcripts in cervical carcinomas (Figure 10) (Table 8; see supplementary data files for additional information).

We classified the differentially expressed genes in functional categories based on Gene Ontology terms (GO) [176]. GO analysis is a powerful bioinformatics tool suited for the analysis of DNA microarray and SAGE data, and allows one to identify families of genes that may play significant roles related to specific molecular or biological processes in expression profiles.

We used the EASE software to annotate the 167 deregulated genes according to the information provided by the GO Consortium [177]. We observed that 30% of deregulated transcripts are involved in biological processes related to cell growth and/ or maintenance, 44% are related to DNA/ protein metabolism, and 17% are related to signal transduction. Approximately 24% of these deregulated genes are related to molecular functions associated with DNA binding, more specifically with transcription factor activity (7%) and transcripts associated with hydrolyse activity (22%) (Figure 11).

Table 8. Commonly differentially expressed transcripts among invasive cervical carcinomas

Gene name	Description	Entrez Gene ID	Modulation p value
Cell growth and/or maintenance			
CDC14B	CDC14 cell division cycle 14 homolog B	8555	▲ p=0.0015
DLC2	dynein light chain 2	140735	▲ p=0.0088
CCNA1	Cyclin A1	8900	▲ p=0.0068
RAB7	Member RAS oncogene family	7879	▲ p=0.0001
PSEN2	Presenilin 2 (Alzheimer disease 4)	5664	▲ p=0.0049
MSH2	MutS homolog 2, colon cancer, nonpolyposis type 1	4436	▲ p=0.0011
APOC1	Apolipoprotein C-1	341	▲ p=0.0050
SEPT8	Septine 8	23179	▼ p=0.0015
NPC1	Niemann-Pick disease, type C1 gene-like 1	29881	▼ p=0.0030
RRAGD	Ras-related GTP binding D	58528	▼ p=0.0051
Signal transduction			
RGS3	Regulator of G-protein signaling 3	5998	▲ p=0.0003
INPP4B	Inositol polyphosphate-4-phosphatase, type II	8821	▲ p=0.0079
RALB	v-ral simian leukemia viral oncogene homolog B	5899	▲ p=0.0092
PPP2R5A	Protein phosphatase 2, regulatory subunit B	5525	▲ p=0.0060
DDR2	Discoidin domain receptor family, member 2	4921	▲ p=0.0004
KLRC2	Killer cell lectine-like receptor subfamily C	3822	▲ p=0.0003
ARHQ	Ras homolog gene family, member Q	23433	▼ p=0.0009
PTPRT	Protein tyrosine phosphatase, receptor type, T	11122	▼ p=0.0017
PTK7	Protein tyrosine kinase 7	5754	▼ p=0.0073
Transcription factor activity			
EZH2	Enhancer of zeste homolog 2 (Drosophila)	2146	▲ p=0.0012
GTF2H1	General transcription factor IIH, polypeptide 1	2965	▲ p=0.0011
TFAP2A	Transcription factor AP-2	7020	▲ p=0.0033
SIN3B	SIN3 homolog B, transcriptional regulator (yeast)	23309	▲ p=0.0087
KLF2	Kruppel-like factor 2 (lung)	10365	▲ p=0.0018
ZNF450	Zinc finger protein 450	9841	▲ p=0.0087
ZNF9	Zinc finger protein 9 (a cellular retroviral protein)	7555	▲ p=0.0092
HLX1	H2.0-like home box 1 (Drosophila)	3142	▲ p=0.0007
NAB1	NGF1-A binding protein 1 (EGR1 binding protein 1)	4664	▼ p=0.0002
NFIX	Nuclear factor I/X (CCAAT-binding transcription factor)	4784	▼ p=0.0083
Apoptosis			
BI1	BAX inhibitor 1 (Testis enhanced gene transcript)	7009	▲ p=0.0095
Hydrolase activity			
PSMC3	Proteasome (prosome, macropain)	5702	▲ p=0.0014
PON3	Paraoxonase 3	5446	▲ p=0.0037
DF	D component of complement (adipsin)	1675	▲ p=0.0013
CAPN2	Calpain 2	824	▼ p=0.0010
ADAH	Acyloxyacyl hydrolase (neutrophil)	313	▼ p=0.0066
Metabolism			
GM2A	GM2 ganglioside activator protein	2760	▲ p=0.0094
ARF4	ADP-ribosylation factor 4	378	▲ p=0.0003
PSPH	Phosphoserine phosphatase	5723	▲ p=0.0044
CA3	Carbonic anhydrase III	761	▼ p=0.0033
Miscellaneous			
CENPC1	Centromere protein C1	1060	▲ p=0.0008
INSL3	Insulin-like 3 (Leydig cell)	3640	▲ p=0.0070
BRD4	Bromodomain containing 4	23476	▲ p=0.0000
TOPORS	Topoisomerase 1 binding, arginine/serine-rich	10210	▲ p=0.0019

▲ Up-regulated gene in invasive cervical carcinomas.

▼ Down regulated gene in invasive cervical carcinomas.

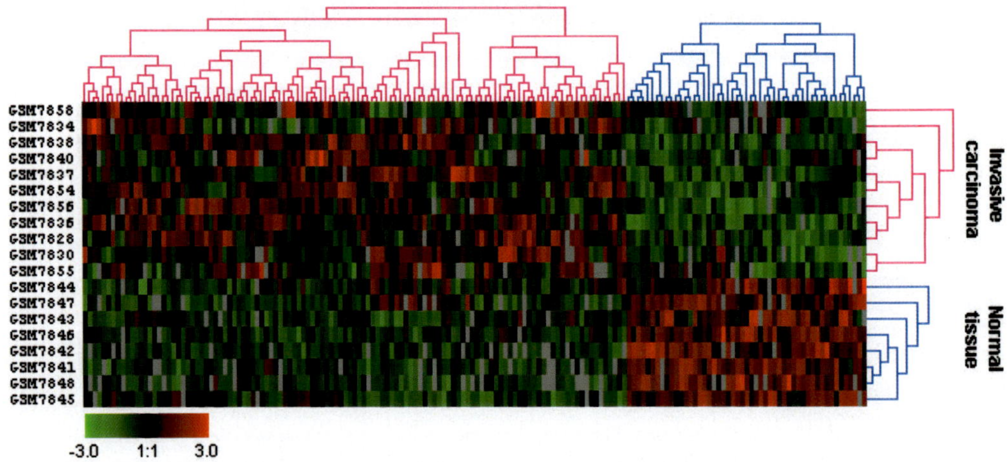

Figure 10. Hierarchical clustering of the most commonly different expressed genes between normal cervical tissue (blue cluster) and invasive cervical carcinoma (fuchsia cluster) groups ($p < 0.01$). Color scale at bottom of picture is used to represent expression level: low expression is represented by green, and high expression is represented by red.

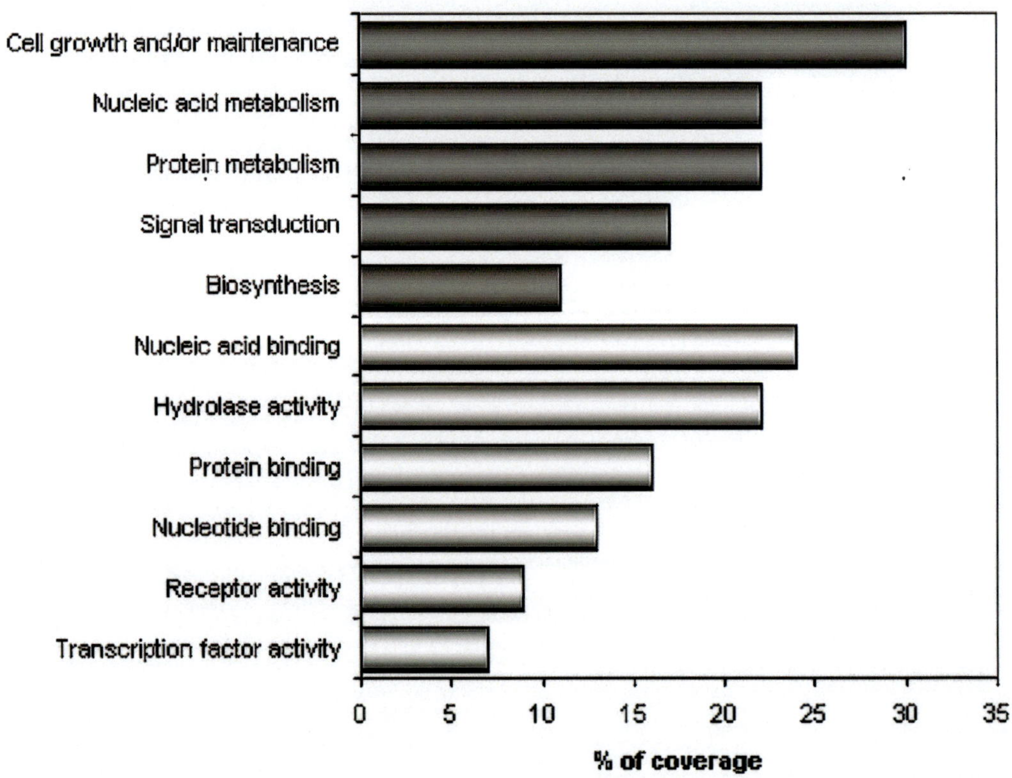

Figure 11. GO classification of 167 deregulated transcripts in cervical carcinoma identified by DNA microarray. Percent of coverage representing the percentage of genes annotated with a specific GO term related to Biological Processes (black bars) and Molecular Function (white bars).

Transcripts involved in cell growth and maintenance showed up-regulated gene expression patterns (Table 8). Besides activating oncogenic mutations and loss of tumor suppressor genes such as p53 and Rb, alterations in cell cycle gene expression are common features during tumor progression. Overexpression of cyclin A1 (CCNA1) was found in acute myeloid leukemia, and CCNA1 induced leukemia in a transgenic mouse model [178,179]. Recently, significant CCNA1 expression was detected in ovarian and endometrial cancer [180]. Furthermore, has been shown that CCNA1 interacts with Rb and E2F-1, and can activate the proto-oncogene B-Myb by phosphorylation in leukemic cell line model [178,181].

It is well known that tumorigenic growth depends on the evasion of normal homeostatic control mechanisms such as apoptotic death pathways. Recently, the anti-apoptotic protein Bax inhibitor-1 (BI1 or TEGT), was shown to represent a novel regulator of cell death pathways controlled by Bcl2 and Bax [182]. It was demonstrated that BI1 overexpression in mammalian cells suppressed apoptosis induced by Bax. Moreover, high expression of the anti-apoptotic protein BI1 has been demonstrated in several human cancers [183,184].

The Ral family of small G proteins are activated in response to several mitogenic regulatory cascades, and RAL activation has been implicated as a contributing factor to oncogenic RAS-induced cellular transformation [185]. RAL proteins has been involved in tumor-cell proliferation/survival, invasion, as well as metastatic process [186]. In addition, expression of constitutively active RalB can stimulate cell migration in bladder and prostate cell lines [187]. However, the role of RALB overexpression in cervical carcinogenesis remains unknown.

Our statistical analysis showed high expression levels of these transcripts in cervical carcinoma compared with normal counterparts. These genes could be involved in cell proliferation (CCNA1), antiapoptotic (BI1) and metastatic (RALB) signaling pathways during malignant transformation. Additional analysis and validation of the identified genes will be required to determine the clinical value, and to determine whether they may constitute novel targets for translational research.

SNPs and Risk of Cervical Cancer Development

Cancer is the consequence of several genetic and epigenetic changes in a certain group of cells and also in the surrounding stroma and the blood vessels [188]. According to published results, 291 cancer related genes have been reported, accounting for 1% of the total human genes [189]. Ninety percent of these cancer genes display somatic mutations in cancer stages, 20% show germline mutations (affecting cancer and normal tissue) and 10% show both kind of mutations [188].

It is being increasingly recognized that genetic predisposition as a result of the presence of some polymorphisms and mutations in the low penetrance genes also play an important role in determining the risk of cancer development [190]. The participation of large-scale and intermediate-size structural variation (ISV) in human genetic diseases and disease resistance/susceptibility conditions is in the initial stages and much more data is needed to be fully understood [191].

In the post-genomic era, single nucleotide polymorphisms (SNPs) are being studied to understand the biological basis of complex traits and multifactorial diseases. Despite the tremendous efforts for the identification of millions of new SNPs, the main priority would be focused in the association of this genetic variation in relation to the risk of disease development, using molecular epidemiology tools. Only a few cancer susceptibility genes were identified using classical case-control designs. This limited success could be mainly explained by the use of small sample sizes (reducing the statistical power and bringing high percentages of false positive associations), limitations in the search and selection of putative genes or sequences and the kind of analytic approach employed.

Identify those genes involved in the development and progression of malignant diseases is essential to fully understand cancer biology, for the development of new therapeutics intended for disease treatment and to find methods for early cancer detection and prevention. The use of polymorphic markers, in particular SNPs, assures to provide a comprehensive tool for studying the human genome in order to identify those genes or genomic regions contributing to reach the cancer phenotype.

After HPV infection, the progression from normal mucosa to cervical cancer involves a high number of environmental and host factors. Recently, family and population-based studies have demonstrated the importance of the hereditary component in cervical cancer, associated with genetic susceptibility [192]. Consequently, SNP markers should be considered for determining which combinations of genetic factors are involved in precancerous changes to cervical cancer.

A limited amount of data appeared in the scientific literature reporting the association of particular SNPs with cervical cancer development. Recently, some SNPs located in the FAS and FAS ligand gene promoter regions were tightly associated with cervical carcinogenesis [193]. Resistance to apoptosis signaling is a characteristic of cancer in which FAS/FAS ligand signaling plays an important role [193]. Other SNPs from the TNF-alpha promoter region have recently been shown to be associated with susceptibility to cervical disease [194]. Some of these polymorphisms have been reported to influence transcription of this protein. Distorted levels of TNF-alpha in the cervix might influence local immune response, thus affecting persistence of human papillomavirus [194]. Also, an SNP located at -1607 bp in the promoter region of the Matrix metalloproteinase-1 (MMP-1) creates Ets binding sites. MMP-1 polymorphisms might influence the ability of cancer invasion via transcriptional activity of this gene [195]. Furthermore, specific combinations of polymorphisms in p53, p21 and IRF-1 were significantly linked to cervical cancer in a set of Korean women [196].

In brief, at present only a limited number of SNPs have been studied in relation to cervical cancer development. The efforts should be directed in order to identify the genetic component bringing susceptibility to HPV infection and predisposition to develop cervical cancer, studying SNPs in those genes related with these processes. Also, a high-throughput technology should be used to obtain the accurate genotyping of several polymorphisms in large samples. In this sense, any project designed to study the so called low penetrance genes should propose a series of experiences in samples belonging to identified populations and providing knowledge of the mechanisms involved in cervical cancer susceptibility, allowing the identification of those groups in excess risk of cervical cancer development.

CONCLUSION

Alterations at the cellular genome level, affecting the function and expression of genes involved in the control of cell growth/ differentiation are considered crucial events for the development and progression of cancer. A critical property of the malignant phenotype is the deregulation of cell signalling, which commonly occurs through over-expression or mutation of proto-oncogenes and inactivation of tumor suppressor genes. An altered oncogenic activity is a characteristic mainly associated with many malignant and pre-malignant phenotypes, and the activation of several oncogenes has been found linked with many tumors, including cervical cancer. Cervical cancer development proceeds via a succession of genetic changes that involved high-penetrance genes (oncogenes, tumor-suppressor and stability genes), mutations triggered by different environmental co-factors such as HPV and co-infections (perhaps HSV and *C. trachomatis*). However, the acquisition of malignant transformation capability directly depends on host genetics background, defined by low-penetrance genes (genetics polymorphisms), immunological and physiological conditions.

Numerous molecular genetic changes have been reported as relevant in cervical carcinogenesis, such as anomalies affecting cell proliferation, apoptosis and invasion. Preinvasive cervical lesions such as HGSIL/ in situ carcinoma are known to have acquired a myriad of genomic and transcriptomic changes, but as their name implies they are not yet invasive. The development of the ability to invade surrounding tissues is perhaps the most critical event in cancer progression. Identifying the key and most common gene expression abnormalities involved in the transition steps from preinvasion to a fully invasive phenotype is an extremely important topic of research. Studies on this area may provide clues to better diagnose premalignant lesions at high-risk of progression and may aid in achieving a better understanding of critical early molecular mechanisms involved in cervical cancer evolution.

Despite the significant advances in the past years, functional genomics will provide one of the most important contributions in cervical cancer research. Future progress is expected in many directions, ranging from the HPV-host cell molecular interaction to elucidation of transcriptional regulatory networks of transformed cells. One powerful approach aimed at studying transcriptional regulatory networks is the genome-wide expression profiling (particularly the 5' SAGE platform) coupled to chromatin immunoprecipitation with promoter DNA microarrays (known as ChIP-on-ChIP assay), which identifies direct target gene under given set of conditions. Among the major advantages of the 5'-end Serial Analysis of Gene Expression (5' SAGE) methodology, is the generation of quantitative and qualitative sequence information of all transcripts being expressed by the cancerous or normal cells. A second major advantage of this methodology is the capability to globally identify transcriptional start sites (TSS) of expressed transcripts. Identification of the TSS is essential in establishing the full-length cDNA sequence of a gene and analyzing its promoter region providing insights on non-coding sequences features. ChIP-on-ChIP is performed with cells grown under a variety of conditions. Expression profiling is conducted on identical populations to determine the expression levels of each transcript. Expression profiling is subsequently performed on knockdown cells that have been treated with siRNA. Computational methods are then used to extract correlations between binding and gene expression and to generate novel putative transcriptional regulatory networks.

REFERENCES

[1] Parkin DM, Bray F, Ferlay J, Pisani P. Global Cancer Statistics, 2002. *CA Cancer J Clin* 2005,55:74-108.

[2] Czene K, Lichtenstein P, Hemminki K. Environmental and heritable causes of cancer among 9.6 million individuals in the Swedish family-cancer database. *Int J Cancer* 2002, 9:260-266.

[3] Beral V. Cancer of the cervix: a sexually transmitted infection?. *Lancet* 1974,1:1037-1040.

[4] Bosch FX, Lorincz A, Muñoz N, Meijer CJLM, Shah KV. The causal relation between human papillomavirus and cervical cancer. *J Clin Pathol* 2002,55:244-265.

[5] zur Hausen H. Human papillomaviruses and their possible role in squamous cell carcinomas. *Curr Top Microbiol Immunol* 1977,78:1-30.

[6] Stoler MH. Human papillomaviruses and cervical neoplasia: a model for carcinogenesis. *Int J Gynecol Pathol* 2000,19:16-28.

[7] zur Hausen H. Papillomaviruses and cancer: from basic studies to clinical application. *Nat Rev Cancer* 2002,2:342-350.

[8] Scheffner M, Romanczuk H, Munger K, Huibregtse JM, Mietz JA, Howley PM. Functions of human papillomavirus proteins. *Curr Top Microbiol Immunol* 1994,186:83-99.

[9] Ferber MJ, Thorland EC, Brink AA, Rapp AK, Phillips LA, McGovern R, Gostout BS, Cheung TH, Chung TK, Fu WY, Smith DI. Preferential integration of human papillomavirus type 18 near the c-myc locus in cervical carcinoma. *Oncogene* 2003,22:7233-7242.

[10] Brison O. Gene amplification and tumor progression. *Biochim Biophys Acta* 1993,1155:25-41.

[11] Bernard HU, Chan SY, Manos MM, Ong CK, Villa LL, Delius H, Peyton CL, Bauer HM, Wheeler CM. Identification and assessment of known and novel human papillomaviruses by polymerase chain reaction amplification, restriction fragment length polymorphisms, nucleotide sequence, and phylogenetic algorithms. *J Infect Dis* 1994,170:1077-1085.

[12] zur Hausen H. Papillomavirus infections - a major cause of human cancers. *Biochim Biophys Acta* 1996,1288:F55-78.

[13] Walboomers JM, Jacobs MV, Manos MM, Bosch FX, Kummer JA, Shah KV, Snijders PJ, Peto J, Meijer CJ, Munoz N. Human papillomavirus is a necessary cause of invasive cervical cancer worldwide. *J Pathol* 1999,189:12-19.

[14] Franco EL. Viral etiology of cervical cancer: a critique of the evidence. *Rev Infect Dis* 1991,13:1195-1206.

[15] Hildesheim A, Mann V, Brinton LA, Szklo M, Reeves WC, Rawls WE. Herpes simplex virus type 2: a possible interaction with human papillomavirus types 16/18 in the development of invasive cervical cancer. *Int J Cancer* 1991,49:335-340.

[16] Bernard C, Mougin C, Madoz L, Drobacheff C, Van Landuyt H, Laurent R, Lab M. Viral co-infections in human papillomavirus-associated anogenital lesions according to the serostatus for the human immunodeficiency virus. *Int J Cancer* 1992,52:731-737.

[17] Smith JS, Herrero R, Bosetti C, Munoz N, Bosch FX, Eluf-Neto J, Castellsague X, Meijer CJ, Van den Brule AJ, Franceschi S, Ashley R. International Agency for Research on Cancer (IARC) Multicentric Cervical Cancer Study Group. Herpes simplex virus-2 as a human papillomavirus cofactor in the etiology of invasive cervical cancer. *J Natl Cancer Inst* 2002,94:1604-1613.

[18] Silins I, Ryd W, Strand A, Wadell G, Tornberg S, Hansson BG, Wang X, Arnheim L, Dahl V, Bremell D, Persson K, Dillner J, Rylander E. Chlamydia trachomatis infection and persistence of human papillomavirus. *Int J Cancer 2005*,116:110-115.

[19] Castellsague X, Diaz M, de Sanjose S, Munoz N, Herrero R, Franceschi S, Peeling RW, Ashley R, Smith JS, Snijders PJ, Meijer CJ, Bosch FX. International Agency for Research on Cancer (IARC) Multicenter Cervical Cancer Study Group. Worldwide human papillomavirus etiology of cervical adenocarcinoma and its cofactors: implications for screening and prevention. *J Natl Cancer Inst* 2006,98:303-315.

[20] Boyle DC, Smith JR. Infection and cervical intraepithelial neoplasia. *Int J Gynecol Cancer* 1999,9:177-186.

[21] Paavonen J. Sexual dysfunction associated with treatment of cervical cancer. *Sex Transm Infect* 1999,75:375-376.

[22] World Health Organization. Sexually transmitted diseases. *Press Release-WHO* 1995:64.

[23] De Schryver A, Meheus A. Epidemiology of sexually transmitted diseases: the global picture. *Bull World Health Organ* 1990,68:639-654.

[24] Markowska J, Fischer N, Filas V, Fischer Z, Breborowicz J, Markowski M. The role of Chlamydia trachomatis infection in cervical cancer development. *Eur J Gynaecol Oncol* 1999,20:144-146.

[25] Kiviat NB, Wolner-Hanssen P, Peterson M, Wasserheit J, Stamm WE, Eschenbach DA, Paavonen J, Lingenfelter J, Bell T, Zabriskie V, et al. Localization of Chlamydia trachomatis infection by direct immunofluorescence and culture in pelvic inflammatory disease. *Am J Obstet Gynecol* 1986,154:865-873.

[26] Koskela P, Anttila T, Bjorge T, Brunsvig A, Dillner J, Hakama M, Hakulinen T, Jellum E, Lehtinen M, Lenner P, Luostarinen T, Pukkala E, Saikku P, Thoresen S, Youngman L, Paavonen J. Chlamydia trachomatis infection as a risk factor for invasive cervical cancer. *Int J Cancer* 2000,85:35-39.

[27] Gopalkrishna V, Aggarwal N, Malhotra VL, Koranne RV, Mohan VP, Mittal A, Das BC. Chlamydia trachomatis and human papillomavirus infection in Indian women with sexually transmitted diseases and cervical precancerous and cancerous lesions. *Clin Microbiol Infect* 2000,6:88-93.

[28] Wallin KL, Wiklund F, Luostarinen T, Angstrom T, Anttila T, Bergman F, Hallmans G, Ikaheimo I, Koskela P, Lehtinen M, Stendahl U, Paavonen J, Dillner J. A population-based prospective study of Chlamydia trachomatis infection and cervical carcinoma. *Int J Cancer* 2002,101:371-374.

[29] Schlott T, Eiffert H, Bohne W, Landgrebe J, Brunner E, Spielbauer B, Knight B. Chlamydia trachomatis modulates expression of tumor suppressor gene caveolin-1 and oncogene C-myc in the transformation zone of non-neoplastic cervical tissue. *Gynecol Oncol* 2005,98:409-419.

[30] Durst M, Gissmann L, Ikenberg H, zur Hausen H. A papillomavirus DNA from a cervical carcinoma and its prevalence in cancer biopsy samples from different geographic regions. *Proc Natl Acad Sci USA* 1983,80:3812-3815.

[31] Vonka V, Kanka J, Hirsch I, Zavadova H, Krcmar M, Suchankova A, Rezacova D, Broucek J, Press M, Domorazkova E, et al. Prospective study on the relationship between cervical neoplasia and herpes simplex type-2 virus. II. Herpes simplex type-2 antibody presence in sera taken at enrollment. *Int J Cancer* 1984,33:61-66.

[32] Guibinga GH, Coutlee F, Kessous A, et al. Role of herpes simplex type 2 in genital cancers: review of the evidence. *Arch STD HIV Res* 1995,9:164-179.

[33] Castle PE, Escoffery C, Schachter J, Rattray C, Schiffman M, Moncada J, Sugai K, Brown C, Cranston B, Hanchard B, Palefsky JM, Burk RD, Hutchinson ML, Strickler HD. Chlamydia trachomatis, herpes simplex virus 2, and human T-cell lymphotrophic virus type 1 are not associated with grade of cervical neoplasia in Jamaican colposcopy patients. *Sex Transm Dis* 2003,30:575-580.

[34] Pérez LO, Barbisan G, Abba MC, Laguens RM, Dulout FN, Golijow CD. Herpes Simplex Virus and Human Papillomavirus Infection in Cervical Disease in Argentine Women. *Int J Gyn Pathol* 2005,25:42-47.

[35] Yamakawa Y, Forslund O, Chua KL, Dillner L, Boon ME, Hansson BG. Detection of the BC 24 transforming fragment of the herpes simplex virus type 2 (HSV-2) DNA in cervical carcinoma tissue by polymerase chain reaction (PCR). *APMIS* 1994,102:401-406.

[36] Tran-Thanh D, Provencher D, Koushik A, Duarte-Franco E, Kessous A, Drouin P, Wheeler CM, Dubuc-Lissoir J, Gauthier P, Allaire G, Vauclair R, Dipaolo JA, Gravitt P, Franco E, Coutlee F. Herpes simplex virus type II is not a cofactor to human papillomavirus in cancer of the uterine cervix. *Am J Obstet Gynecol* 2003,188:129-34.

[37] Pisani S, Imperi M, Seganti L, Superti F, Tinari A, Bucci M, Degener AM. Effect of HSV-2 infection on the expression of HPV 16 genes in CaSki cells. *Int J Immunopathol Pharmacol* 2004,17:65-70.

[38] Vogelstein B, Kinzler K. The multistep nature of cancer. *Trend Genet* 1993,9:138-141.

[39] Ross D. *Introduction to oncogenes and molecular cancer medicine*. Springer, New York, USA 1998.

[40] Todd R, Wong D. Oncogenes. *Anticancer Res* 1999,19:4729-4746.

[41] Mouron SA, Abba MC, Guerci A, Gomez MA, Dulout FN, Golijow CD. Association between activated K-ras and c-erbB-2 oncogenes with "high-risk" and "low-risk" human papillomavirus types in preinvasive cervical lesions. *Mutat Res* 2000,469:127-134.

[42] Golijow CD, Abba MC, Mouron SA, Gomez MA, Dulout FN. c-myc gene amplification detected in preinvasive intraepithelial cervical lesions. *Int J Gynecol Cancer* 2001,11:462-465.

[43] zur Hausen H. Papillomavirus causing cancer: evasion from host-cell control in early events in carcinogenesis. *J Natl Cancer Inst* 2000,9:690-698.

[44] Golijow CD, Abba M, Mouron SA, Gomez MA, Guercci A, Dulout FN. Detection of c-erbB-2 gene amplification in cervical scrapes positive for human papillomavirus (HPV). *Cancer Invest* 2001,19:678-683.

[45] Sherbet GV, Patil D. Genetic abnormalities of cell proliferation, invasion and metastasis, with special reference to gynaecological cancers. *Anticancer Res* 2003,23:1357-1371.

[46] Mammas IN, Zafiropoulos A, Spandidos DA. Involvement of the ras genes in female genital tract cancer. *Int J Oncol* 2005,26:1241-1255.

[47] Moodley M. Update on pathophysiologic mechanisms of human papillomavirus. *Curr Opin Obstet Gynecol* 2005,17:61-64.

[48] Busmanis I. Biomarkers in carcinoma of the cervix: emphasis on tissue-related factors and their potential prognostic factors. *Ann Acad Med Singapore* 1998,27:671-675.

[49] Soh LT, Heng D, Lee IW, Ho TH, Hui KM. The relevance of oncogenes as prognostic markers in cervical cancer. *Int J Gynecol Cancer* 2002,12:465-474.

[50] Graflund M, Sorbe B, Sigurdardottir S, Karlsson MG. Relation between HPV-DNA and expression of p53, bcl-2, p21WAF-1, MIB-1, HER-2/neu and DNA ploidy in early cervical carcinoma: correlation with clinical outcome. *Oncol Rep* 2004,12:169-176.

[51] Colby WW, Chen EY, Smith DH, Levinson AD. Identification and nucleotide sequence of a human locus homologous to the v-myc oncogene of avian myelocytomatosis virus MC29. *Nature* 1983,301:722-725.

[52] Koskinen PJ, Alitalo K. Role of myc amplification and overexpression in cell growth, differentiation and death. *Semin Cancer Biol* 1993,4:3-12.

[53] Galaktionov K, Chen X, Beach D. 1996. Cdc25 cell-cycle phosphatase as a target of c-myc. *Nature 382(6591)*:511-7.

[54] Zanet J, Pibre S, Jacquet C, Ramirez A, de Alboran IM, Gandarillas A. Endogenous Myc controls mammalian epidermal cell size, hyperproliferation, endoreplication and stem cell amplification. *J Cell Sci* 2005,118:1693-1704.

[55] Facchini LM, Penn LZ. The molecular role of Myc in growth and transformation: recent discoveries lead to new insights. *FASEB J* 1998,12:633-651.

[56] Donzelli M, Bernardi R, Negri C, Prosperi E, Padovan L, Lavialle C, Brison O, Scovassi AI. Apoptosis-prone phenotype of human colon carcinoma cells with a high level amplification of the c-myc gene. *Oncogene* 1999,18:439-448.

[57] Riou GF, Bourhis J, Le MG. The c-myc proto-oncogene in invasive carcinomas of the uterine cervix: clinical relevance of overexpression in early stages of the cancer. *Anticancer Res* 1990,10:1225-1231.

[58] Schwab M. Oncogene amplification in neoplastic development and progression of human cancers. *Crit Rev Oncog* 1990,2:35-51.

[59] Schwab M, Amler LC. Amplification of cellular oncogenes: a predictor of clinical outcome in human cancer. *Genes Chromosomes Cancer* 1990,1:181-193.

[60] DePinho RA, Schreiber-Agus N, Alt FW. myc family oncogenes in the development of normal and neoplastic cells. *Adv Cancer Res* 1991,57:1-46.

[61] Heerdt BG, Molinas S, Deitch D, Augenlicht LH. Aggressive subtypes of human colorectal tumors frequently exhibit amplification of the c-myc gene. *Oncogene* 1991,6:125-129.

[62] Kreipe H, Feist H, Fischer L, Felgner J, Heidorn K, Mettler L, Parwaresch R. Amplification of c-myc but not of c-erbB-2 is associated with high proliferative capacity in breast cancer. *Cancer Res* 1993,53:1956-1961.

[63] Abou-Elella A, Gramlich T, Fritsch C, Gansler T. c-myc amplification in hepatocellular carcinoma predicts unfavorable prognosis. *Mod Pathol* 1996,9:95-98.

[64] Jenkins RB, Qian J, Lieber MM, Bostwick DG. Detection of c-myc oncogene amplification and chromosomal anomalies in metastatic prostatic carcinoma by fluorescence in situ hybridization. *Cancer Res* 1997,57:524-531.

[65] Masramon L, Arribas R, Tortola S, Perucho M, Peinado MA. Moderate amplifications of the c-myc gene correlate with molecular and clinicopathological parameters in colorectal cancer. *Br J Cancer* 1998,77:2349-2356.

[66] Christoph F, Schmidt B, Schmitz-Drager BJ, Schulz WA. Over-expression and amplification of the c-myc gene in human urothelial carcinoma. *Int J Cancer* 1999,84:169-173.

[67] Nair SA, Nair MB, Jayaprakash PG, Rajalekshmy TN, Nair MK, Pillai MR. ras and c-myc oncoproteins during tumor progression in the uterine cervix. *Tumori* 1998,84:583-588.

[68] Brewer CA, Liao SY, Wilczynski SP, Pastorekova S, Pastorek J, Zavada J, Kurosaki T, Manetta A, Berman ML, DiSaia PJ, Stanbridge EJ. A study of biomarkers in cervical carcinoma and clinical correlation of the novel biomarker MN. *Gynecol Oncol* 1996,63:337-344.

[69] Aoyama C, Peters J, Senadheera S, Liu P, Shimada H. Uterine cervical dysplasia and cancer: identification of c-myc status by quantitative polymerase chain reaction. *Diagn Mol Pathol* 1998,7:324-330.

[70] Brychtova S, Brychta T, Sedlakova E, Kolar Z. 2004. Proto-oncogene c-myc in uterine cervix carcinogenesis. *Neoplasma.* 51(2):84-9.

[71] Zhang A, Maner S, Betz R, Angstrom T, Stendahl U, Bergman F, Zetterberg A, Wallin KL. Genetic alterations in cervical carcinomas: frequent low-level amplifications of oncogenes are associated with human papillomavirus infection. *Int J Cancer* 2002,101:427-33.

[72] Ferber MJ, Thorland EC, Brink AA, Rapp AK, Phillips LA, McGovern R, Gostout BS, Cheung TH, Chung TK, Fu WY, Smith DI. Preferential integration of human papillomavirus type 18 near the c-myc locus in cervical carcinoma. *Oncogene* 2003,22:7233-7242.

[73] Bhattacharya N, Singh RK, Mondal S, Roy A, Mondal R, Roychowdhury S, Panda CK. Analysis of molecular alterations in chromosome 8 associated with the development of uterine cervical carcinoma of Indian patients. *Gynecol Oncol* 2004,95:352-362.

[74] Herrick J, Conti C, Teissier S, Thierry F, Couturier J, Sastre-Garau X, Favre M, Orth G, Bensimon A. Genomic organization of amplified MYC genes suggests distinct mechanisms of amplification in tumorigenesis. *Cancer Res* 2005,65:1174-1179.

[75] Subramanyam D, Krishna S. c-Myc substitutes for Notch1-CBF1 functions in cooperative transformation with papillomavirus oncogenes. *Virology* 2006,347:191-198.

[76] Semba K, Kamata N, Toyoshima K, Yamamoto T. A v-erbB-related protooncogene, c-erbB-2, is distinct from the c-erbB-1/epidermal growth factor-receptor gene and is amplified in a human salivary gland adenocarcinoma. *Proc Natl Acad Sci USA* 1985,82:6497-6501.

[77] Hudziak RM, Schlessinger J, Ullrich A. Increased expression of the putative growth factor receptor p185HER2 causes transformation and tumorigenesis of NIH 3T3 cells. *Proc Natl Acad Sci USA* 1987,84:7159-7163.

[78] Dougall WC, Qian X, Peterson NC, Miller MJ, Samanta A, Greene MI. The neu-oncogene: signal transduction pathways, transformation mechanisms and evolving therapies. *Oncogene* 1994,9:2109-2123.

[79] Slamon DJ, Godolphin W, Jones LA, Holt JA, Wong SG, Keith DE, Levin WJ, Stuart SG, Udove J, Ullrich A, et al. Studies of the HER-2/neu proto-oncogene in human breast and ovarian cancer. *Science* 1989,244:707-712.

[80] Tiwari RK, Borgen PI, Wong GY, Cordon-Cardo C, Osborne MP. HER-2/neu amplification and overexpression in primary human breast cancer is associated with early metastasis. *Anticancer Res* 1992,12:419-425.

[81] Lönn U, Lonn S, Nylen U, Friberg S, Stenkvist B. Gene amplification detected in carcinoma cells from human urinary bladder washings by the polymerase chain reaction method. *Cancer* 1993,71:3605-3610.

[82] Medl M, Sevelda P, Czerwenka K, Dobianer K, Hanak H, Hruza C, Klein M, Leodolter S, Mullauer-Ertl S, Rosen A, et al. DNA amplification of HER-2/neu and INT-2 oncogenes in epithelial ovarian cancer. *Gynecol Oncol* 1995,59:321-326.

[83] Dellas A, Torhorst J, Gaudenz R, Mihatsch MJ, Moch H. DNA copy number changes in cervical adenocarcinoma. *Clin Cancer Res* 2003,9:2985-2991.

[84] Rosty C, Couturier J, Vincent-Salomon A, Genin P, Freneaux P, Sigal-Zafrani B, Sastre-Garau X. Overexpression/amplification of HER-2/neu is uncommon in invasive carcinoma of the uterine cervix. *Int J Gynecol Pathol* 2004,23:13-17.

[85] Chavez-Blanco A, Perez-Sanchez V, Gonzalez-Fierro A, Vela-Chavez T, Candelaria M, Cetina L, Vidal S, Duenas-Gonzalez A. HER2 expression in cervical cancer as a potential therapeutic target. *BMC Cancer* 2004,4:59.

[86] Kim YT, Kim SW, Yoon BS. Expression of c-erbB-2 oncoprotein and the prognosis of patients with cervical carcinoma. *Int J Gynaecol Obstet* 2005,92:151-152.

[87] Al Moustafa AE, Foulkes WD, Benlimame N, Wong A, Yen L, Bergeron J, Batist G, Alpert L, Alaoui-Jamali MA. E6/E7 proteins of HPV type 16 and ErbB-2 cooperate to induce neoplastic transformation of primary normal oral epithelial cells. *Oncogene* 2004, 23:350-358.

[88] Woods Ignatoski KM, Dziubinski ML, Ammerman C, Ethier SP. Cooperative interactions of HER-2 and HPV-16 oncoproteins in the malignant transformation of human mammary epithelial cells. *Neoplasia* 2005,7:788-798.

[89] Bos JL. ras oncogenes in human cancer: a review. *Cancer Res* 1989,49:4682-4689

[90] Mizuuchi H, Nasim S, Kudo R, Silverberg SG, Greenhouse S, Garrett CT. Clinical implications of K-ras mutations in malignant epithelial tumors of the endometrium. *Cancer Res* 1992,52:2777-2781.

[91] Slebos RJ, Kibbelaar RE, Dalesio O, Kooistra A, Stam J, Meijer CJ, Wagenaar SS, Vanderschueren RG, van Zandwijk N, Mooi WJ, et al. K-ras oncogene activation as a prognostic marker in adenocarcinoma of the lung. *N Engl J Med* 1990,323:561-565.

[92] Pochylski T, Kwasniewska A. Absence of point mutation in codons 12 and 13 of K-RAS oncogene in HPV-associated high grade dysplasia and squamous cell cervical carcinoma. *Eur J Obstet Gynecol Reprod Biol* 2003,111:68-73.

[93] Prokopakis P, Sourvinos G, Koumantaki Y, Koumantakis E, Spandidos DA. K-ras mutations and HPV infection in cervicitis and intraepithelial neoplasias of the cervix. *Oncol Rep* 2002,9:129-133.

[94] Stenzel A, Semczuk A, Rozynskal K, Jakowicki J, Wojcierowski J. "Low-risk" and "high-risk" HPV-infection and K-ras gene point mutations in human cervical cancer: a study of 31 cases. *Pathol Res Pract* 2001,197:597-603.

[95] Kotnis A, Sarin R, Mulherkar R. Genotype, phenotype and cancer: role of low penetrance genes and environment in tumour susceptibility. *J Biosci* 2005,30:93-102.

[96] Hanahan D, Weinberg RA. The hallmarks of cancer. *Cell* 2000,100:57-70.

[97] Balmain A, Gray J, Ponder B. The genetics and genomics of cancer. *Nat Genet* 2003,33:238-44.

[98] Ewart-Toland A, Balmain A. The genetics of cancer susceptibility: from mouse to man. *Toxicol Pathol* 2004,32:26-30.

[99] Pietsch EC, Humbey O, Murphy ME. Polymorphisms in the p53 pathway. *Oncogene* 2006,25:1602-1611.

[100] Schlecht NF, Franco EL, Rohan TE, Kjaer SK, Schiffman MH, Moscicki AB, Duffy SW, Marsh International Collaborative Group. Repeatability of sexual history in longitudinal studies on HPV infection and cervical neoplasia: determinants of reporting error at follow-up interviews. *J Epidemiol Biostat* 2001,6:393-407.

[101] Hemminki K, Dong C, Vaittinen P. Familial risks in cervical cancer: is there a hereditary component? *Int J Cancer* 1999,82:775-781.

[102] Horng JT, Hu KC, Wu LC, Huang HD, Lin FM, Huang SL, Lai HC, Chu TY. Identifying the combination of genetic factors that determine susceptibility to cervical cancer. *IEEE Trans Inf Technol Biomed* 2004,8:59-66.

[103] Engle LJ, Simpson CL, Landers JE. Using high-throughput SNP technologies to study cancer. *Oncogene* 2006,25:1594-1601.

[104] Levine AJ. p53, the cellular gatekeeper for growth and division. *Cell* 1997,88:323-331.

[105] Matlashewski GJ, Tuck S, Pim D, Lamb P, Schneider J, Crawford LV. Primary structure polymorphism at amino acid residue 72 of human p53. *Mol Cell Biol* 1987,7:961-963.

[106] Beckman G, Birgander R, Sjalander A, Saha N, Holmberg PA, Kivela A, Beckman L. Is p53 polymorphism maintained by natural selection?. *Hum Hered* 1994,44:266-270.

[107] Storey A, Thomas M, Kalita A, Harwood C, Gardiol D, Mantovani F, Breuer J, Leigh IM, Matlashewski G, Banks L. Role of a p53 polymorphism in the development of human papillomavirus-associated cancer. *Nature* 1998, 393:229-34.

[108] van Duin M, Snijders PJ, Vossen MT, Klaassen E, Voorhorst F, Verheijen RH, Helmerhorst TJ, Meijer CJ, Walboomers JM. Analysis of human papillomavirus type 16 E6 variants in relation to p53 codon 72 polymorphism genotypes in cervical carcinogenesis. *J Gen Virol* 2000,81:317-325.

[109] Gudleviciene Z, Didziapetriene J, Ramael M, Uleckiene S, Valuckas KP. Human papillomavirus and p53 polymorphism in Lithuanian cervical cancer patients. *Gynecol Oncol* 2006. In Press.

[110] Helland A, Langerod A, Johnsen H, Olsen AO, Skovlund E, Borresen-Dale AL. p53 polymorphism and risk of cervical cancer. *Nature* 1998,396:530-531.

[111] Klug SJ, Wilmotte R, Santos C, Almonte M, Herrero R, Guerrero I, Caceres E, Peixoto-Guimaraes D, Lenoir G, Hainaut P, Walboomers JM, Munoz N. TP53 polymorphism, HPV infection, and risk of cervical cancer. *Cancer Epidemiol Biomarkers Prev* 2001,10:1009-1012.

[112] Koushik A, Platt RW, Franco EL. p53 codon 72 polymorphism and cervical neoplasia: a meta-analysis review. *Cancer Epidemiol Biomarkers Prev* 2004,13:11-22.

[113] Zehbe I, Voglino G, Wilander E, Delius H, Marongiu A, Edler L, Klimek F, Andersson S, Tommasino M. p53 codon 72 polymorphism and various human papillomavirus 16 E6 genotypes are risk factors for cervical cancer development. *Cancer Res* 2001,61:608-611.

[114] de Araujo Souza PS, Villa LL. Genetic susceptibility to infection with human papillomavirus and development of cervical cancer in women in Brazil. *Mutat Res* 2003,544:375-383.

[115] Hildesheim A, Wang SS. Host and viral genetics and risk of cervical cancer: a review. *Virus Res* 2002,89:229-240.

[116] Beskow AH, Moberg M, Gyllensten UB. HLA class II allele control of HPV load in carcinoma in situ of the cervix uteri. *Int J Cancer* 2005,117:510 514.

[117] Ferrera A, Olivo A, Alaez C, Melchers WJ, Gorodezky C. HLA DOA1 and DOB1 loci in Honduran women with cervical dysplasia and invasive cervical carcinoma and their relationship to human papillomavirus infection. *Hum Biol* 1999,71:367-379.

[118] Zoodsma M, Nolte IM, Schipper M, Oosterom E, van der Steege G, de Vries EG, te Meerman GJ, van der Zee AG. Analysis of the entire HLA region in susceptibility for cervical cancer: a comprehensive study. *J Med Genet* 2005a,42:e49.

[119] Zoodsma M, Nolte IM, Te Meerman GJ, De Vries EG, Van der Zee AG. HLA genes and other candidate genes involved in susceptibility for (pre)neoplastic cervical disease. *Int J Oncol* 2005b,26:769-784.

[120] Riggins GJ, Strausberg RL. Genome and genetic resources from the Cancer Genome Anatomy Project. *Hum Mol Genet* 2001,10:663-667.

[121] Edgar R, Domrachev M, Lash AE. Gene Expression Omnibus: NCBI gene expression and hybridization array data repository. *Nucl Acids Res* 2002,30:207-210.

[122] Rhodes DR, Yu J, Shanker K, Deshpande N, Varambally R, Ghosh D, Barrette T, Pandey A, Chinnaiyan AM. ONCOMINE: a cancer microarray database and integrated data-mining platform. *Neoplasia* 2004,6:1-6.

[123] Alazawi W, Pett M, Arch B, Scott L, Freeman T, Stanley MA, Coleman N. Changes in cervical keratinocyte gene expression associated with integration of human papillomavirus 16. *Cancer Res* 2002;62:6959-6965.

[124] Kitahara O, Katagiri T, Tsunoda T, Harima Y, Nakamura Y. Classification of sensitivity or resistance of cervical cancers to ionizing radiation according to

expression profiles of 62 genes selected by cDNA microarray analysis. *Neoplasia* 2002;4:295-303.

[125] Wong YF, Selvanayagam ZE, Wei N, Porter J, Vittal R, Hu R, Lin Y, Liao J, Hu R, Lin Y, Liao J, Shih JW, Cheung TH, Lo KWK, Yim SF, Yip SK, Ngong DT, Siu N, Chan LKY, Chan CS, Kong T, Kutlina E, McKinnon RD, Denhardt DT, Chin K, Chung TKH. Expression genomics of cervical cancer: molecular classification and prediction of radiotherapy response by DNA microarray. *Clin Cancer Res* 2003, 9:5486-5492.

[126] Fujimoto T, Nishikawa A, Iwasaki M, Akutagawa N, Teramoto M, Kudo R. Gene expression profiling in two morphologically different uterine cervical carcinoma cell lines derived from a single donor using a human cancer cDNA array. *Gynecol Oncol* 2004;93:446-453.

[127] Contag SA, Gostaut BS, Clayton AC, Dixon MH, McGovern RM, Calhoun ES. Comparison of gene expression in squamous cell carcinoma and adenocarcinomas of the uterine cervix. *Gynecol Oncol* 2004;95:610-617.

[128] Thierry F, Benotmane MA, Demeret C, Mori M, Teissier S, Desaintes C. A genomic approach reveals a novel mitotic pathway in papillomavirus carcinogenesis. *Cancer Res* 2004;64:895-903.

[129] Seo M, Bae SM, Kim Y, Kim YW, Hur SY, Ro DY, Lee JM, Namkoong SE, Kim CK, Ahn WS. New approaches to pathogenic gene function discovery with human squamous cell cervical carcinoma by gene ontology. *Gynecologic Oncology* 2005, 96:621-629.

[130] Tewari D, Monk BJ, Al-Ghazi MS, Parker R, Heck JD, Burger RA, Fruehauf JP. Gene expression profiling of in vitro radiation resistance in cervical carcinoma: a feaseibility study. *Gynecol Oncol* 2005;99:84-91.

[131] Pérez-Plasencia C, Riggins G, Vázquez-Ortiz G, Moreno J, Arreola H, Hidalgo A, Piña-Sanchez P, Salcedo M. Characterization of the global profile of gene expressed in cervical epithelium by Serial Análisis of Gene Expresión (SAGE). *BMC Genomics* 2005, 6:130.

[132] Abba MC, Gomez MA, Golijow CD. Human papillomavirus genotype distribution in cervical infections among woman in La Plata, Argentina. *Rev Argent Microbiol* 2003,35:74-79.

[133] Evander M, Edlund K, Bodun E. Comparison of a one-step and two-step polymerase chain reaction with the degenerate general primers in a population-based study of *Human Papillomavirus* infection in young Swedish women. *J Clin Microbiol* 1992,30:987–992.

[134] Gómez MA, Abba MC, Golijow CD. Detección y genotipificación del *Papillomavirus Humano* (HPV) por PCR-LIS-SSCP. *Rev Arg Microbiol* 2001,1:22-27.

[135] Snijders PS, van den Brule AJ, Jacobs MV, Pol RP, Meijer CS. HPV DNA detection and typing in cervical scrapes. *Methods Mol Med* 2005,119:101-114.

[136] Lin H, Moh JS, Ou YC, Shen SY, Tsai YM, ChangChien CC, Liu JM, Ma YY. A simple method for the detection and genotyping of high-risk human papillomavirus using seminested polymerase chain reaction and reverse hybridization. *Gynecol Oncol* 2005,96:84-91.

[137] Abba MC, Mourón SA, Gómez MA, Dulout FN and Golijow CD. Association Human Papillomavirus viral load with HPV-16 and high-grade intraepithelial lesion. *Int J Gynecol Cancer* 2003,13:154-158.

[138] Caballero OL, Villa LL, Simpson AJ. Low stringency-PCR (LS-PCR) allows entirely internally standardized DNA quantitation. *Nucl Acids Res* 1995,23:192-193.

[139] Swan DC, Tucker RA, Tortolero-Luna G, Mitchell MF, Wideroff L, Unger ER, Nisenbaum RA, Reeves WC, Icenogle JP. Human papillomavirus (HPV) DNA copy number is dependent on grade of cervical disease and HPV type. *J Clin Microbiol* 1999,37:1030-1034.

[140] Abba MC, Golijow CD. Herpes simplex virus genotyping: multiple optional PCR based RFLP systems and a single-stranded conformation polymorphism method. *J Virol Methods* 2004,118:73-76.

[141] Morré SA, van Valkengoed IGM, DE Jong A, Boeke AJ, van Eijk JT, Meijer CJ, van den Brule AJ. Mailed, home-obtained urine specimens: a reliable screening approach for detecting asymptomatic Chlamydia trachomatis infections. *J Clin Microbiol* 1999,37:976-980.

[142] Abba MC, Laguens RM, Dulout FN, Golijow CD. C-myc activation in cervical carcinomas and high-risk HPV infections. *Mutation Res* 2004,557:151-158.

[143] Ward RL, Santiago F, Hawkins NJ, Coomber D, O'Connor T, Todd AV. A rapid PCR ELISA for the detection of activated K-*ras* in colorectal cancer. *J Clin Pathol Mol Pathol* 1995,48:273-277.

[144] Mourón SA, Abba MC, Güercci A, Gómez MA, Dulout FN, Golijow CD. Association between activated K-ras and c-erbB-2 oncogenes with "high-risk" and "low-risk" HPV types in non-cancerous cervical samples. *Mutation Res* 2000,469:127-134.

[145] Abba MC, Gómez MA, Golijow CD. Allele typing of HLA-DQA1 by non-isotopic PCR-LIS-SSCP. *Braz J Med Biol Res* 2001,34:867-869.

[146] Saeed AI, Sharov V, White J, Li J, Liang W, Bhagabati N, Braisted J, Klapa M, Currier T, Thiagarajan M, Sturn A, Snuffin M, Rezantsev A, Popov D, Ryltsov A, Kostukovich E, Borisovsky I, Liu Z, Vinsavich A, Trush V, Quackenbush J. TM4: a free, open-source system for microarray data management and analysis. *Biotechniques* 2003,34:374-378.

[147] Dennis G, Sherman BT, Hosack DA, Yang J, Gao W, Lane HC, Lempicki RA. DAVID: Database for Annotation, Visualization, and Integrated Discovery. *Genome Biol* 2003,4:R60.

[148] Galloway DA, McDougall JK. The oncogenic potential of herpes simplex viruses: evidence for a hit and run mechanism. *Nature* 1981,302:21-24.

[149] Belland RJ, Scidmore MA, Crane DB, Hogan DM, Whitmire W, McClarty G, Caldwell HD. Chlamydia trachomatis cytotoxicity associated with complete and partial cytotoxin genes. *Proc Natl Acad Sci USA* 2001, 98:13984-13989.

[150] Chiarini F, Pisani S, Gallinelli C, Papi E, Seganti L, Degener AM, Pierangeli A, Gentile V, Brunori S, Di Silverio F. Simultaneous detection of HPV and other sexually transmitted agents in chronic urethritis. *Minerva Urol Nefrol* 1998,50:225-231.

[151] Prozialeck WC, Fay MJ, Lamar PC, Pearson CA, Sigar I, Ramsey KH. *Chlamydia trachomatis* disrupts N-cadherin-dependent cell-cell junctions and sequesters beta-catenin in human cervical epithelial cells. *Infect Immun* 2002,70:2605-2613.

[152] Donzelli M, R. Bernardi, C. Negri, E. Prosperi, L. Padovan, C. Lavialle, O. Brison, A.I. Scovassi. Apoptosis-prone phenotype of human colon carcinoma cells with a high level amplification of the c-*myc* gene. *Oncogene* 1999,18:439-448.

[153] Brewer C, Liao S, Wilczynski S, Pastorekova S, Pastorek J, Zavada J, Kurosaki T, Manetta A, Berman M, DiSaia P, Stanbridge E. A study of biomarkers in cervical carcinoma and clinical correlation of the novel biomarker MN. *Gynecol Oncol* 1996,63:337-344.

[154] Yin XY, Grove L, Datta NS, Long MW, Prochownik EV. C-myc overexpression and p53 loss cooperate to promote genomic instability. *Oncogene* 1999,18:1177-1184.

[155] Adjei AA. Blocking oncogenic ras signaling for cancer therapy. *J Nat Cancer Inst* 2001,93:1062-1074.

[156] Luscher B. Function and regulation of the transcription factors of the Myc/Max/Mad network. *Gene* 2001,277:1-14.

[157] Sastre-Garau X, Favre M, Couturier J, Orth G. Distinct patterns of alteration of *myc* genes associated with integration of *Human Papillomavirus* type 16 or type 45 DNA in two genital tumors. *J Gen Virol* 2000,81:1983-1993.

[158] Herrick J, Conti C, Teissier S, Thierry F, Couturier J, Sastre-Garau X, Favre M, Orth G, Bensimon A. Genomic organization of amplified MYC genes suggests distinct mechanisms of amplification in tumorigenesis. *Cancer Res* 2005,65:1174-1179.

[159] Schlott T, Eiffert H, Bohne W, Landgrebe J, Brunner E, Spielbauer B, Knight B. Chlamydia trachomatis modulates expression of tumor suppressor gene caveolin-1 and oncogene C-myc in the transformation zone of non-neoplastic cervical tissue. *Gynecol Oncol* 2005,98:409-419.

[160] Saffari B, Jones LA, El-Naggar A, Felix JC, George J, Press M. Amplification and overexpression of *HER-2/neu. c-erbB-2* in endometrial cancers: correlation with overall survival. *Cancer Res* 1995,55:5693-5698.

[161] Mitra AB, Murty VV, Pratap M, Sodhani P, Chaganti RS. *erbB-2 HER-2/neu* oncogene is frequently amplified in squamous cell carcinoma of the uterine cervix. *Cancer Res* 1994,54:637-639.

[162] Press MF, Pike M, Hung G, Zhou JY, Ma Y, George J, Dietz-Band J, James W, Slamon D, Batsakis J, El-Naggar AK. Amplification and overexpression of *HER-2/neu* in carcinomas of the salivary gland: correlation with poor prognosis, *Cancer Res* 1994,54:5675-5682.

[163] Sharma S, Pratap M, Sawhney V, Khan Y, Bhambhani S, Mitra A. Frequent amplification of c-erbB-2 (HER-2/neu) oncogene in cervical carcinoma as detected by non-fluorescence in situ hybridization technique on paraffin sections. *Oncology* 1999,56:83-87.

[164] Depowski PL, Brien TP, Sheehan CE, Stylos S, Johnson RL, Ross J. Prognostic significance of p34cdc2 cyclindependent kinase and MIBI overexpression, and *HER-2/neu* gene amplification detected by fluorescence in situ hybridization in breast cancer. *Am J Clin Pathol* 1999,112:459-469.

[165] Tiwari RK, Borgen PI, Wong GY, Cordon CC, Osborne MP. *HER-2/neu* amplification and overexpression in primary human breast cancer is associated with early metastasis. *Anticancer Res* 1992,12:419-425.

[166] Dellas A, Torhorst J, Jliang F, Proffitt J, Schultheiss E, Holzgreve W, Sauter G, Mihatsch M, Moch H. Prognostic value of genomic alterations in invasive cervical squamous cell carcinoma of clinical stage IB detected by comparative genomic hybridisation. *Cancer Res* 1999,59:3475-3479.

[167] Tenti P, Romagnoli S, Sillini E, Pellegata S, Zappatore R, Spinillo A, Zara C, Panzani N, Carnevali L. Analysis and clinical implications of K-*ras* gene mutations and infection with human papillomavirus types 16 and 18 in primary adenocarcinoma of the uterine cervix. *Int J Cancer* 1995, 64:9-13.

[168] Grendys EC, Barnes WA, Weitzel J, Sparkowski J, Schlegel R. Identification of H-, K- and N-*ras* point mutations in stage IB cervical carcinoma. *Gynecol Oncol* 1997,65:343-347.

[169] Parker MF, Arroyo GF, Geradts J, Sabichi AL, Park RC, Taylor RR, Birrer MJ. Molecular characterization of adenocarcinoma of the cervix. *Gynecol Oncol* 1997,64:242-251.

[170] Stenzel A, Semczuk A, Rozynskal K, Jakowicki J, Wojcierowski J. "Low-risk" and "high-risk" HPV-infection and K-ras gene point mutations in human cervical cancer: a study of 31 cases. *Pathol Res Pract* 2001,197:597-603.

[171] Prokopakis P, Sourvinos G, Koumantaki Y, Koumantakis E, Spandidos DA. K-ras mutations and HPV infection in cervicitis and intraepithelial neoplasias of the cervix. *Oncol Rep* 2002,9:129-133.

[172] Mammas IN, Zafiropoulos A, Koumantakis E, Sifakis S, Spandidos DA. Transcriptional activation of H- and N-ras oncogenes in human cervical cancer. *Gynecol Oncol* 2004,92:941-948.

[173] Ferrera A, Olivo A, Alaez C, Melchers WJ, Gorodezky C. HLA DOA1 and DOB1 loci in Honduran women with cervical dysplasia and invasive cervical carcinoma and their relationship to human papillomavirus infection. *Hum Biol* 1999,71:367-379.

[174] Maciag PC, Schlecht NF, Souza PSA, Franco EL, Villa LL, Petzl-Erler ML. Major histocompatibility complex class II polymorphisms and risk of cervical cancer and human papillomavirus infection in Brazilian women. *Cancer Epidemiol Biomark Prev* 2000,9:1183-1191.

[175] Konya J, Dillner J. Immunity to oncogenic human papillomaviruses. *Adv Cancer Res* 2001,82:205-238.

[176] Ashburner M, Ball CA, Blake JA, Botstein D, Butler H, Cherry JM, Davis AP, Dolinski K, Dwight SS, Eppig JT, Harris MA, Hill DP, Issel-Tarver L, Kasarskis A, Lewis S, Matese JC, Richardson JE, Ringwald M, Rubin GM, Sherlock G. Gene ontology: tool for the unification of biology. The Gene Ontology Consortium. *Nat Genet* 2000,25:25-29.

[177] Hosack DA, Dennis G, Sherman BT, Lane HC, Lempicki RA. Identifying biological themes within lists of genes with EASE. *Genome Biol* 2003,4:R70.

[178] Yang R, Muller C, Huynh V, Fung YK, Yee AS, Koeffler HP. Functions of cyclin A1 in the cell cycle and its interactions with transcription factor E2F-1 and Rb family of proteins. *Mol Cell Biol* 1999,19:2400-2407.

[179] Liao C, Wang XY, Wei HQ, Li SQ, Merghoub T, Pandolfi PP, Wolgermuth DJ. Altered myelopoiesis and the development of acute myeloid leukaemia in transgenic mice overexpressing cyclin A1. *Proc Natl Acad Sci USA* 2001,98:6853-6858.

[180] Muller-Tidow C, Diederichs S, Schrader MG, Vogt U, Miller K, Berdel WE, Serve H. Cyclin A1 is highly expressed in aggressive testicular germ cell tumors. *Cancer Lett* 2003,190:89-95.

[181] Muller-Tidow C, Wang W, Idos GE, Diederichs S, Yang R, Readhead C, Berdel WE, Serve H, Saville M, Watson R, Koeffler HP. Cyclin A1 directly interacts with B-myb and cyclin A1/cdk2 phosphorylate B-myb at functionally important serine and threonine residues: tissue-specific regulation of B-myb function. *Blood* 2001,97:2091-2097.

[182] Xu Q, Reed JC. Bax inhibitor-1, a mammalian apoptosis suppressor identified by functional screening in yeast. *Mol Cell* 1998,1:337-346.

[183] Grzmil M, Thelen P, Hemmerlein B, Schweyer S, Voigt S, Mury D, Burfeind P. Bax inhibitor-1 is overexpressed in prostate cancer and its specific down-regulation by RNA interference leads to cell death in human prostate carcinoma cells. *Am J Pathol* 2003,163:543-552.

[184] Grzmil M, Kaulfuss S, Thelen P, Hemmerlein B, Schwever S, Obenauer S, Kang TW, Burfeind P. Expression and functional analysis of Bax inhibitor-1 in human breast cáncer cells. *J Pathol* 2006,208:340-349.

[185] Reuther GW, Der CJ. The Ras branch of small GTPases: Ras family members don't fall far from the tree. *Curr Opin Cell Biol* 2000,12:157-165.

[186] Chien Y, White MA. RAL GTPases are linchpin modulators of human tumour-cell proliferation and survival. *EMBO* 2003,4:800-806.

[187] Oxford G, Owens CR, Titus BJ, Foreman TL, Herlevsen MC, Smith SC, Theodorescu D. RalA and RalB: antagonistic relatives in cancer cell migration. *Cancer Res* 2005,65:7111-7120.

[188] Kotnis A, Sarin R, Mulherkar R. Genotype, phenotype and cancer: role of low penetrance genes and environment in tumour susceptibility. *J Biosci* 2005,30:93-102.

[189] Futreal PA, Coin L, Marshall M, Down T, Hubbard T, Wooster R, Rahman N, Stratton MR. A census of human cancer genes. *Nat Rev Cancer* 2004,4:177-183.

[190] Houlston RS, Peto J. The search for low-penetrance cancer susceptibility alleles. *Oncogene* 2004,23:6471-6476.

[191] Newman TL, Rieder MJ, Morrison VA, Sharp AJ, Smith JD, Sprague LJ, Kaul R, Carlson CS, Olson MV, Nickerson DA, Eichler EE. High-throughput genotyping of intermediate-size structural variation. *Hum Mol Genet* 2006,15:1159-1167.

[192] Magnusson PK, Lichtenstein P, Gyllensten UB. Heritability of cervical tumours. *Int J Cancer* 2000,88:698-701.

[193] Lai HC, Lin WY, Lin YW, Chang CC, Yu MH, Chen CC, Chu TY. Genetic polymorphisms of FAS and FASL (CD95/CD95L) genes in cervical carcinogenesis: An analysis of haplotype and gene-gene interaction. *Gynecol Oncol* 2005,99:113-118.

[194] Deshpande A, Nolan JP, White PS, Valdez YE, Hunt WC, Peyton CL, Wheeler CM. TNF-alpha promoter polymorphisms and susceptibility to human papillomavirus 16-associated cervical cancer. *J Infect Dis* 2005,191:969-976.

[195] Nishioka Y, Sagae S, Nishikawa A, Ishioka S, Kudo R. A relationship between Matrix metalloproteinase-1 (MMP-1) promoter polymorphism and cervical cancer progression. *Cancer Lett* 2003,200:49-55.

[196] Lee SA, Kim JW, Roh JW, Choi JY, Lee KM, Yoo KY, Song YS, Kang D. Genetic polymorphisms of GSTM1, p21, p53 and HPV infection with cervical cancer in Korean women. *Gynecol Oncol* 2004,93:14-18.

In: New Research on Cervical Cancer
Editor: George Z. Rolland, pp. 109-127
ISBN 1-60021-300-6

Chapter 4

SMALL CELL CARCINOMA OF THE UTERINE CERVIX: A SIBLING OF SMALL CELL LUNG CARCINOMA?

***Haodong Xu*[1,*] *and Hanlin L. Wang*[2]**

[1]Department of Pathology and Laboratory Medicine, University of Rochester Medical Center, Rochester, NY 14642, USA;

[2] Lauren V. Ackerman Laboratory of Surgical Pathology, Department of Pathology and Immunology, Washington University School of Medicine, MO 63110-1093, USA.

ABSTRACT

Small cell carcinoma is a unique type of neuroendocrine tumor. It occurs most commonly in the lungs and is only rarely seen in extrapulmonary sites including the uterine cervix. Irrespective of anatomic location, the diagnosis of this highly aggressive malignant neoplasm is usually based on its classic histopathologic features. Sometimes, immunohistochemical stains, and occasionally, electron microscopic examination, may be needed to confirm the diagnosis. No specific biomarkers have been identified to distinguish small cell lung carcinoma (SCLC) from its extrapulmonary counterparts. However, primary small cell carcinoma of the uterine cervix (SCCC) is distinct in that it typically occurs in middle-aged women and is etiopathogenetically associated with high risk types of human papillomavirus (HPV), particularly type 18. This is in contrast with SCLC, which is typically seen in older individuals and associated with cigarette smoking. SCCC also differs from SCLC in chromosomal alterations as well as molecular

* Correspondence concerning this article should be addressed to:
Haodong Xu, M.D., Ph.D., Department of Pathology and Laboratory Medicine, Box 626, University of Rochester Medical Center, 601 Elmwood Avenue, Rochester, NY 14642, USA. 585-275-0857 (phone); 585-273-3736 (fax); Haodong_Xu@urmc.rochetser.edu (email).
Hanlin L. Wang, M.D., Ph.D., Lauren V. Ackerman Laboratory of Surgical Pathology, Department of Pathology and Immunology, Campus Box 8118, Washington University School of Medicine, 660 South Euclid Avenue, St. Louis, MO 63110-1093, USA. 314-362-0127 (phone); 314-747-2040 (fax); hwang@path.wustl.edu (email).

mechanisms that regulate the expression of tumor suppressor genes, in particular, *Rb* and *p53*. In SCCC, these two tumor suppressors are likely inactivated at the protein level via interaction with HPV oncoproteins, whereas in SCLC they are inactivated at the genetic level through gene mutations. Furthermore, c-kit proto-oncoprotein and bcl-2 anti-apoptotic protein that may bear therapeutic significance are frequently overexpressed in SCLC but infrequently in SCCC. This chapter discusses current understanding of the etiology, pathogenesis and clinicopathologic features for SCCC and emphasizes the distinction from SCLC.

Keywords: small cell carcinoma, uterine cervix.

INTRODUCTION

Primary small cell carcinoma of the uterine cervix (SCCC) is a rare malignancy, accounting for only 0.5-2% of all cervical cancers (Straughn *et al.*, 2001; Conner *et al.*, 2002). Similar to small cell lung carcinoma (SCLC), SCCC is occasionally associated with paraneoplastic syndromes (Jones *et al.*, 1976; Lojek *et al.*, 1980; Sutton *et al.*, 1988; Kothe *et al.*, 1990; Iemura *et al.*, 1991), is difficult to manage, and usually follows an aggressive clinical course with death within a few years after diagnosis (Gersell *et al.*, 1988; Walker *et al.*, 1988; Perrin and Ward 1995; Krystal *et al.*, 2000; Wang *et al.*, 2000; Straughn *et al.*, 2001; Conner *et al.*, 2002; Soria *et al.*, 2003; Weed *et al.*, 2003). Histologically, SCCC is indistinguishable from SCLC (Albores-Saavedra *et al.*, 1997; Nicholson *et al.*, 2002). Characteristic morphologic features include small size of the tumor cells (less than three times the diameter of a small mature lymphocyte), hyperchromatic nuclei and scant cytoplasm. Nucleoli are typically inconspicuous or absent. Mitotic activity is brisk and necrosis is common. Histopathologic diagnosis of small cell carcinoma is usually made based on evaluation of hematoxylin-eosin staining and is independent of the extent of neuroendocrine differentiation. However, neuroendocrine markers including chromogranin, synaptophysin and CD56 are commonly used to assist the diagnosis and occasionally, electron microscopic studies to search for neurosecretory granules may be needed.

Despite different anatomic location, the morphologic spectrum and the degree of neuroendocrine differentiation of both SCCC and SCLC are indistinguishable. No specific biomarkers have been identified to distinguish one from the other. However, SCCC typically occurs in women around 40 years of age (Gersell *et al.*, 1988; Ambros *et al.*, 1991; Abeler *et al.*, 1994; Perrin and Ward 1995; Straughn *et al.*, 2001; Conner *et al.*, 2002; Masumoto *et al.*, 2003; Weed *et al.*, 2003; Wang and Lu, 2004a), and is etiologically associated with high risk types of human papillomavirus (HPV) (Ambros *et al.*, 1991; Stoler *et al.*, 1991; Abeler *et al.*, 1994; Lizano *et al.*, 1997; Mannion *et al.*, 1998; Wistuba *et al.*, 1999; Masumoto *et al.*, 2003). This is in contrast with SCLC which is typically seen in older individuals and is associated with cigarette smoking (Cook *et al.*, 1993; Nicholson *et al.*, 2002; Rachtan 2002; Videtic *et al.*, 2003). These dissimilarities raise the possibility that the pathogenetic mechanisms underlying the development of these two morphologically similar tumors may be divergent. In fact, differences in cytogenetic and molecular alteration, proto-oncogene activation, tumor suppressor gene inactivation, and anti-apoptotic molecule expression have been observed between these two types of cancer. This chapter reviews the clinicopathologic features and current understanding of the etiology and pathogenesis for SCCC, and focuses the discussion on the distinction from SCLC.

CLINICOPATHOLOGIC FEATURES

Clinical Features

Primary SCCC is an uncommon malignancy, accounting for 0.5-2% of all cervical cancers (Straughn *et al.*, 2001; Conner *et al.*, 2002). Although SCCC occurs over a wide age range, the reported mean ages are between 36 and 47 years (Gersell *et al.*, 1988; Ambros *et al.*, 1991; Straughn *et al.*, 2001; Conner *et al.*, 2002; Chan *et al.*, 2003; Hoskins *et al.*, 2003; Weed *et al.*, 2003; Ishida *et al.*, 2004; Viswanathan *et al.*, 2004; Wang and Lu 2004a; Wang and Lu 2004b; Tsunoda *et al.*, 2005). Therefore, the patients with SCCC are in general younger than those with SCLC. In a recent large series, the ages of the patients with SCLC range from 30 to 87 years with a mean age of 64 years (Nicholson *et al.*, 2002). In our own data, the patients with SCCC are 25 years younger, on average, than those with SCLC (Wang and Lu, 2004a).

The most frequent clinical presentation of SCCC is abnormal vaginal bleeding or postcoital spotting, reported in 88% of patents. Other less common manifestations include vaginal discharge and pelvic mass (Straughn *et al.*, 2001). At the time of diagnosis, most patients are in an early stage (FIGO I and IIA) (Viswanathan *et al.*, 2004; Wang and Lu 2004). These patients are usually managed with either radical hysterectomy or definite radiotherapy. Because of its unfavorable prognosis, particularly for those with more advanced disease, multimodality therapy has increasingly become the treatment of choice. These may include combined chemotherapy and radiotherapy, and possible surgery depending on the extent of disease (Levenson *et al.*, 1981; Remick and Ruckdeschel 1992; Galanis *et al.*, 1997; Sykes *et al.*, 1999; Hoskins *et al.*, 2003; Sengoz *et al.*, 2003; Kim *et al.*, 2004; Viswanathan *et al.*, 2004).

Paraneoplastic syndromes have been recognized to be associated with small cell carcinoma, especially SCLC, for a long time. The paraneoplastic endocrine disorders are caused by ectopic production of peptide hormones, whereas the paraneoplastic neurological complications are related to antibody-mediated damage to the nervous system. SCCC has been reported to be associated with Cushing's syndrome (Jones *et al.*, 1976; Lojek *et al.*, 1980; Iemura *et al.*, 1991), hyponatremia (Kothe *et al.*, 1990), and Lambert-Eaton-syndrome (Sutton *et al.*, 1988).

Prognosis

Similar to SCLC, SCCC is characterized by frequent and early nodal and distant metastasis, is difficult to manage, and usually follows an aggressive clinical course with death within a few years after diagnosis (Gersell *et al.*, 1988; Perrin and Ward 1995; Krystal *et al.*, 2000; Wang *et al.*, 2000; Straughn *et al.*, 2001; Conner *et al.*, 2002; Soria *et al.*, 2003; Weed *et al.*, 2003). The overall survival rates have been reported to be 43% and 29% at 2 and 5 years, respectively (Viswanathan *et al.*, 2004). The patient survival appears to correlate with tumor size and clinical stage (Chan *et al.*, 2003; Viswanathan *et al.*, 2004). Interestingly, the study by Straughn *et al.* (2001) showed that the expression of a neuroendocrine marker chromogranin by tumor cells was a poor prognostic factor, but the expression of other two neuroendocrine markers synaptophysin and neuron-specific enolase had no impact on survival. It is also interesting to note that smoking was found to be a significant independent prognostic factor for survival in the study by Chan *et al.* (2003). However, this finding was not confirmed by a later study by Viswanathan *et al.* (2004).

Pathology

Histologically, SCCC is indistinguishable from SCLC (Figure 1). The diagnostic criteria are adopted from those used for SCLC (Albores-Saavedra *et al.*, 1997; Nicholson *et al.*, 2002). Characteristic features include small size of the tumor cells (less than three times the diameter of a small mature lymphocyte), hyperchromatic round or fusiform nuclei, dispersed granular chromatin, inconspicuous or no nucleoli, nuclear molding, scant cytoplasm, high nuclear-to-cytoplasmic ratio, frequent mitotic figures, and extensive necrosis. In small biopsy specimens, "crush artifact" may be evident, which can make histologic interpretation difficult. In well preserved specimens, tumor cells may form rosettes and exhibit prominent peripheral palisading.

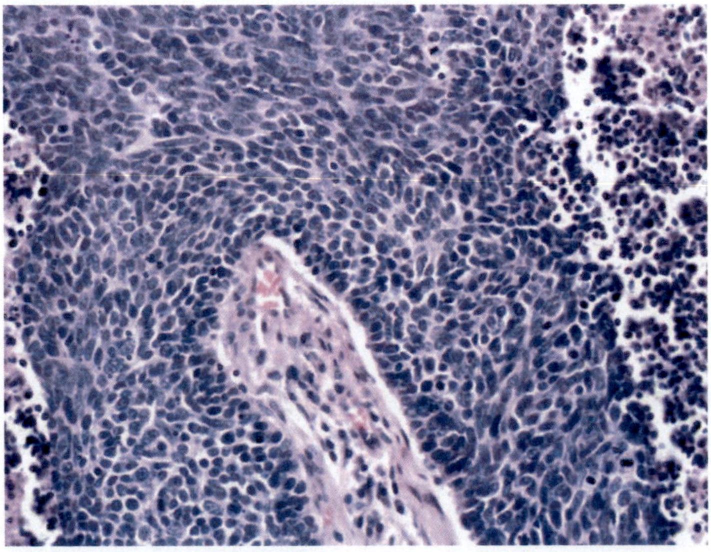

Figure 1. Small cell carcinoma of the uterine cervix, which is indistinguishable histologically from small cell lung carcinoma (original magnification ×400).

Routine hematoxylin-eosin staining alone is usually sufficient for the diagnosis of small cell carcinoma, and the diagnosis is independent of the extent of neuroendocrine differentiation. However, neuroendocrine markers, such as chromogranin, synaptophysin and CD56, are commonly used to aid the diagnosis in clinical setting. More than 85% of small cell carcinomas diagnosed with hematoxylin-eosin staining express one or more neuroendocrine markers by immunohistochemistry (Straughn *et al.*, 2001; Albores-Saavedra *et al.*, 2005). Positive cytokeratin staining, especially with a paranuclear "dot-like" pattern, is very helpful in the distinction from lymphoma or other small round blue cell tumors. Immunohistochemical stains for neuroendocrine markers and cytokeratin are particularly useful when the diagnostic material is a small biopsy with marked crush artifact. With the availability of these diagnostic markers, electron microscopy, which has been frequently used in the past, has become less and less important as a diagnostic tool. Only occasionally may electron microscopy be needed to search for neurosecretory granules in tumor cells to confirm the diagnosis.

No specific biomarkers have been identified to distinguish SCCC from SCLC or other extrapulmonary counterparts in daily practice. Thyroid transcription factor-1 (TTF-1) is highly expressed in more than 90% of SCLC (Ordonez, 2000), but extrapulmonary small cell carcinomas, including SCCC, also express TTF-1, although at a lower frequency. Clinical history and imaging studies are thus imperative in the investigation of tumor origin.

Etiology and Pathogenesis

As discussed above, SCCC is similar to SCLC in morphology, neuroendocrine differentiation, and biological behavior. However, they appear to differ in etiology and pathogenesis. In this regard, the role of HPV infection, chromosomal alterations, and regulation of important cellular proteins have been extensively investigated.

HPV Infection

Numerous epidemiological and experimental studies have established a strong etiopathogenetic relationship between HPV infection and the development of cervical cancers (Sherr, 1996; zur Hausen, 1996; Furumoto and Irahara, 2002). The carcinogenic effect of the "high risk" HPVs, as defined by their documented association with invasive carcinomas (Lorincz *et al.*, 1992), is thought to be mainly mediated by two viral oncoproteins, E6 and E7 (Watanabe *et al.*, 1989; Jeon *et al.*, 1995), through their action of inactivating the functions of two important cellular tumor suppressors, p53 and Rb (Munger and Howley 2002). It has been demonstrated that the E6 oncoprotein binds to p53 to promote its degradation by an ubiqitin-proteasomal pathway (Scheffner *et al.*, 1990; Werness *et al.*, 1990; Scheffner *et al.*, 1993), whereas the E7 oncoprotein forms a complex with Rb, leading to its functional inactivation as well as accelerated degradation (Dyson *et al.*, 1989; Boyer *et al.*, 1996). These synergistic effects result in a deregulated cell cycle control and are thus believed to be critically important in HPV-induced carcinogenesis (Hawley-Nelson *et al.*, 1989; Munger *et al.*, 1989; Ishiji 2000; Giarre *et al.*, 2001; Helt *et al.*, 2002).

As in cervical squamous cell carcinoma and adenocarcinoma, high risk types of HPV have been implicated in the carcinogenesis in SCCC (Ambros *et al.*, 1991; Stoler *et al.*, 1991; Abeler *et al.*, 1994; Lizano *et al.*, 1997; Mannion *et al.*, 1998; Wistuba *et al.*, 1999; Wang and Lu, 2004a). Using sensitive broad-spectrum HPV DNA amplification and line probe assay for genotyping, we detected the presence of high risk HPV in all 22 SCCCs we examined (Wang and Lu, 2004a), among which type 18 was the most prevalent, demonstrated in 18 cases (82%). On the contrary, a recent study by Brouchet *et al.* (Brouchet *et al.*, 2005) showed no single HPV-positive cell in 122 lung carcinomas, including 9 cases of SCLC, by immunohistochemistry and *in situ* hybridization. In a review of 85 studies containing 2468 bronchial carcinomas subjected to HPV detection, HPV DNA was reported in 536 cases (21.7%), ranging from 0% to 100% among different studies. However, none of these studies included SCLC (Syrjanen, 2002). These available data thus suggest that conventional oncogenic HPVs are unlikely to play a critical role in the development of lung carcinomas.

Cytogenetics

Loss of heterozygosity (LOH) involving markers on the short arm of chromosome 3 is one of the most frequent acquired genetic changes observed in lung cancer (Sekido *et al.*, 1998). This abnormality was first detected by cytogenetic studies showing 3p deletions and later confirmed by allele loss and comparative genome hybridization (CGH) analyses (Brauch *et al.*, 1987; Kok *et al.*, 1987; Naylor *et al.*, 1987; Brauch *et al.*, 1990). These LOH sites are candidates to harbor tumor suppressor genes (TSGs).

Allelic loss of chromosome 3p has been detected in nearly all SCLCs examined (Sekido *et al.*, 1998). The specific homozygous deletion and LOH have been mapped to the region of 3p14-25 (Hibi *et al.*, 1992), which supports the hypothesis that the 3p arm carries several TSGs including *FHIT* (fragile histidine gene), *RASSFIA* (RAS effector homologue), *RARB* (retinoic acid receptor β) and *FUS1*. However, available data suggest that allelic losses involving chromosome 3p (any region) are a less frequent event in SCCC, observed in 3 of 8 cases in one study, with only one occurring in the restricted region 3p14-21 (Wistuba *et al.*, 1999). Furthermore, allelic losses involving the *FHIT* gene locus, the candidate TSG at 3p14.2 that spans the FRA3B fragile site, are detected in 100% SCLCs (Fong *et al.*, 1997), but not in SCCCs (Wistuba *et al.*, 1999).

In addition to chromosomal 3p deletion, losses of chromosomal 4q, 5q, 10q, 13q and 17q, and gains of chromosomal 3q, 5p, 8q and 17q detected by CGH (Levin *et al.*, 1994; Ried *et al.*, 1994; Levin *et al.*, 1995; Petersen *et al.*, 1997; Schwendel *et al.*, 1997) and cytogenetic techniques (Whang-Peng *et al.*, 1982; Testa *et al.*, 1997) have been reported in SCLC. On the contrary, LOH involving markers on the chromosomes 5q22 (*APC-MCC* region), 9p21 (*CDKN2* gene), 13q (*Rb* gene) and 17p (*p53* gene) have been detected in rare cases of SCCC (Mannion *et al.*, 1998; Wistuba *et al.*, 1999). Overall, SCCC and SCLC exhibit different profiles of chromosomal abnormality, although the number of SCCC investigated is very small.

Tumor Suppressors p53 and Rb

Mutations of tumor suppressor genes are common during tumorigenesis of lung cancer and mutational inactivation of the *Rb* and *p53* tumor suppressors are identified in up to 90% of SCLC (Gouyer *et al.*, 1998; Sekido *et al.*, 2003). Together with retinoblastoma, SCLC is the most common neuroendocrine tumor that harbors *Rb* gene mutations, detected in almost all cases (Sherr and McCormick 2002). In SCCC, however, inactivation of p53 and Rb functions appears to be mediated via a different mechanism: accelerated protein degradation by interaction with HPV oncoproteins (Wang and Lu 2004a).

To study the direct roles of *Rb* and *p53* genes in the development of SCLC *in vivo*, Meuwissen *et al.* (2003) used the Cre-loxP system to generate lung epithelium-specific deletion of *Rb* and *p53* genes in mice. The authors report that conditional somatic inactivation of both *Rb* and *p53* alleles in pulmonary epithelial cells leads to the development of multiple tumors with histopathology and immunophenotype closely mirroring human SCLC. On the other hand, a recent *in vivo* study by Carraresi *et al.* (2006) directly tested the role of HPV E6 and E7 oncoproteins in SCLC carcinogenesis. Using an HPV-E6/E7 transgenic mouse model, where the induction of overexpression of E6 and E7 oncoproteins is driven by cytokeratin 5 promoter to direct gene expression in the basal cells of stratified epithelium, the authors found that the induced SCLCs lacked expression of p53 and Rb proteins. These two studies provide direct evidence to support the notion that inactivation of p53 and Rb tumor suppressor functions either at the gene level via mutations or at the protein level through interaction with HPV oncoproteins leads to the development of small cell carcinoma.

Under physiologic conditions, p53 promotes cell cycle arrest at the late G1 phase and prevents the propagation of genetically damaged cells (Levine 1997). Deletions or point mutations, which are most commonly found in lung cancers (Olivier *et al.*, 2002), ultimately result in deregulation of cell growth control and increased rate of cell proliferation. It is important to note, however, that the mechanism by which HPV E6 oncoprotein deregulates p53 is via a direct protein–protein interaction to induce accelerated degradation of the p53 protein (Scheffner *et al.*, 1990; Werness *et al.*, 1990; Scheffner *et al.*, 1993). This mechanism is different from that occurring in many other types of human cancers where mutations of the *p53* gene are the targeting events (Levine 1997). Although there have been a number of studies on p53 in SCCC, the reported data have been inconclusive and conflicting (Holm *et al.*, 1993; Pao *et al.*, 1994; Mannion *et al.*, 1998; Herrington *et al.*, 1999; Wistuba *et al.*, 1999; Straughn *et al.*, 2001; Zarka *et al.*, 2003). For example, Pao *et al.* (1994) found no mutations in the *p53* gene in 12 SCCCs, even though these tumors were free of HPV infection. Similarly, Mannion *et al.* (1998) failed to detect loss of heterozygosity (LOH) at the 17p/*p53* locus in 10 SCCCs in which high risk types of HPV were detected in 6 of 8 informative cases. However, in the study by Wistuba *et al.* (1999), *p53* gene mutations and loss of heterozygosity at the 17p/*p53* locus were demonstrated in 6 of 8 SCCCs, among which 4 cases were positive for HPV 18 or 16. The results of p53 protein expression in SCCC also varied widely (Holm *et al.*, 1993; Herrington *et al.*, 1999; Straughn *et al.*, 2001; Zarka *et al.*, 2003; Wang and Lu, 2004a). In our own series of 22 SCCCs, which all harbored high risk types of HPV (Wang and Lu, 2004a), p53 protein was essentially undetectable by immunohistochemistry in all the cases. These findings are not unexpected, however, given the fact that HPV E6 oncoprotein facilitates p53 protein degradation (Scheffner *et al.*, 1990; Werness *et al.*, 1990; Scheffner *et al.*, 1993). As controls, in HPV-negative colorectal and bladder small cell carcinomas, p53 was overexpressed in about one half of the cases (Wang and Lu, 2004a), a frequency similar to that reported in SCLC (Gemba *et al.*, 2000).

The tumor suppressor Rb is a nuclear phosphoprotein that plays a key role in regulating the cell cycle (Sherr 1996). Loss of its function via mutational or epigenetic mechanisms has been reported in a variety of human malignancies. In SCLC, mutational inactivation of the *Rb* gene occurs in approximately 90% of the cases (Kaye, 2002). This is in marked contrast with SCCC where Rb gene mutation has been shown to be an uncommon event, although there are only two published studies in this regard. In the study by Pao *et al.* (1994), no Rb mutation was found in 12 SCCCs. In the study by Wistuba *et al.* (1999), loss of heterozygosity at 13q/Rb region was observed in only 1 of 5 cases they examined. Nevertheless, the results from our own study (Wang and Lu, 2004a) and the study by Herrington *et al.* (1999) demonstrate a high frequency of loss of Rb nuclear protein expression in SCCC. These findings are in line with the notion that HPV oncoprotein preferentially interacts with the hypophosphorylated Rb protein, the active form, resulting in a functional inactivation as well as accelerated protein degradation.

Tumor Suppressor p16

The p16 protein is also a key cell cycle regulator that functions as a tumor suppressor. As a result, it is a common target of inactivation in human cancers (Clurman and Groudine, 1998). It has been recently reported, however, that in HPV-related cervical cancers, p16 protein is paradoxically overexpressed as detected by immunohistochemistry (Kim *et al.*, 1998; Sano *et al.*, 1998; Sano *et al.*, 1998; Keating *et al.*, 2001; Klaes *et al.*, 2001; Milde-Langosch *et al.*, 2001; Riethdorf *et al.*, 2002; Agoff *et al.*, 2003; Ishikawa *et al.*, 2003; Masumoto *et al.*, 2003; Negri *et al.*, 2003; Ishikawa *et al.*, 2006). These unexpected findings are thought to result from a negative feedback control mechanism second to Rb deregulation (Li *et al.*, 1994; Khleif *et al.*, 1996; Klaes *et al.*, 2001). It has been well established that there exists an inverse relationship between the expression of p16 and the presence of functional Rb in many cell systems and that Rb represses the transcription of the *p16* gene (Li *et al.*, 1994; Khleif *et al.*, 1996). However, once the inhibitory effect of Rb is abolished, the transcriptional activity and the protein expression level of p16 are expected to increase. Similar to what has been observed in HPV-related cervical squamous cell carcinoma and adenocarcinoma (Kim *et al.*, 1998; Sano *et al.*, 1998; Sano *et al.*, 1998; Keating *et al.*, 2001; Klaes *et al.*, 2001; Milde-Langosch *et al.*, 2001; Riethdorf *et al.*, 2002; Agoff *et al.*, 2003; Ishikawa *et al.*, 2003; Negri *et al.*, 2003), we demonstrate that p16 protein is also overexpressed in the nuclei of tumor cells in over 90% of SCCCs that harbor HPV DNA (Wang and Lu, 2004a). Similar results have also been reported by Masumoto *et al.* (2003), who examined 10 cases of SCCC and found all the cases overexpressing p16 and harboring HPV 18 and 16. The observation that in a small subset of p16-overexpressing tumors, the loss of nuclear Rb expression is not evident may suggest that Rb protein is deregulated through two different mechanisms in HPV-related tumors. That is, in the majority of the tumors, Rb deregulation is achieved through accelerated protein degradation as evidenced by negative nuclear staining. In others, Rb is inactivated by the HPV E7 oncoprotein at the functional level and thus the nuclear Rb protein remains detectable immunohistochemically.

The *p16* gene mutations have been found frequently in non-small cell carcinomas of the lung, but only rarely in SCLC. However, p16 protein overexpression has been consistently detected in SCLC (Zhang *et al.*, 2005). This is also likely caused by downregulation of Rb protein (Igarashi *et al.*, 2004), apparently secondary to its gene mutations (Sherr and McCormick, 2002).

Other Potential Tumor Suppressors

As discussed earlier, four genes located in chromosome 3p, *FHIT*, *RASSF1*, *RARB* and *FUS1*, are of particular interest as potential tumor suppressors in SCLC. Deletions of the loci containing these genes in chromosome 3p have been well documented in SCLC, but not in SCCC. *FHIT* encodes the enzyme diadenosine triphosphophate hydrolase (Pekarsky *et al.*, 2002), which is thought to serve an indirect role in proapoptosis and cell cycle control. *RASSF1* encodes a microtubule-binding protein (Rong *et al.*, 2004) that interacts with and stabilizes microtubules, and subsequently induces G1 and G2/M arrest. Loss of RASSF1 function allows tumor cells to grow more rapidly. The third potential tumor suppressor gene is *RARB*. Through its encoded retinoic acid receptor β, retinoids suppress activator protein-1 (Lin *et al.*, 2000) and promote apoptosis (Liu *et al.*, 1996). *FUS1*, the fourth potential tumor suppressor, is located at 3p21.3 (Kondo *et al.*, 2001). Although its specific function has not been elucidated, myristoylation of its protein seems to be necessary for tumor suppression (Uno *et al.*, 2004). Experimental studies have shown that all these four genes are commonly deleted or inactivated in SCCC cell lines (Sozzi *et al.*, 1996; Virmani *et al.*, 2000; Burbee *et al.*, 2001). Transfection of wild-type *FHIT* (Siprashvili *et al.*, 1997), RASSF1 (Dammann *et al.*, 2000), or FUS1 (Ito *et al.*, 2004) into tumor cells results in restoration of regulatory control and growth inhibition.

Proto-Oncoprotein c-kit

The tyrosine kinase receptor, c-kit, is mutated and activated in most gastrointestinal stromal tumors and may serve a role in SCLC biology as well. Its ligand, stem cells factor, is expressed and secreted by SCLC tumor cells, binds to c-kit, and causes receptor activation. This process forms an autocrine loop to stimulate cancer cell growth. The c-kit receptor is overexpressed in the majority of SCLCs (Wang and Lu, 2004b; LaPoint *et al.*, 2006). In addition, mutations of the *c-kit* gene have been identified in 10% of SCLCs, although these observations have not been unanimously confirmed (Sekido *et al.*, 1993; Burger *et al.*, 2003; Tamborini *et al.*, 2004; Sihto *et al.*, 2005). Interestingly, the frequency of c-kit protein overexpression in SCCC is much lower than that in SCLC (Wang and Lu, 2004b; Ohwada *et al.*, 2006). The molecular mechanisms for this difference are currently unknown, however.

Anti-Apoptotic Molecule bcl-2

There is accumulating evidence that tumor cells acquire the ability to escape the regulatory mechanisms by which normal cells would undergo programmed cell death (apoptosis) under such conditions as DNA damage. A key member of the apoptotic pathway is the *bcl-2* proto-oncogene product. Bcl-2 protects cells from apoptotic process and is thus likely to play a critical role in determining therapeutic response in cancer cells. A human SCLC cell line transfected with *bcl-2* showed higher resistance to certain anti-cancer agents by inhibiting apoptosis (Ohmori *et al.*, 1993; Ziegler *et al.*, 1997). Transfection of antisense oliogodeoxynucletides targeting the *bcl-2* mRNA into SCLC cells also showed a reduction in viability by reducing bcl-2 protein levels to facilitate apoptosis. Furthermore, ABT-737, a small-molecule inhibitor of the bcl-2 family proteins, induces regression of solid tumors including SCLC in *in vitro* and xenograft animal models (Oltersdorf *et al.*, 2005).

Several studies have documented a high frequency (75-100%) of bcl-2 protein expression in SCLC (Jiang *et al.*, 1995; Jiang *et al.*, 1996; Kaiser *et al.*, 1996; LaPoint *et al.*, 2006). However, bcl-2 expression has been detected in only one of four cases of SCCC examined thus far (Zarka *et al.*, 2003). These observations, together with the findings of a lower frequency of c-kit expression in SCCC in comparison with SCLC, signify the differences in etiopathogenetic mechanisms involved in the development of these two morphologically identical neoplasms.

CONCLUSION

SCCC, usually occurring in younger women, is etiologically associated with high risk types of HPV, particularly type 18. SCLC, on the other hand, is typically seen in older individuals and is associated with cigarette smoking. SCCC is much less well studied than SCLC, probably due to its rarity. Nevertheless, the available data indicate that chromosomal alterations are more frequently detected in SCLC than in SCCC. The molecular mechanisms by which the tumor suppressor genes *p53* and *Rb* are deregulated also differ in these two types of small cell carcinoma. In SCLC, deregulation occurs at the genetic level via gene mutations, whereas in SCCC, the tumor suppressor functions of these two genes are inactivated at the protein level through interaction with viral oncoproteins. Given these etiopathogenetic differences, it is not surprising that some critical cell regulators may show different expression patterns in SCCC and SCLC. Examples include c-kit proto-oncoprotein and bcl-2 anti-apoptotic molecule, which are more frequently overexpressed in SCLC than in SCCC. Therefore, despite the fact that SCCC and SCLC share identical histopathology and similar clinical course, they differ greatly at the molecular level, which may have implications in the future development of tumor-specific targeted therapies.

REFERENCES

Abeler VM, Holm R, Nesland JM and Kjorstad KE. Small cell carcinoma of the cervix. A clinicopathologic study of 26 patients. *Cancer.* 1994; 73:672-677.

Agoff SN, Lin P, Morihara J, Mao C, Kiviat NB and Koutsky LA. p16(INK4a) expression correlates with degree of cervical neoplasia: a comparison with Ki-67 expression and detection of high-risk HPV types. *Mod Pathol.* 2003; 16:665-673.

Albores-Saavedra J, Gersell D, Gilks CB, Henson DE, Lindberg G, Santiago H, Scully RE, Silva E, Sobin LH, Tavassoli FJ, Travis WD and Woodruff JM. Terminology of endocrine tumors of the uterine cervix: results of a workshop sponsored by the College of American Pathologists and the National Cancer Institute. *Arch Pathol Lab Med.* 1997; 121:34-39.

Albores-Saavedra J, Latif S, Carrick KS, Alvarado-Cabrero I and Fowler MR. CD56 reactivity in small cell carcinoma of the uterine cervix. *Int J Gynecol Pathol.* 2005; 24:113-117.

Ambros RA, Park JS, Shah KV and Kurman RJ. Evaluation of histologic, morphometric, and immunohistochemical criteria in the differential diagnosis of small cell carcinomas of the cervix with particular reference to human papillomavirus types 16 and 18. *Mod Pathol.* 1991; 4:586-593.

Boyer SN, Wazer DE and Band V. E7 protein of human papilloma virus-16 induces degradation of retinoblastoma protein through the ubiquitin-proteasome pathway. *Cancer Res.* 1996; 56:4620-4624.

Brauch H, Johnson B, Hovis J, Yano T, Gazdar A, Pettengill OS, Graziano S, Sorenson GD, Poiesz BJ, Minna J, et al. Molecular analysis of the short arm of chromosome 3 in small-cell and non-small-cell carcinoma of the lung. *N Engl J Med.* 1987; 317:1109-1113.

Brauch H, Tory K, Kotler F, Gazdar AF, Pettengill OS, Johnson B, Graziano S, Winton T, Buys CH, Sorenson GD, et al. Molecular mapping of deletion sites in the short arm of chromosome 3 in human lung cancer. *Genes Chromosomes Cancer.* 1990; 1:240-246.

Brouchet L, Valmary S, Dahan M, Didier A, Galateau-Salle F, Brousset P and Degano B. Detection of oncogenic virus genomes and gene products in lung carcinoma. *Br J Cancer.* 2005; 92:743-746.

Burbee DG, Forgacs E, Zochbauer-Muller S, Shivakumar L, Fong K, Gao B, Randle D, Kondo M, Virmani A, Bader S, Sekido Y, Latif F, Milchgrub S, Toyooka S, Gazdar AF, Lerman MI, Zabarovsky E, White M and Minna JD. Epigenetic inactivation of RASSF1A in lung and breast cancers and malignant phenotype suppression. *J Natl Cancer Inst.* 2001; 93:691-699.

Burger H, den Bakker MA, Stoter G, Verweij J and Nooter K. Lack of c-kit exon 11 activating mutations in c-KIT/CD117-positive SCLC tumour specimens. *Eur J Cancer.* 2003; 39:793-799.

Carraresi L, Martinelli R, Vannoni A, Riccio M, Dembic M, Tripodi S, Cintorino M, Santi S, Bigliardi E, Carmellini M and Rossini M. Establishment and characterization of murine small cell lung carcinoma cell lines derived from HPV-16 E6/E7 transgenic mice. *Cancer Lett.* 2006; 231:65-73.

Chan JK, Loizzi V, Burger RA, Rutgers J and Monk BJ. Prognostic factors in neuroendocrine small cell cervical carcinoma: a multivariate analysis. *Cancer.* 2003; 97:568-574.

Clurman BE and Groudine M The CDKN2A tumor-suppressor locus--a tale of two proteins. *N Engl J Med.* 1998; 338:910-2.

Conner MG, Richter H, Moran CA, Hameed A and Albores-Saavedra J. Small cell carcinoma of the cervix: a clinicopathologic and immunohistochemical study of 23 cases. *Ann Diagn Pathol.* 2002; 6:345-348.

Cook RM, Miller YE and Bunn PA, Jr. Small cell lung cancer: etiology, biology, clinical features, staging, and treatment. *Curr Probl Cancer.* 1993; 17:69-141.

Dammann R, Li C, Yoon JH, Chin PL, Bates S and Pfeifer GP. Epigenetic inactivation of a RAS association domain family protein from the lung tumour suppressor locus 3p21.3. *Nat Genet.* 2000; 25:315-319.

Dyson N, Howley PM, Munger K and Harlow E. The human papilloma virus-16 E7 oncoprotein is able to bind to the retinoblastoma gene product. *Science.* 1989; 243:934-937.

Fong KM, Biesterveld EJ, Virmani A, Wistuba I, Sekido Y, Bader SA, Ahmadian M, Ong ST, Rassool FV, Zimmerman PV, Giaccone G, Gazdar AF and Minna JD FHIT and FRA3B 3p14.2 allele loss are common in lung cancer and preneoplastic bronchial lesions and are associated with cancer-related FHIT cDNA splicing aberrations. *Cancer Res.* 1997; 57:2256-2267.

Furumoto H and Irahara M. Human papilloma virus (HPV) and cervical cancer. *J Med Invest.* 2002; 49:124-133.

Galanis E, Frytak S and Lloyd RV. Extrapulmonary small cell carcinoma. *Cancer.* 1997; 79:1729-36.

Gemba K, Ueoka H, Kiura K, Tabata M and Harada M. Immunohistochemical detection of mutant p53 protein in small-cell lung cancer: relationship to treatment outcome. *Lung Cancer.* 2000; 29:23-31.

Gersell DJ, Mazoujian G, Mutch DG and Rudloff MA. Small-cell undifferentiated carcinoma of the cervix. A clinicopathologic, ultrastructural, and immunocytochemical study of 15 cases. *Am J Surg Pathol.* 1988; 12:684-698.

Giarre M, Caldeira S, Malanchi I, Ciccolini F, Leao MJ and Tommasino M Induction of pRb degradation by the human papillomavirus type 16 E7 protein is essential to efficiently overcome p16INK4a-imposed G1 cell cycle Arrest. *J Virol.* 2001; 75:4705-4712.

Gouyer V, Gazzeri S, Bolon I, Drevet C, Brambilla C and Brambilla E. Mechanism of retinoblastoma gene inactivation in the spectrum of neuroendocrine lung tumors. *Am J Respir Cell Mol Biol.* 1998; 18:188-196.

Hawley-Nelson P, Vousden KH, Hubbert NL, Lowy DR and Schiller JT. HPV16 E6 and E7 proteins cooperate to immortalize human foreskin keratinocytes. *Embo J.* 1989; 8:3905-3910.

Helt AM, Funk JO and Galloway DA. Inactivation of both the retinoblastoma tumor suppressor and p21 by the human papillomavirus type 16 E7 oncoprotein is necessary to inhibit cell cycle arrest in human epithelial cells. *J Virol.* 2002; 76:10559-1068.

Herrington CS, Graham D, Southern SA, Bramdev A and Chetty R. Loss of retinoblastoma protein expression is frequent in small cell neuroendocrine carcinoma of the cervix and is unrelated to HPV type. *Hum Pathol.* 1999; 30:906-910.

Hibi K, Takahashi T, Yamakawa K, Ueda R, Sekido Y, Ariyoshi Y, Suyama M, Takagi H, Nakamura Y and Takahashi T. Three distinct regions involved in 3p deletion in human lung cancer. *Oncogene.* 1992; 7:445-449.

Holm R, Abeler VM, Skomedal H and Nesland JM. Overexpression of p53 protein and c-erbB-2 protein in small cell carcinoma of the cervix uteri. *Zentralbl Pathol.* 1993; 139:153-156.

Hoskins PJ, Swenerton KD, Pike JA, Lim P, Aquino-Parsons C, Wong F and Lee N Small-cell carcinoma of the cervix: fourteen years of experience at a single institution using a combined-modality regimen of involved-field irradiation and platinum-based combination chemotherapy. *J Clin Oncol.* 2003; 21:3495-3501.

Iemura K, Sonoda T, Hayakawa A, Abe S, Nemoto N, Adachi I, Tsuda H and Teshima S. Small cell carcinoma of the uterine cervix showing Cushing's syndrome caused by ectopic adrenocorticotropin hormone production. *Jpn J Clin Oncol.* 1991; 21:293-298.

Igarashi T, Jiang SX, Kameya T, Asamura H, Sato Y, Nagai K and Okayasu I. Divergent cyclin B1 expression and Rb/p16/cyclin D1 pathway aberrations among pulmonary neuroendocrine tumors. *Mod Pathol.* 2004; 17:1259-1267.

Ishida GM, Kato N, Hayasaka T, Saito M, Kobayashi H, Katayama Y, Sasou S, Yaegashi N, Kurachi H and Motoyama T. Small cell neuroendocrine carcinomas of the uterine cervix: a histological, immunohistochemical, and molecular genetic study. *Int J Gynecol Pathol* 2004; 23:366-372.

Ishiji T. Molecular mechanism of carcinogenesis by human papillomavirus-16. *J Dermatol.* 2000; 27:73-86.

Ishikawa M, Fujii T, Masumoto N, Saito M, Mukai M, Nindl I, Ridder R, Fukuchi T, Kubushiro K, Tsukazaki K and Nozawa S. Correlation of p16INK4A overexpression with human papillomavirus infection in cervical adenocarcinomas. *Int J Gynecol Pathol.* 2003; 22:378-385.

Ishikawa M, Fujii T, Saito M, Nindl I, Ono A, Kubushiro K, Tsukazaki K, Mukai M and Nozawa S. Overexpression of p16 INK4a as an indicator for human papillomavirus oncogenic activity in cervical squamous neoplasia. *Int J Gynecol Cancer.* 2006; 16:347-353.

Ito I, Ji L, Tanaka F, Saito Y, Gopalan B, Branch CD, Xu K, Atkinson EN, Bekele BN, Stephens LC, Minna JD, Roth JA and Ramesh R. Liposomal vector mediated delivery of the 3p FUS1 gene demonstrates potent antitumor activity against human lung cancer in vivo. *Cancer Gene Ther.* 2004; 11:733-739.

Jeon S, Allen-Hoffmann BL and Lambert PF. Integration of human papillomavirus type 16 into the human genome correlates with a selective growth advantage of cells. *J Virol.* 1995; 69:2989-2997.

Jiang SX, Kameya T, Sato Y, Yanase N, Yoshimura H and Kodama T. Bcl-2 protein expression in lung cancer and close correlation with neuroendocrine differentiation. *Am J Pathol.* 1996; 148:837-846.

Jiang SX, Sato Y, Kuwao S and Kameya T. Expression of bcl-2 oncogene protein is prevalent in small cell lung carcinomas. *J Pathol.* 1995; 177:135-138.

Jones HW, Plymate S, Gluck FB, Miles PA and Greene JF. Small cell nonkeratinizing carcinoma of the cervix associated with ACTH production. *Cancer.* 1976; 38:1629-1635.

Kaiser U, Schilli M, Haag U, Neumann K, Kreipe H, Kogan E and Havemann K. Expression of bcl-2--protein in small cell lung cancer. *Lung Cancer.* 1996; 15:31-40.

Kaye FJ. RB and cyclin dependent kinase pathways: defining a distinction between RB and p16 loss in lung cancer. *Oncogene.* 2002; 21:6908-6914.

Keating JT, Cviko A, Riethdorf S, Riethdorf L, Quade BJ, Sun D, Duensing S, Sheets EE, Munger K and Crum CP. Ki-67, cyclin E, and p16INK4 are complimentary surrogate biomarkers for human papilloma virus-related cervical neoplasia. *Am J Surg Pathol.* 2001; 25:884-891.

Khleif SN, DeGregori J, Yee CL, Otterson GA, Kaye FJ, Nevins JR and Howley PM. Inhibition of cyclin D-CDK4/CDK6 activity is associated with an E2F-mediated induction of cyclin kinase inhibitor activity. *Proc Natl Acad Sci U S A.* 1996; 93:4350-4354.

Kim JH, Lee SH, Park J, Kim HY, Lee SI, Nam EM, Park JO, Kim K, Jung CW, Im YH, Kang WK, Lee MH and Park K. Extrapulmonary small-cell carcinoma: a single-institution experience. *Jpn J Clin Oncol.* 2004; 34:250-254.

Kim YT, Cho NH, Park SW and Kim JW. Underexpression of cyclin-dependent kinase (CDK) inhibitors in cervical carcinoma. *Gynecol Oncol.* 1998; 71:38-45.

Klaes R, Friedrich T, Spitkovsky D, Ridder R, Rudy W, Petry U, Dallenbach-Hellweg G, Schmidt D and von Knebel Doeberitz M. Overexpression of p16(INK4A) as a specific marker for dysplastic and neoplastic epithelial cells of the cervix uteri. *Int J Cancer.* 2001; 92:276-284.

Kok K, Osinga J, Carritt B, Davis MB, van der Hout AH, van der Veen AY, Landsvater RM, de Leij LF, Berendsen HH, Postmus PE, et al. Deletion of a DNA sequence at the chromosomal region 3p21 in all major types of lung cancer. *Nature.* 1987; 330:578-581.

Kondo M, Ji L, Kamibayashi C, Tomizawa Y, Randle D, Sekido Y, Yokota J, Kashuba V, Zabarovsky E, Kuzmin I, Lerman M, Roth J and Minna JD. Overexpression of candidate tumor suppressor gene FUS1 isolated from the 3p21.3 homozygous deletion region leads to G1 arrest and growth inhibition of lung cancer cells. *Oncogene.* 2001; 20:6258-6262.

Kothe MJ, Prins JM, de Wit R, Velden KV and Schellekens PT. Small cell carcinoma of the cervix with inappropriate antidiuretic hormone secretion. Case report. *Br J Obstet Gynaecol.* 1990; 97:647-648.

Krystal GW, Honsawek S, Litz J and Buchdunger E. The selective tyrosine kinase inhibitor STI571 inhibits small cell lung cancer growth. *Clin Cancer Res.* 2000; 6:3319-3326.

LaPoint R, Bourne P, Wang H and Xu H. Coexpression of c-kit and bcl-2 in small cell carcinoma and large cell neuroendocrine carcinoma of the lung. *Mod Pathol.* 2006; 19:312A.

Levenson RM, Jr., Sauerbrunn BJ, Ihde DC, Bunn PA, Jr., Cohen MH and Minna JD. Small cell lung cancer: radionuclide bone scans for assessment of tumor extent and response. *Am J Roentgenol.* 1981; 137:31-35.

Levin NA, Brzoska P, Gupta N, Minna JD, Gray JW and Christman MF. Identification of frequent novel genetic alterations in small cell lung carcinoma. *Cancer Res.* 1994; 54:5086-5091.

Levin NA, Brzoska PM, Warnock ML, Gray JW and Christman MF. Identification of novel regions of altered DNA copy number in small cell lung tumors. *Genes Chromosomes Cancer.* 1995; 13:175-185.

Levine AJ. p53, the cellular gatekeeper for growth and division. *Cell.* 1997; 88:323-331.

Li Y, Nichols MA, Shay JW and Xiong Y. Transcriptional repression of the D-type cyclin-dependent kinase inhibitor p16 by the retinoblastoma susceptibility gene product pRb. *Cancer Res.* 1994; 54:6078-6082.

Lin F, Xiao D, Kolluri SK and Zhang X. Unique anti-activator protein-1 activity of retinoic acid receptor beta. *Cancer Res.* 2000; 60:3271-3280.

Liu Y, Lee MO, Wang HG, Li Y, Hashimoto Y, Klaus M, Reed JC and Zhang X. Retinoic acid receptor beta mediates the growth-inhibitory effect of retinoic acid by promoting apoptosis in human breast cancer cells. *Mol Cell Biol.* 1996; 16:1138-1149.

Lizano M, Berumen J, Guido MC, Casas L and Garcia-Carranca A. Association between human papillomavirus type 18 variants and histopathology of cervical cancer. *J Natl Cancer Inst.* 1997; 89:1227-1231.

Lojek MA, Fer MF, Kasselberg AG, Glick AD, Burnett LS, Julian CG, Greco FA and Oldham RK. Cushing's syndrome with small cell carcinoma of the uterine cervix. *Am J Med.* 1980; 69:140-144.

Lorincz AT, Reid R, Jenson AD, Greenberg MD, Lancaster W and Kurman RJ. Human papillomavirus infection of the cervix: relative risk associations of 15 common anogenital types. *Obstet Gynecol.* 1992; 79:328-337.

Mannion C, Park WS, Man YG, Zhuang Z, Albores-Saavedra J and Tavassoli FA. Endocrine tumors of the cervix: morphologic assessment, expression of human papillomavirus, and evaluation for loss of heterozygosity on 1p,3p, 11q, and 17p. *Cancer.* 1998; 83:1391-1400.

Masumoto N, Fujii T, Ishikawa M, Saito M, Iwata T, Fukuchi T, Susumu N, Mukai M, Kubushiro K, Tsukazaki K and Nozawa S. P16 overexpression and human papillomavirus infection in small cell carcinoma of the uterine cervix. *Hum Pathol.* 2003; 34:778-783.

Meuwissen R, Linn SC, Linnoila RI, Zevenhoven J, Mooi WJ and Berns A. Induction of small cell lung cancer by somatic inactivation of both Trp53 and Rb1 in a conditional mouse model. *Cancer Cell.* 2003; 4:181-189.

Milde-Langosch K, Riethdorf S, Kraus-Poppinghaus A, Riethdorf L and Loning T. Expression of cyclin-dependent kinase inhibitors p16MTS1, p21WAF1, and p27KIP1 in HPV-positive and HPV-negative cervical adenocarcinomas. *Virchows Arch.* 2001; 439:55-61.

Munger K and Howley PM. Human papillomavirus immortalization and transformation functions. *Virus Res.* 2002; 89:213-228.

Munger K, Mitchell M and Baylis C. Differences between the sexes and the effects of surgery and anesthesia on the urinary excretion rate of eicosinoids in the rat. *Prostaglandins.* 1989; 37:379-388.

Naylor SL, Johnson BE, Minna JD and Sakaguchi AY. Loss of heterozygosity of chromosome 3p markers in small-cell lung cancer. *Nature.* 1987; 329:451-454.

Negri G, Egarter-Vigl E, Kasal A, Romano F, Haitel A and Mian C. p16INK4a is a useful marker for the diagnosis of adenocarcinoma of the cervix uteri and its precursors: an immunohistochemical study with immunocytochemical correlations. *Am J Surg Pathol.* 2003; 27:187-193.

Nicholson SA, Beasley MB, Brambilla E, Hasleton PS, Colby TV, Sheppard MN, Falk R and Travis WD. Small cell lung carcinoma (SCLC): a clinicopathologic study of 100 cases with surgical specimens. *Am J Surg Pathol.* 2002; 26:1184-1197.

Ohmori T, Podack ER, Nishio K, Takahashi M, Miyahara Y, Takeda Y, Kubota N, Funayama Y, Ogasawara H, Ohira T, et al. Apoptosis of lung cancer cells caused by some anti-cancer agents (MMC, CPT-11, ADM) is inhibited by bcl-2. *Biochem Biophys Res Commun.* 1993; 192:30-36.

Ohwada M, Wada T, Saga Y, Tsunoda S, Jobo T, Kuramoto H, Konno R and Suzuki M. C-kit overexpression in neuroendocrine small cell carcinoma of the uterine cervix. *Eur J Gynaecol Oncol.* 2006; 27:53-55.

Olivier M, Eeles R, Hollstein M, Khan MA, Harris CC and Hainaut P. The IARC TP53 database: new online mutation analysis and recommendations to users. *Hum Mutat.* 2002; 19:607-614.

Oltersdorf T, Elmore SW, Shoemaker AR, Armstrong RC, Augeri DJ, Belli BA, Bruncko M, Deckwerth TL, Dinges J, Hajduk PJ, Joseph MK, Kitada S, Korsmeyer SJ, Kunzer AR, Letai A, Li C, Mitten MJ, Nettesheim DG, Ng S, Nimmer PM, O'Connor JM, Oleksijew A, Petros AM, Reed JC, Shen W, Tahir SK, Thompson CB, Tomaselli KJ, Wang B, Wendt MD, Zhang H, Fesik SW and Rosenberg SH. An inhibitor of Bcl-2 family proteins induces regression of solid tumours. *Nature.* 2005; 435:677-681.

Ordonez NG. Value of thyroid transcription factor-1, E-cadherin, BG8, WT1, and CD44S immunostaining in distinguishing epithelial pleural mesothelioma from pulmonary and nonpulmonary adenocarcinoma. *Am J Surg Pathol.* 2000; 24:598-606.

Pao CC, Kao SM, Chen JH, Tang GC, Chang PY and Tan TT. State of mutational alterations of p53 and retinoblastoma susceptibility genes in papillomavirus-negative small cell cervical carcinomas. *J Surg Oncol.* 1994; 57:87-93.

Pekarsky Y, Palamarchuk A, Huebner K and Croce CM. FHIT as tumor suppressor: mechanisms and therapeutic opportunities. *Cancer Biol Ther.* 2002; 1:232-236.

Perrin L and Ward B. Small cell carcinoma of the cervix. *Int J Gynecol Cancer.* 1995; 5:200-203.

Petersen I, Langreck H, Wolf G, Schwendel A, Psille R, Vogt P, Reichel MB, Ried T and Dietel M. Small-cell lung cancer is characterized by a high incidence of deletions on chromosomes 3p, 4q, 5q, 10q, 13q and 17p. *Br J Cancer.* 1997; 75:79-86.

Rachtan J. Smoking, passive smoking and lung cancer cell types among women in Poland. *Lung Cancer.* 2002; 35:129-136.

Remick SC and Ruckdeschel JC. Extrapulmonary and pulmonary small-cell carcinoma: tumor biology, therapy, and outcome. *Med Pediatr Oncol.* 1992; 20:89-99.

Ried T, Petersen I, Holtgreve-Grez H, Speicher MR, Schrock E, du Manoir S and Cremer T. Mapping of multiple DNA gains and losses in primary small cell lung carcinomas by comparative genomic hybridization. *Cancer Res.* 1994; 54:1801-1806.

Riethdorf L, Riethdorf S, Lee KR, Cviko A, Loning T and Crum CP. Human papillomaviruses, expression of p16, and early endocervical glandular neoplasia. *Hum Pathol.* 2002; 33:899-904.

Rong R, Jin W, Zhang J, Sheikh MS and Huang Y. Tumor suppressor RASSF1A is a microtubule-binding protein that stabilizes microtubules and induces G2/M arrest. *Oncogene.* 2004; 23:8216-8230.

Sano T, Oyama T, Kashiwabara K, Fukuda T and Nakajima T. Expression status of p16 protein is associated with human papillomavirus oncogenic potential in cervical and genital lesions. *Am J Pathol.* 1998; 153:1741-1748.

Sano T, Oyama T, Kashiwabara K, Fukuda T and Nakajima T. Immunohistochemical overexpression of p16 protein associated with intact retinoblastoma protein expression in cervical cancer and cervical intraepithelial neoplasia. *Pathol Int.* 1998; 48:580-585.

Scheffner M, Huibregtse JM, Vierstra RD and Howley PM The HPV-16 E6 and E6-AP complex functions as a ubiquitin-protein ligase in the ubiquitination of p53. *Cell.* 1993; 75:495-505.

Scheffner M, Werness BA, Huibregtse JM, Levine AJ and Howley PM. The E6 oncoprotein encoded by human papillomavirus types 16 and 18 promotes the degradation of p53. *Cell.* 1990; 63:1129-1136.

Schwendel A, Langreck H, Reichel M, Schrock E, Ried T, Dietel M and Petersen I. Primary small-cell lung carcinomas and their metastases are characterized by a recurrent pattern of genetic alterations. *Int J Cancer.* 1997; 74:86-93.

Sckido Y, Fong KM and Minna JD. Molecular genetics of lung cancer. *Annu Rev Med.* 2003; 54:73-87.

Sekido Y, Fong KM and Minna JD. Progress in understanding the molecular pathogenesis of human lung cancer. *Biochim Biophys Acta.* 1998; 1378:F21-59.

Sekido Y, Takahashi T, Ueda R, Takahashi M, Suzuki H, Nishida K, Tsukamoto T, Hida T, Shimokata K, Zsebo KM, et al. Recombinant human stem cell factor mediates chemotaxis of small-cell lung cancer cell lines aberrantly expressing the c-kit protooncogene. *Cancer Res.* 1993; 53:1709-1714.

Sengoz M, Abacioglu U, Salepci T, Eren F, Yumuk F and Turhal S. Extrapulmonary small cell carcinoma: multimodality treatment results. *Tumori.* 2003; 89:274-277.

Sherr CJ. Cancer cell cycles. *Science.* 1996; 274:1672-1677.

Sherr CJ and McCormick F. The RB and p53 pathways in cancer. *Cancer Cell.* 2002; 2:103-12.

Sihto H, Sarlomo-Rikala M, Tynninen O, Tanner M, Andersson LC, Franssila K, Nupponen NN and Joensuu H KIT and platelet-derived growth factor receptor alpha tyrosine kinase gene mutations and KIT amplifications in human solid tumors. *J Clin Oncol.* 2005; 23:49-57.

Siprashvili Z, Sozzi G, Barnes LD, McCue P, Robinson AK, Eryomin V, Sard L, Tagliabue E, Greco A, Fusetti L, Schwartz G, Pierotti MA, Croce CM and Huebner K. Replacement of Fhit in cancer cells suppresses tumorigenicity. *Proc Natl Acad Sci U S A.* 1997; 94:13771-13776.

Soria JC, Johnson BE and Chevalier TL. Imatinib in small cell lung cancer. *Lung Cancer.* 2003; 41 Suppl 1:S49-53.

Sozzi G, Veronese ML, Negrini M, Baffa R, Cotticelli MG, Inoue H, Tornielli S, Pilotti S, De Gregorio L, Pastorino U, Pierotti MA, Ohta M, Huebner K and Croce CM. The FHIT gene 3p14.2 is abnormal in lung cancer. *Cell.* 1996; 85:17-26.

Stoler MH, Mills SE, Gersell DJ and Walker AN. Small-cell neuroendocrine carcinoma of the cervix. A human papillomavirus type 18-associated cancer. *Am J Surg Pathol.* 1991; 15:28-32.

Straughn JM, Jr., Richter HE, Conner MG, Meleth S and Barnes MN. Predictors of outcome in small cell carcinoma of the cervix--a case series. *Gynecol Oncol.* 2001; 83:216-220.

Sutton GP, Siemers E, Stehman FB and Ehrlich CE. Eaton-Lambert syndrome as a harbinger of recurrent small-cell carcinoma of the cervix with improvement after combination chemotherapy. *Obstet Gynecol.* 1988; 72:516-518.

Sykes AJ, Shanks JH and Davidson SE. Small cell carcinoma of the uterine cervix: a clinicopathological review. *Int J Oncol.* 1999; 14:381-386.

Syrjanen KJ. HPV infections and lung cancer. *J Clin Pathol.* 2002; 55:885-891.

Tamborini E, Bonadiman L, Negri T, Greco A, Staurengo S, Bidoli P, Pastorino U, Pierotti MA and Pilotti S. Detection of overexpressed and phosphorylated wild-type kit receptor in surgical specimens of small cell lung cancer. *Clin Cancer Res.* 2004; 10:8214-8219.

Testa JR, Liu Z, Feder M, Bell DW, Balsara B, Cheng JQ and Taguchi T. Advances in the analysis of chromosome alterations in human lung carcinomas. *Cancer Genet Cytogenet.* 1997; 95:20-32.

Tsunoda S, Jobo T, Arai M, Imai M, Kanai T, Tamura T, Watanabe J, Obokata A and Kuramoto H. Small-cell carcinoma of the uterine cervix: a clinicopathologic study of 11 cases. *Int J Gynecol Cancer.* 2005; 15:295-300.

Uno F, Sasaki J, Nishizaki M, Carboni G, Xu K, Atkinson EN, Kondo M, Minna JD, Roth JA and Ji L. Myristoylation of the fus1 protein is required for tumor suppression in human lung cancer cells. *Cancer Res.* 2004; 64:2969-2976.

Videtic GM, Stitt LW, Dar AR, Kocha WI, Tomiak AT, Truong PT, Vincent MD and Yu EW. Continued cigarette smoking by patients receiving concurrent chemoradiotherapy for limited-stage small-cell lung cancer is associated with decreased survival. *J Clin Oncol.* 2003; 21:1544-1549.

Virmani AK, Rathi A, Zochbauer-Muller S, Sacchi N, Fukuyama Y, Bryant D, Maitra A, Heda S, Fong KM, Thunnissen F, Minna JD and Gazdar AF. Promoter methylation and silencing of the retinoic acid receptor-beta gene in lung carcinomas. *J Natl Cancer Inst.* 2000; 92:1303-1307.

Viswanathan AN, Deavers MT, Jhingran A, Ramirez PT, Levenback C and Eifel PJ. Small cell neuroendocrine carcinoma of the cervix: outcome and patterns of recurrence. *Gynecol Oncol.* 2004; 93:27-33.

Walker AN, Mills SE and Taylor PT. Cervical neuroendocrine carcinoma: a clinical and light microscopic study of 14 cases. *Int J Gynecol Pathol.* 1988; 7:64-74.

Wang HL and Lu DW. Overexpression of c-kit protein is an infrequent event in small cell carcinomas of the uterine cervix. *Mod Pathol.* 2004a; 17:732-738.

Wang HL and Lu DW. Detection of human papillomavirus DNA and expression of p16, Rb, and p53 proteins in small cell carcinomas of the uterine cervix. *Am J Surg Pathol.* 2004b; 28:901-908.

Wang WL, Healy ME, Sattler M, Verma S, Lin J, Maulik G, Stiles CD, Griffin JD, Johnson BE and Salgia R. Growth inhibition and modulation of kinase pathways of small cell lung cancer cell lines by the novel tyrosine kinase inhibitor STI 571. *Oncogene.* 2000; 19:3521-3528.

Watanabe S, Kanda T and Yoshiike K. Human papillomavirus type 16 transformation of primary human embryonic fibroblasts requires expression of open reading frames E6 and E7. *J Virol.* 1989; 63:965-969.

Weed JC, Jr., Graff AT, Shoup B and Tawfik O. Small cell undifferentiated (neuroendocrine) carcinoma of the uterine cervix. *J Am Coll Surg.* 2003; 197:44-51.

Werness BA, Levine AJ and Howley PM. Association of human papillomavirus types 16 and 18 E6 proteins with p53. *Science.* 1990; 248:76-79.

Whang-Peng J, Kao-Shan CS, Lee EC, Bunn PA, Carney DN, Gazdar AF and Minna JD. Specific chromosome defect associated with human small-cell lung cancer; deletion 3p(14-23). *Science.* 1982; 215:181-182.

Wistuba, II, Thomas B, Behrens C, Onuki N, Lindberg G, Albores-Saavedra J and Gazdar AF. Molecular abnormalities associated with endocrine tumors of the uterine cervix. *Gynecol Oncol.* 1999; 72:3-9.

Zarka TA, Han AC, Edelson MI and Rosenblum NG. Expression of cadherins, p53, and BCL2 in small cell carcinomas of the cervix: potential tumor suppressor role for N-cadherin. *Int J Gynecol Cancer.* 2003; 13:240-243.

Zhang H, Liu J, Cagle PT, Allen TC, Laga AC and Zander DS. Distinction of pulmonary small cell carcinoma from poorly differentiated squamous cell carcinoma: an immunohistochemical approach. *Mod Pathol.* 2005; 18:111-118.

Ziegler A, Luedke GH, Fabbro D, Altmann KH, Stahel RA and Zangemeister-Wittke U. Induction of apoptosis in small-cell lung cancer cells by an antisense oligodeoxynucleotide targeting the Bcl-2 coding sequence. *J Natl Cancer Inst.* 1997; 89:1027-1036.

zur Hausen H. Papillomavirus infections--a major cause of human cancers. *Biochim Biophys Acta.* 1996; 1288:F55-78.

In: New Research on Cervical Cancer
Editor: George Z. Rolland, pp. 129-147
ISBN 1-60021-300-6

Chapter 5

THE PROTEIN P16^{INK4A} AS A RELIABLE INDICATOR OF THE HPV-INDUCED CARCINOGENESIS

Galina M. Volgareva[1,*], Larisa E. Zavalishina[2], Daria A. Golovina[1], Yulia Y. Andreeva[2], Andrey N. Petrov[2], Valeria D. Ermilova[1], Anatoliy A. Petrenko[1], Alexey N. Katargin[1], Maria V. Bateva[2], Natalia P. Kisseljova[1] and Georgy A. Frank[2]

[1]N.N. Blokhin Cancer Research Center of the Russian Academy of Medical Sciences;
[2]P.A. Gertzen Research Institute of Oncology, the Russian Ministry of Health, Russia

ABSTRACT

The protein p16^{INK4a}, an inhibitor of cycline-dependent kinases CDKs 4/6, is encoded by the tumor suppressor gene *INK4a.* In various tumors its control function over a cell passing through G1/S check-point is broken due to mutational or epigenetic events. Cervical carcinomas stay by themselves with this respect. Owing to the pRb inactivation by the HPV E7 oncoprotein cells uncontrollably pass to the S- cell cycle stage. In the *RB* signal pathway p16^{INK4a} acts upstream of pRb. In cells of HPV-positive cervical dysplasia and carcinomas it looses the role of the G1/S check-point controller. The content of p16^{INK4a} increases drastically. The feed-back loop between pRb inactivation by the oncoprotein E7 and the sharp growth of the p16^{INK4a} amount had been demonstrated in in vitro systems. However details of this feed-back loop in primary dysplasia and carcinoma remain not quite clear. None the less the given phenomenon was taken as the basis of the proposal to use detection of p16^{INK4a} for early diagnostics of cervical cancer. We had demonstrated formerly that the share of p16^{INK4a}-positive cells increases in the following row: LSIL → HSIL → invasive carcinoma. However in line with the communications of other research groups we had registered some samples of HSIL and invasive squamous

* Correspondence concerning this article should be addressed to Kashirskoye shosse, 24, 115478 Moscow, Russia.

carcinomas either containing very small numbers of p16^{INK4a}-positive cells or fully lacking them (the "negative" samples). Thus in the present study correspondence of expression of the HPV E7 oncogene and cellular gene *INK4a* was evaluated in squamous cervical carcinomas at two levels. The virus oncogene expression was studied by two methods: RT-PCR and immunochemistry with HPV16 E7-specific antibodies. To study an expression of the gene *INK4a* two kinds of experiments were performed: semi-quantitative RT-PCR including the development of the PCR product by Southern blot hybridization with the radio-active probe; immunochemistry with the p16^{INK4a}-specific antibodies. For RNA isolation both total tumor samples and tumor cell populations enriched by microdissections were used. Expression levels of the HPV *E7* oncogene greatly varied from sample to sample; in most carcinomas they were accompanied with the 3-30-fold rise of the *INK4a* m-RNA amount in comparison with that in normal tissue. So transcription of the gene *INK4a* contributes to the cervical cancer-specific overexpression of its protein product p16^{INK4a}. The gene *INK4a* transcription in specimens with a predominantly cytoplasmic location of p16^{INK4a} was not less active than that in the carcinomas expressing p16^{INK4a} in majority of nuclei. Thus both variants of staining with p16^{INK4a}-specific antibodies are to be regarded as positively stained. The results obtained are in accordance with the notion that the HPV *E7* oncogene has some influence on the gene *INK4a* transcription activation. However in "negative" samples some different links of the feed-back loop seem to be disturbed. There exist rare cervical carcinomas harboving HPV DNA and expressing the oncogene E7 at both the m-RNA and the protein level while fully lacking the *INK4a* expression at the both levels.

Keywords: tumor suppressor *INK4a*, protein p16^{INK4a}, subcellular location, HPV oncogene E7, correspondence of expression at the m-RNA and the protein level.

INTRODUCTION

Human papilloma viruses (HPV) of the certain types, the so-called high risk types (HR-HPV) were found to be aetiological agents of cervical cancer [1-3]. HPV-negative squamous cell cervical carcinomas are extremely rare [4].

Efficiency of early diagnostics of cervical cancer has increased significantly with the introduction of cytological analysis of vaginal smear cells known as Papanicolaou test or Pap test [5]. However even under application of Pap test probability of both false-positive and false-negative diagnoses is still high [6]. Attempts to detect DNA of HR-HPV by PCR in these materials did not result in working out of a more reliable test for the cancer prediction. Cancer in situ and invasive cervical carcinoma are known to originate in only a small part of women with HPV-positive low-grade squamous intraepithelial lesions (LSIL) [2]. Thus despite high sensitivity of PCR specificity of the given approach turned out to be low. Nowaday attempts to improve early diagnostics of cervical cancer are mostly concentrated on the search of such host cell genes expression of which in dysplastic and cancerous cervical epithelium under the influence of HR-HPV oncoproteins gets greatly and irreversibly altered. The number of genes – potential candidates for the role of markers for diagnostics and therapy of cervical carcinogenesis as had been detected by expression microarray techniques makes up many dozens [7,8].

The gene *INK4a* (*CDKN2A, MTS1, INK4a/ARF*) is one of them. Its protein product p16^{INK4a} is an inhibitor of cycline-D-dependent kinases Cdk 4/6 [9]. The protein p16^{INK4a} was found to prevent phosphorylation of the retinoblastoma susceptibility gene product (pRb). Being tumor suppressor pRb in underphosphorylated state blocks cells in the G1 stage precluding them from replicating DNA [10]. Thus as an inhibitor of the pRb phosphorylation p16^{INK4a} displays its action in a proliferation signal transduction pathway upstream of pRb. The gene *INK4a* is a bona fide tumor suppressor as had been demonstrated in experiments with knock-out mice [11,12]. p16^{INK4a} is an important component of the *RB/INK4a* signal pathway which in its turn is the component of a more complex signal network [13].

In many tumor types the *RB/INK4a* signal pathway is damaged by one of the following mechanisms: mutations in the gene *RB*, hyperphosphorylation of pRb owing to overexpression of cycline D; mutations in *CDK4* and *CDK6* genes which preclude their protein products from binding to the inhibitors (p16^{INK4} being one of them); overexpression of the genes *CDK4* and *CDK6*; the gene *INK4a* point mutations, deletions in this gene or methylation of its promotor region [10,14]. Either of those events leads to the slackening of the genetic control over a cell transition from the G1 cell cycle stage to the S stage.

Cervical carcinomas stay by themselves with this respect. In the course of oncogenesis in HR-HPV-harboring cervical epithelium cells the *RB/INK4a* signal pathway gets hampered by an unified mode.

As had been shown in cell cultures in vitro, the HR-HPV oncoprotein E7 is capable of binding to the protein pRb [15]. This interaction is equivalent to the inactivating mutation of the gene *RB*: it leads to the dissociation of the complexes of pRb with E2F transcriptional factors [16]. The release of the E2F transcriptional factors stimulates cells to pass from the G1 stage to the stage of DNA replication. Apart from the dissociation of the pRb/E2F complexes the E7 binding to the protein pRb causes the sharp decrease in the protein pRb stability and its rapid proteosomal degradation [17]. In cell cultures there exists a negative feed-back regulatory loop involving the *RB* gene status, on the one hand, and the transcription activity of the p16^{INK4a}-encoding gene, on the other: the active pRb suppresses the gene *INK4a* transcription [18-20]. Existence of this correlation, - abrogation of the pRb function → overexpression of p16^{INK4a}, - was shown at the protein level as well [18,19].

Those observations were confirmed in primary carcinomas. The content of the protein E7 HPV in cervical epithelium cells at the stages of high-grade squamous intraepithelial lesions (HSIL) and carcinoma sharply increases while the level of the protein pRb decreases drastically and the predominant majority of invasive cancer cells lack the latter [21-23]. Several research groups including us demonstrated in immunohistochemical studies a manyfold growth of the gene *INK4a* expression in primary cervical dysplasia and carcinomas in comparison with that in normal epithelium [24-30]. In our study the portion of the p16^{INK4a}-positive specimens increased in a row: LSIL → HSIL → carcinomas [30]. The sum total of those results allows one to regard the procedure of immunohistochemical detection of the protein p16^{INK4a} as a promising optional test for early diagnostics of cervical cancer and the detection of p16^{INK4a}-positive cells – as an indication of the HPV-induced carcinogenesis [21-30].

As regards the rare HPV-negative cervical cancers, the *RB/INK4a* pathway damaging events in their cells may probably belong to any of the numerous types mentioned above. Overexpression of p16^{INK4a} may occur in their cells also in case they had acquired the state of uncontrollable proliferation due to the *RB* gene mutation. This suggestion is confirmed with some experimental data. Thus the p16^{INK4} overproduction was found in the HPV-negative RB-mutant cell line C33A [19, 26]. In the study carried out on cervical adenocarcinomas K. Milde-Langosch et al. registered moderate and strong expression of the protein p16^{INK4a} in HPV-negative specimens [27].

By the present moment the number of publications on p16^{INK4a} detection in HPV-positive dysplastic and cancerous epithelium of cervix uteri obtained in numerous laboratories all over the world reached many dozens. Immunochemical staining with p16^{INK4a}-specific antibodies was communicated to sufficiently improve interobserver agreement in the diagnosis of cervical intraepithelial neoplasia [29]. LSILs which expressed p16^{INK4a} in numerous cells were shown to have a significantly higher tendency to progress to HSILs than p16^{INK4a}-negative cases; so p16^{INK4a} may have the potential to support the interpretation of low-grade dysplastic lesion [31]. J.-L. Wang et al. communicated the presence of p16^{INK4a}-positive cells in early (morphologically normal, sometimes with the signs of inflammation) biopsy to correlate well with a significantly higher speed of disease progression [32]. This study was carried out on the group of patients having HSILs or invasive carcinomas of cervix uteri. For every of them several preceding diagnostic biopsy materials were available including ones lacking any features of premalignant alterations. When the time interval for disease progression from initial biopsy to HSIL or invasive cancer was compared with states of p16^{INK4a}- expression, cases stained positive for p16^{INK4a} progressed within 64.2 months as compared with 122.3 months among those stained negatively.

When attempting to compare in immunohistochemical studies prognostic values of several cellular markers of cervical carcinogenesis, for example, p16^{INK4a}, p14^{ARF}, p53 и PCNA [32], Ki67, cyclin E and p16^{INK4a} [33], p16^{INK4a}, CDC6 and MCM5 [34], the investigators invariably show p16^{INK4a} to be the reliable [32] or the most reliable [33,34] one.

Cytological versions of the test aimed for p16^{INK4a} detection were worked out and are currently being specified [34-39]. In this connection the results of the study by S. Nieh et al. [35,39] seem to be of primary importance. The investigators compared (1) results of common Pap test, (2) data of immunocytochemical analysis of the same smear stained with p16^{INK4a}-specific antibodies, (3) results of histological and immunohistological analyses of follow-up cervical biopsies as well as (4) results of HR-HPV DNA detection on smears by in situ hybridization. The study was done on the group of women with atypical squamous cells of undetermined significance (abbreviated as ASCUS - [40]) in Pap test for whom follow-up cervical biopsy materials were available. Detection of p16^{INK4a}-positive cells on the ASCUS-containing smear turned out to be a highly sensitive (sensitivity - 95%) and specific (specificity – 96%) indicator of a possible origination of HSIL or carcinoma in a given patient later on, a more efficient one than the data on HR-HPV DNA detection on ASCUS-containing cytological smears [39].

Thus more and more experimental evidences are being obtained that immunohisto-/cytochemical detection of the protein p16^{INK4a} is a promising supplementary test for early diagnostics of cervical cancer. Simultaneously the demand is growing for a cytological version of the test to carry out wide-scale preventive examinations of healthy women. It seems important in this connection to timely remove ambiguities and equivocalities which may influence interpretation of the immunocytochemical p16^{INK4a} detection data in a diagnostic laboratory.

One of such difficulties is due to the ability of some commercially available p16^{INK4a}-specific monoclonal antibodies to stain not only dysplastic and cancerous cervical epithelium but normal one as well. Such effects were described by R. Klaes et al. in particular on the grounds of the comparison they carried out of several p16^{INK4a}-specific monoclonal antibodies produced by different firms [26]. The ability of a certain antibody to stain normal cells may be the evidence of its high sensitivity enabling one to detect amounts of p16^{INK4a} commonly present in normal epithelial cells of cervix uteri. However under conditions of a diagnostic laboratory a capacity of an antibody for staining of normal cells may significantly hamper the discrimination of dysplastic and cancerous cells, on the one hand, from normal ones, on the other. For the purposes of practical diagnostics in this respect monoclonal antibody produced by hybridoma cell clone E6H4 obtained by R. Klaes et al. [26] distributed at present by DakoCytomation has acquired a very good reputation as is confirmed with the fact that many research groups use it. One has to state that varying abilities of different p16^{INK4a}-specific monoclonal antibodies to stain normal epithelial cells of cervix uteri makes it rather difficult to compare the results obtained by research groups who had detected the given protein with different antibodies.

Additional difficulties arise from the fact that different research groups use diverse approaches of semiquantitative data registration. The opinion was expressed to score as positively stained with p16^{INK4a}-specific antibodies only those dysplasia and carcinoma specimens in which not less than 25% of cells got stained [37,38]. Such point of view deserves a reserved attitude, in our opinion: in the previous on-line work we presented several specimens of HSILs and cancer in situ in which p16^{INK4a}-positive cells made up a significantly smaller portion [30].

It remains not quite clear as well whether or not specimens are to be regarded as positively stained when only a cytoplasm gets stained and no signs of the p16^{INK4a} protein can be seen in cellular nuclei. The decision to score an exclusively nuclear staining when detecting a protein which displays its function within a nucleus, - and that is just the case with the protein p16^{INK4a}, - would seem not unreasonable. The corresponding trend to fully disregard an exclusively cytoplasmic staining was founded in immunohistochemical studies dedicated to p16^{INK4a} unmasking in tumors of different types [41-43]. In this connection the question seems to be of primary importance whether on Pap-smears the staining with a p16^{INK4a}-specific antibody is to be regarded as positive when displayed exclusively in a cytoplasm.

Data are not quite homogeneous on whether a strict correlation exists between a p16^{INK4a}-positive staining of dysplastic and cancerous cervical cells, on the one hand, and positive results of detection of HR-HPV DNA in these cells, on the other. Communications on existence of such a correlation are numerous [25,26,34,44,45]. However J.L. Wang et al. doubt it so far as approximately every fourth HPV-positive dysplasia in their study was found p16^{INK4a}-negative [46]. In our previous investigation every p16^{INK4a}-positive dysplastic and neoplastic cervical squamous epithelial specimen contained HR-HPV DNA while about 16 % of the HR-HPV-positive HSILs and 1 invasive cancer (out of 21 studied) were found absolutely p16^{INK4a}-negative [30]. According to the other research groups data p16^{INK4a}-negative adenocarcinoma incidence may reach 43 % and that of squamous cell cancer – about 10 % (the summary is presented in [30]). More communications have recently appeared proving that overexpression of $p16^{INK4a}$ is found in less than 100 % of HR-HPV positive HSILs and carcinomas of cervix uteri [32, 47,48]. Thus the fact of the $p16^{INK4a}$-negative HR-HPV-positive neoplasia and carcinoma existence is to be mentioned also among the points which may hamper the use of immunohisto-/cytochemical detection of the protein $p16^{INK4a}$ in early diagnostics of cervical cancer.

The aim of the present study is specifying of diagnostic potentialities of the protein $p16^{INK4a}$ immunohistochemical detection in cervical cancer as well as of criteria of the given reaction registration.

We have tried to find answers to the following questions:

1. Is the viral oncogene *E7* expression accompanied with the $p16^{INK4a}$ – encoding gene *INK4a* overexpression always indeed?
2. Are the specimens in which predominates an exclusively cytoplasmic staining and stained nuclei are rare to be scored as positively stained? Or, on the contrary, are only those specimens to be regarded as positive in which $p16^{INK4a}$ is detected in the majority of nuclei?

The expression of the genes *INK4a* and *E7* was evaluated at two levels: the level of m-RNA and that of the protein.

MATERIALS AND METHODS

Specimens were used of 15 invasive squamous cell carcinomas taken from patients who underwent surgical treatment in the N.N. Blokhin Cancer Research Center of the Russian Academy of Medical Sciences, Moscow, Russia. Six specimens of adjacent morphologically normal cervical tissues from those women were used also. All the specimens were collected according to the regulations of the N.N. Blokhin Cancer Research Center. Fourteen of the specimens were harboring HPV type 16 DNA as had been determined by PCR, the fifteenth had turned out HPV 18 positive.

Cervical cancer cell lines C33A, HT3, SiHa, CaSki and HeLa originated from the American Type Culture Collection. Cells of SiHa and CaSki cell lines harbor high risk HPV type 16, HeLa – type 18, HT3-type 30; cells of the line C33A is HPV-negative RB-mutant [19, 49]. The cells were maintained in DMEM medium with the addition of 10 % of fetal calf serum. For the immunocytochemical detection of $p16^{INK4a}$ in the course of regular culture reseedings cell suspension was placed on the HistoBond adhesive coated slide (SMT Geraetehandel GmbH, Germany). Then smears were prepared; after drying they were fixed in neutral formalin, washed in running water and processed similarly to the deparaffinized histological slides.

For immunohistochemical studies neutral formalin-fixed paraffin embedded materials were used. Serial sections (4-5 μm thick) were transferred on HistoBond slides. Sections were immersed in xylene to remove paraffin and then rehydrated through graded alcohol. The first of the cuts was stained with hematoxylin-eosin to confirm the diagnosis. Two or three independent pathologists (Y.Y.A., V.D.E., G.A.F) performed diagnosis verification. Next slides were stained with antibodies.

To detect p16^{INK4a} the procedures of epitope retrieval, endogenous peroxidase activity blocking, blocking of nonspecific binding and incubating with the p16^{INK4a}-specific monoclonal antibodies (CINtec^{TM} Histology Kit, DakoCytomation) were conducted according to Klaes et al [26]. To detect the oncoprotein E7 HPV16 the rabbit polyclonal HPV 16 E7-specific serum was used kindly provided by Dr. W. Zwerschke; all the procedures were similar to those described by the serum originators [21]. In both cases to visualize the results the slides which had been exposed to the primary antibody were treated with the EnVision^{TM}+Dual Link DakoCytomation reagent. The reaction was developed with either AEC or DAB chromogen. The slides were counterstained with Mayer's hematoxylin. For a positive control in immunochemical tests with both p16^{INK4a} – and E7-specific antibodies sections of HPV16-positive HSIL or carcinoma specimens were used which had been stained diffusely with the p16^{INK4a}-specific antibody.

For microdissecting the carcinoma specimen was transferred from the liquid nitrogen depository into the cryostat precooled down to -20°C. The sections (5 μm thick) were placed on glass slides and ethanol fixed. The details of the fixation procedure were as follows: 1-2 min in 70% ethanol; 1-2 min in Mayer's hematoxylin; rinsing with running water for 30-60 sec; rinsing with 70 % ethanol; rinsing in 95% ethanol (twice); rinsing in 100 % ethanol; immersing into xylene for 1 min; air-drying (until xylene evaporates). Then a homogeneous zone was selected under the microscope containing not less than 90 % of cancerous cells while practically lacking stromal elements. This zone was marked off, then the drop of lyzing buffer solution was placed onto it (the RNeasy® Micro Kit "Qiagen" intended for isolation of total RNA from microdissected tissues) and the procedure of RNA isolation on spin columns carried out according to the directions of the kit manufacturer.

To perform RT-PCR RNA was isolated from frozen tissues by guanidine isothiocyanate homogenization procedure followed by ultracentrifugation (30000 rpm, 16h, 19°C) through a cesium chloride cushion according to the protocol described earlier [50]. One microgram of total RNA was treated with DNase (DNase I Amp.Grade, "Invitrogen") and used in reverse transcription with random hexanucleotide primers ("Lytekh", Russia) and Super Script II reverse transcriptase ("Invitrogene") according to the directions of the enzyme manufacturer.

To equalize cDNA preparations the PCR with GAPDH- gene specific primers was performed. The following primers were used: forward, 5'-ACC ACA GTC CAT GCC ATC AC-3'; reverse, 5'-TCC ACC ACC CTG TTG CTG TA-3'. The length of the amplification product was 450 bp. The reaction mixture composition was as follows: PCR buffer (0,016 M $(NH_4)_2SO_4$; 0,06 M tris-HCl, pH 8,8; Tween-20, 0,1%); 2,0 мM $MgCl_2$; 200 μM each of dNTPs; 8 pM each of the primers; 0,7u Taq-DNA-polymerase (Research Institute of Bioorganic Chemistry, Russia). The amplification program was like this: 94°C – 5 min, 28 cycles of 94°C – 30 sec, 58°C – 30 sec, 72°C – 60 sec; final extension for 2 min.

The INK4a gene-specific primers and PCR conditions were used as described by T.T. Nguyen et al. [51]: sense, 5'-AGC CTT CGG CTG ACT GGC TGG-3' (exon I); antisense, 5'-GCG CTG CCC ATC ATC ATG AC-3' (exon II). The size of the amplification product was 140 bp. The reaction mixture composition was as follows: PCR-buffer; 2,0 мM $MgCl_2$; 400 μM of each of the four dNTPs; 16 pM of each primer; 1 u of Taq-DNA-polymerase. The cycle number was 35. The amplified DNA fragment was detected by means of electrophoresis in 2.0 % agarose gel in presence of ethidium bromide (0,5 μg/ml). To perform Southern blot hybridization with the radio-active probe the product of amplification was transferred onto the nylon membrane Hybondand ^{TM}-N+ "Amersham Biosciences" and developed with the ^{32}P-labelled internal oligonucleotide probe. The nucleotide sequence of the probe was as follows: 5'-CTG CCC AAC GCA CCG AAT AGT TAC G-3'. To perform those procedures the protocol recommended by the membrane manufacturers was used.

To compare the amounts of INK4a-specific amplification products in different samples the optical densities of the PCR products separated in agarose gel and visualized either by the ethidium bromide staining or by hybridization with the radio-active probe were processed by the Image Quality computer program.

Analysis of the E7 HPV16 transcripts was performed with the following primers: sense, 5'- CGG ACA GAG CCC ATT ACA AT- 3'; antisense, 5'-GAA CAG ATG GGG CAC ACA AT – 3'. The amplification product length was 144 bp. The oncogene E7 HPV18 was amtlified in PCR with the following primers: sense, 5'-GCC GAE CCA CAA CGT CAG AC– 3'; antisense, 5'- GGT CGT CTG CTG AGC TTT CT – 3' [52]. The composition of the reaction mixture with the both primer pairs was as follows: PCR-buffer; 2,0 mM $MgCl_2$; 400 μM of each of the dNTPs; 16 pM of each primer; 1 u of Taq-DNA-polymerase. The program was like this: 94°C – 4 min; then 35 cycles of three steps: 94°C – 30 sec, 58°C –30 sec, 72°C – 90 sec; concluding elongation for 6 minutes.

Results and Discussion

As we have mentioned above there is no common approach among different investigators to the point whether to score as positive result of staining or not the specimens in which only a cytoplasm is stained while nuclei lack any sign of p16^{INK4a}. We subdivided carcinoma specimens under study into the following five groups according to the quota of nuclei in their cells in which the protein p16^{INK4a} was revealed (the Table):

I. Totally negative carcinomas, - specimens in which the p16^{INK4a}-specific staining was found neither in nuclei nor in a cytoplasm of cells (the specimen №1 in the Table, Fig. 1d). We undertook repeated attempts to stain serial sections of the given specimen as well as of some other ones included into the excerpt described herein (belonging to the groups II-V, - see bellow). For all of them results of repeated stainings coincided with the initial data completely under application of the p16^{INK4a} – specific E6H4 antibodies from several batches at different moments separated from one another with different time intervals. Thus the specimen №1 was shown to be p16^{INK4a}-negative thrice.

II. Carcinomas which contained less than 1 % of stained nuclei while cytoplasmic staining was seen in a predominant majority of cells (specimen №2 in the Table, Fig. 1f).

III. Carcinomas with 1-5 % of stained nuclei and stained cytoplasm in about 100 % of cells (specimens №№3-5 in the Table).

IV. Carcinomas with 5-25% of stained nuclei and about 100 % of stained cytoplasm (specimens №№ 6-8 in the Table).
V. Carcinomas in which over 25 % of nuclei were p16^{INK4a}-positive and cytoplasmic staining was found in about 100 % of cells (specimens №№ 9-15 in the Table, Fig.1h).

Table 1. The genes *INK4a* and HPV *E7* expression in invasive squamous cell carcinomas of cervix uteri.

Specimen	Group	INK4a		*E7*	
		Immunochemical detection	RT-PCR*	Immunochemical detection of E7HPV16	RT-PCR
1	I	0 % of stained cells	-	+	+
2	II	Less than 1% of stained nuclei, cytoplasmic staining in predominant majority of cancer cells	+	+	+
3	III	1- 5% of stained nuclei, cytoplasmic staining in predominant majority of cancer cells	+	+	+
4			+	+	+
5			+	+	+
6	IV	5 - 25% of stained nuclei, cytoplasmic staining in predominant majority of cancer cells	+	+	+
7			+	not tested	+**
8			+	+	+
9	V	Over 25% of stained nuclei, cytoplasmic staining in predominant majority of cancer cells	+	not tested	+
10			+	+	+
11			+ (+)	+	+
12			+ (+)	+	+
13			+ (+)	+	+
14			+ (+)	+	+
15			+ (+)	+	+

*- the data obtained in experiments with purified by microdissections tumor cell populations are presented in parentheses;
**- the given specimen was HPV18-positive, all the rest –HPV16-positive.

We did not find any cervical carcinomas with an exclusively or predominantly nuclear staining.

In cervical cancer cell lines subcellular location of p16^{INK4a} varied: SiHa cells expressed it exclusively in a cytoplasm (Fig.1m) while C33A and HT3 cells – in both cytoplasm and nuclei (Fig.1l). Earlier R. Klaes et al. had described a predominantly cytoplasmic staining of cells of cervical cell lines including the cells C33A, HT3 and SiHa with the same antibody [26]. Thus the results of immunocytochemical study of cervical cancer cell lines are in agreement with those obtained in primary invasive carcinomas: besides a nuclear-cytoplasmic staining type there seem to occur an exclusively cytoplasmic one.

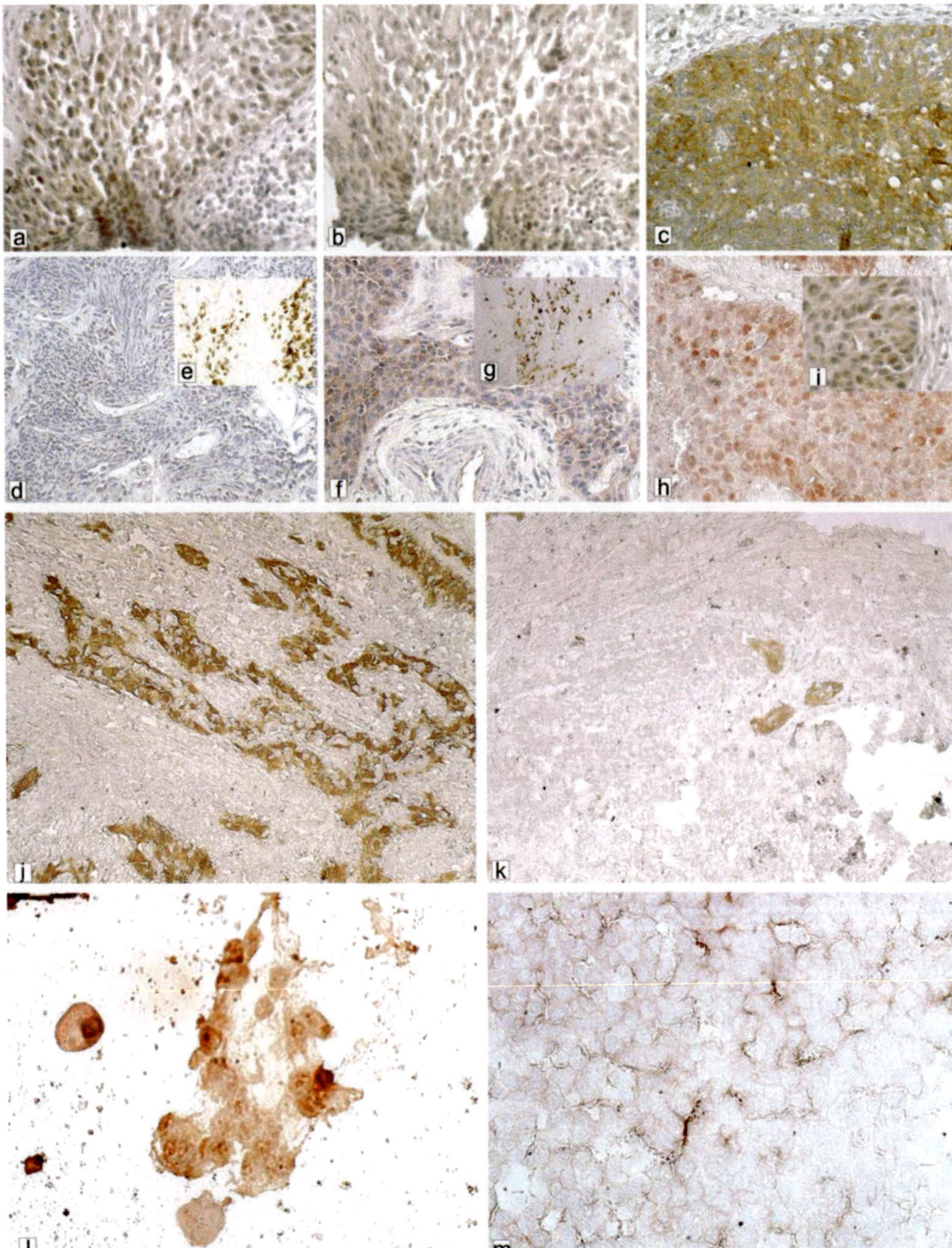

Figure 1. Immunochemical detection of the proteins p16^{INK4a} and E7 HPV16 in primary cervical dysplasia and carcinoma, as well as in cervical cancer cells lines. a, b - serial sections of carcinoma in situ taken for a positive control. a - staining with the p16^{INK4a}-specific antibody; b – staining with the E7 – specific serum. c – HSIL, staining with the p16^{INK4a}-specific antibody; d-i – three invasive carcinomas, staining with the p16^{INK4a}-specific antibodies (d, f and h) and with the E7-specific serum (the latter presented on the incuts,- e, g and i); specimens 1 (d,e), 2 (f,g) and 10 (h,i); j, k – invasive carcinoma, specimen 15, staining with the p16^{INK4a}-specific antibody; l, m - cells of cervical cancer cell lines SiHa (m) and HT3 (l), staining with the p16^{INK4a}-specific antibody.

The fact that just the fifth group of carcinoma specimens turned out to be the most numerous in the present study seems in our previous experience to reflects the actual occurrence of invasive squamous cell carcinomas of cervix uteri in which the protein p16^{INK4a} is found in many nuclei. However carcinomas included into groups I-IV when summarized are not infrequent as well. In several HSIL specimens we also found a similar predominantly cytoplasmic staining with the p16^{INK4a} – specific antibody (Fig. 1c). In veiw of the observation that a predominantly cytoplasmic staining may be found not only in cancerous cervical epithelial cells but in dysplastic ones as well proper evaluation of the results of immunohistochemical test with such specimens becomes an urgent issue for the purposes of diagnostics. Are the results of immunocytochemical analysis of a smear to be scored as positive when cells with an exclusively cytoplasmic p16^{INK4a} expression are found? Is the carcinoma specimen №2 to be regarded as a poorly stained one on the grounds that rare nuclei of this specimen express p16^{INK4a} or is it to be scored as a strongly stained case owing to the fact that p16^{INK4a} was detected in a cytoplasm in the overwhelming majority of its cells?

As we have mentioned above the p16^{INK4a} overexpression in cells of cervical cancer cell lines is accompanied with the INK4a transcription activation [19]. In this connection we analysed on primary carcinomas and cervical cancer cell lines characterized with different staining types the INK4a expression at the level of m-RNA by RT-PCR. Summarized data are presented in the Table and Fig. 2. The INK4a-specific amplification product was detected for all the carcinoma specimens studied with the only exception of the specimen №1. The gene INK4a expression was also registered in the specimens of morphologically normal cervical epithelium (Fig. 2a). The amounts of the PCR-products in the carcinoma tissue was 3-30 times greater when compared with that in the adjacent normal tissue from one and the same patient (Fig. 2a – specimens №№ 5 and 5N, 6 and 6N, 9 and 9N). This result proves that the gene INK4a transcription in carcinomas of cervix uteri undergoes substantial activation in comparison with normal cervical epithelium. The results obtained are in agreement with the notion that the INK4a transcription activation in cervical carcinomas contributes to the phenomenon of the p16^{INK4a} overexpression in these carcinomas.

There seem to be no correlation between the level of the INK4a-specific m-RNA in a cervical carcinoma specimen, on the one hand, and the portion of the p16^{INK4a}-expressing nuclei, on the other. The content of the INK4a-specific m-RNA in specimens expressing p16^{INK4a} in less than 5% of nuclei was not lesser than that in carcinomas with greater shares of stained nuclei (Fig. 2a). In some instances the amount of the INK4a m-RNA turned out to be greater in tissues with the smaller portion of the p16^{INK4a}-containing nuclei (the specimens №№2,4 and 5 in comparison with the specimens №№ 6 and 8).

As to the quantitative indices of the INK4a transcription activation in cervical cancer cells in comparison with normal cervical epithelium, they may be underestimated in a study performed on total tumor specimens containing in addition to cancer cells stromal cell admixtures. The share of stromal cell admixture may vary from moderate to sharply predominating in different cancer specimens (Fig. 1j and 1k, respectively). So for five specimens (№№ 11-15) we evaluated the gene INK4a expression at the level of m-RNA on cancer cell populations enriched by microdissections. Results of RT-PCR were developed by Southern blot hybridization with the radio-active probe (the Table). In all the cases the results obtained with the microdissected cancer tissues were found to qualitatively coincide with those with the total specimens: the gene encoding p16^{INK4a} was actively transcribed.

The gene INK4a expression at the level of m-RNA we evaluated in cells of three HPV-positive cell lines, - HeLa, SiHa and Caski. The specific amplification product was detected in experiments with all three cell lines; the most pronounced expression of the gene was seen in SiHa cells (Fig 2b). A model system "cell line in vitro" possesses an advantage over a model "primary carcinoma, total specimen" as it does not contain any admixture of stromal cells. So when trying to find an answer to a question if it is correct to score an exclusively cytotlasmic staining of cells with p16^{INK4a} – specific antibodies as a positive reaction it becomes an observation of principal importance that the gene encoding this protein is actively transcribed in the SiHa cell line for which an exclusively cytopmasmic type of staining was shown in the immunocytochemical study.

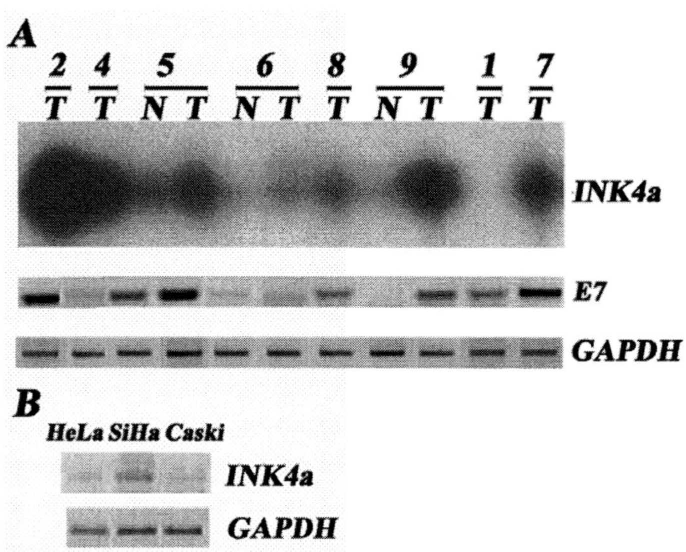

Figure 2. Analysis of expression of *INK4a* and *E7* HPV by RT-PCR in primary squamous cell cervical carcinomas (a) and of cervical cancer cell lines (b). (a) T- cervical carcinomas, N- morphologically normal tissue adjacent to tumor. Specimen numbers are indicated in the upper lines. The top panel electrophoregram after Southern blot hybridization with the *INK4a*-specific radio-active probe. The middle and the bottom panels: electrophoregrams after ethidium bromide staining. The middle panel: results with the *E7*- specific primers. The bottom panel: results with the *GAPDH*-specific primers as a control for stability and concentration of RNA. (b) RNAs isolated from cells of cervical cancer cell lines HeLa, SiHa and CaSki; amplification products visualized by staining with ethidium bromide.

Thus in primary carcinomas of cervix uteri as well as in cells of some cervical cancer cell lines characterized with a predominantly cytoplasmic subcellular localization of p16^{INK4a} an active transcription occurs of the gene encoding this protein. We did not find any carcinomas or cervical cancer cell lines in which p16^{INK4a} would be detected in a cytoplasm while the gene INK4a was transcriptionally inactivated.

Possibility of connection between altered subcellular location of p16^{INK4a} and malignant conversion of epithelial cells was mentioned in the study by A. Di Vinci et al. [53]. These investigators described in several breast carcinoma specimens an exclusively cytoplasmic subcellular location of the protein while in normal epithelial cells and in fibroadenomas it was localized predominantly in nuclei. Quite recently the communication by K.Nilsson and G. Landberg appeared who demonstrated on cell cultures using subcellular fractionation that the functionally active p16^{INK4a} is indeed located both in the cytoplasm and in the nucleus; similar results were obtained in primary basal cell carcinomas and invasive squamous cell carcinomas of the skin; cytoplasmic p16^{INK4a} was shown to be capable of binding cyclin dependent kinase 4/6, which potentially indicated that this protein could have a function in the cytoplasm [54]. In this connection further studies of mechanisms predetermining subcellular location of this protein and its cytoplasmic sequestration in cells of some cancer types seem worthwhile.

The sum total of the results presented herein proves that in addition to the indisputably p16^{INK4a}-positive specimens expressing the protein in numerous nuclei either of the following staining types should be also scored as a positive result of staining: "exclusively cytoplasmic" as well as "predominantly cytoplasmic with a small share of stained nuclei".

Variable as they were in the mode of the p16^{INK4a} expression, all the carcinomas under study were HR-HPV-positive; their cells did express the HPV E7 oncogene (the Table, Figs. 1b, 1e, 1g and 1i). Results of the immunohistochemical test were registered only if the E7-specific antibodies displayed the activity on a section taken for a positive control (Fig.1b). The oncoprotein E7 was found both in nuclei and in a cytoplasm of cancer cells, this result being in agreement with the data communicated by the serum creators [21].

The results obtained when studying the oncogene E7 expression at the level of m-RNA are presented in Fig. 2a and in the Table. Carcinoma specimens differed from each other in amounts of the E7-specific amplification product obtained by RT-PCR (Fig. 2a). However this product was seen in RT-PCR with RNAs from all 15 carcinomas which proves the oncogene E7 transcription in all of them. Other investigators also communicated great variations of the levels of the oncogene E7 expression among invasive carcinomas of cervix uteri [7]. In some instances we found signs of the E7 transcription in the adjoining to cancer normal cervical tissue (specimen №5N in Fig. 2a). Such results may reflect presence of HPV-positive micrometastases in those tissues.

Quantitative correlations between the viral oncogene E7 expression in carcinomas at the level of m-RNA detected by RT-PCR, on the one hand, and at the level of the protein detected by immunochemical method, on the other, could be revealed not for every specimen studied. An explanation of such discrepancies may be found in interference of posttranscriptional mechanisms of the HPV E7 expression regulation [55,56].

As to the specimen №1 for which negative results were obtained when staining with the p16^{INK4a}-specific antibody (Fig. 1d), the INK4a -specific product of amplification was not detected in this case even under the prolonged film exposition with the radio-active membrane. Thus the gene INK4a was not transcribed in this specimen. In the cells of this carcinoma the oncogene E7 HPV was abundantly expressed (Fig. 1e and Fig. 2a). Thus the given specimen does not belong to the rare category of the HPV-negative squamous cell cervical cancers [4]. There exist, in that way, p16^{INK4a}-negative HPV-positive cervical carcinomas in the cells of which the HPV oncogene E7 is actively expressed. Causes are to be studied of breakage of the described above relationship "HR-HPV oncogene E7 expression $\rightarrow$ the protein p16^{INK4a} overexpression" in such carcinomas.

Thus at two levels, m-RNA and protein, on the excerpt of the HR-HPV DNA harboring cervical carcinomas we observed overexpression of the viral oncogene E7, on the one hand, and of the encoding the protein $p16^{INK4a}$ tumor suppressor gene INK4a, on the other. This result is in agreement with the notion of the $p16^{INK4a}$ overexpression in cervical carcinoma cells being the consequence of the event chain triggered by the HPV oncoprotein E7. Those events had been described in cells of the cancer cell lines previously. Interaction of the oncoprotein E7 with pRb seem to originate this chain of events [15]. According to the feed-back loop mechanism alterations in the pRb state entail the strengthened activity of the gene INK4a transcription [18-20]. In primary dysplasia and carcinomas the mechanisms responsible for this overexpression may be more complicated. The reason for such a suggestion is the membership of the gene INK4a/ARF in the complex regulatory network including besides the RB/INK4a pathway the p53 pathway as well [13]. Thus the quite unexpected three-fold increase of the INK4a transcription activity registered by Y.Li at al. in the "in vitro" system after the introduction of the HPV E6 oncogene into it confirms this suggestion [19]. The gene INK4a seems to possess in addition to transcriptional regulatory mechanisms some posttranscriptional ones also. The fact of the sharp variability of the $p16^{INK4a}$ nuclear content in different carcinoma specimens under approximately equal transcriptional activity of the gene INK4a in those specimens demonstrated in the present study testifies to the correctness of this suggestion. Further investigations are needed to clarify whether in the course of tumor progression the mechanisms of the $p16^{INK4a}$ transportation from cytoplasm into nucleus are hampered, whether the stability of the protein itself gets altered, whether these events influence the rate of progression, etc.

Conclusion

When registering results of the immunohistochemical reaction with $p16^{INK5a}$ – specific antibodies those specimens are to be regarded as positively stained in which an exclusively cytoplasmic subcellular location of this protein predominates in addition to specimens traditionally scored as positive in which $p16^{INK4a}$ is found in majority of cellular nuclei. This approach may lead to the increase of the number of the specimens scored as positive. Subcellular location of p16INK4a is likely to be determined by some posttranscriptional mechanisms; in the course of carcinoma progression these mechanisms may get altered.

The data obtained are in agreement with the notion that overexpression of $p16^{INK4a}$ in cervical dysplasia and carcinomas may serve an indicator of the HPV-induced carcinogenesis.

There exist rare HPV-positive invasive carcinomas of cervix uteri in which the HPV oncogene E7 is expressed at the levels both of m-RNA and of the protein but the gene INK4a transcription does not occur. Cells of such carcinomas give negative immunohistochemical reaction with $p16^{INK4a}$-specific antibodies. So $p16^{INK4a}$-negativity is not a sufficient reason to exclude a patient from the high risk group.

REFERENCES

[1] Durst M, Gissmann L, Ikenberg H, zur Hausen H. A papillomavirus DNA from a cervical carcinoma and its prevalence in cancer biopsy samples from different geographic regions.*PNAS* 1983; 80: 3812-3815.

[2] zur Hausen H. Papillomaviruses causing cancer: evasion from host-cell control in early events in carcinogenesis. Review. *J. Natl Cancer Inst.* 2000; 92: 690- 698.

[3] zur Hausen H. Oncogenic DNA viruses. Review. *Oncogene* 2001; 20: 7820-7823.

[4] Morrison C, Catania F, Wakely P, Nuovo GJ. Highly differentiated keratinizing squamous cell cancer of the cervix. A rare, locally aggressive tumor not associated with human papillomavirus or squamous intraepithelial lesions. *Amer J Surg Pathol* 2001; 25: 1310 – 1315.

[5] Papanicolaou GN. *Science* 1942; 95: 438-439.

[6] Jacobs MV, Snijders PJF, Voorharst FJ, Dillner J, Forslund O, Johansson B, won Knebel Doeberitz M, Meijer CJ, Meyer T, Nindl I, Pfister H, Stockfleth E, Strand A, Wadell G, Walboomers JM. Reliable high risk HPV DNA testing by polymerase chain reaction: an intermethod and intramethod comparison. *J. Clin. Pathol* 1999; 52: 498-503.

[7] Rosty C, Sheffer M, Tsafrird D, Stransky N, Tsafrir i, Peter M, de Cremoux P., de La Rochefordiere A, Salmon R, Dorval T, Thiery JP, Counturier J, Radvanyi F, Domany E, Sastre-Garau X. Identification of a proliferation gene cluster associated with HPV E6/E7 expression level and viral DNA load in invasive cervical carcinoma. *Oncogene* 2005; 24, 7094-7104.

[8] Santin AD, Zhan F, Bignotti E, Siegel ER, Cane S, Bellone S, Palmieri M, Anfossi S, Thomas M, Burnett A, Kay HH, Roman JJ, O'Brien TJ, Tian E, Cannon MJ, Shaughnessy J Jr, Pecorelli S. Gene expression profiles of primary HPV16- and HPV18-infected early stage cervical cancers and normal cervical epithelium: identification of novel candidate molecular markers for cervical cancer diagnosis and therapy. *Virology* 2005; 331, 269-291.

[9] Serrano M, Hannon G J, Beach D. A new regulatory motif in cell-cycle control causing specific inhibition of cyclin D/CDK4. *Nature* 1993; 366: 704-707.

[10] Ruas M, Peters G. The p16^{INK4a}/CDKN2A tumor suppressor and its relatives. Review. Biochim Biophys Acta 1998; 1378: 115-177.

[11] Krimpenfort P, Quon KC, Mooi WJ, Loonstra A, Berns A. Loss of p16^{INK4a} confers susceptibility to metastatic melanoma in mice. *Nature* 2001; 413:83-86.

[12] Sharpless NE, Bardeesy N, Lee K-H, Carrasco D, Castrillon DH, Aguirre AJ, Wu EA, Horner JW, DePinho RA. Loss of p16^{INK4a} with retention of p19^{ARF} predisposes mice to tumorigenesis. *Nature* 2001; 413: 86-91.

[13] Lowe SW, Sherr C. Tumor suppression by *Ink4a-Arf*: progress and puzzles. Review.*Curr Opin Genet Dev* 2003; 13: 77-83.

[14] Cobrinik D. Pocket proteins and cell cycle control. Review. *Oncogene* 2005; 24: 2796-2809.

[15] Dyson N, Howley PM, Munger K, Harlow E. The human papilloma virus E7 oncoprotein is able to bind to the retinoblastoma gene product. *Science* 1989; 243: 934-937.

[16] Helt A-M, Galloway DA. Mechanisms by which DNA tumor virus oncoproteins target the Rb family of pocket proteins. *Carcinogenesis* 2003; 24: 159-169.

[17] Boyer SN, Wazer DE, Band V. E7 protein of human papilloma virus-16 induces degradation of retinoblastoma protein through the ubiquitin-proteasome pathway. *Cancer Res* 1996; 56: 4620-4624.

[18] Li Y., Nichols M.A., Shay JW, Xiong Y. Transcriptional repression of the D-type cycline-dependent kinase inhibitor p16 by the retinoblastoma susceptibility gene product pRb. *Cancer Res.* 1994; 54: 6078-6082.

[19] Khleif SN, DeGregori J, Yee C, Otterson GA, Kaye FG, Nevins JR, Howley PM. Inhibition of cycline D-CDK4/CDK6 activity is associated with an E2F-mediated induction of cyclin kinase inhibitor activity. *Proc Natl Acad Sci USA* 1996; 93: 4350-4354.

[20] Kaneko S, Nishioka J, Tanaka M, Nakashima K, Nobori T. Transcriptional regulation of the CDK inhibitor $p16^{INK4a}$ gene by a novel pRB-associated repressor, RBAR1. *Biochem Mol Biol Int* 1999; 47: 205-215.

[21] Fiedler M, Muller-Holzner E, Viertler H-P, Widschwendter A, Laich A, Pfister G, Spoden GA, Jansen-Durr P, Zwerschke W. High level HPV-16 E7 oncoprotein expression correlates with reduced pRb-levels in cervical biopsies. *The FASEB Journal* 2004; 18(10); 1120-1122. Available from: URL: http://www.fasebj.org/cgi/reprint/03-1332fjev1.

[22] 22.Tringer B, Gup CJ, Singh M, Groshong S, Shroyer AL, Heinz DE, Shroyer KR. Evaluation of p16 and Rb expression in cervical squamous and glandular neoplasia. *Hum Pathol* 2004, 35: 689-696.

[23] Fiedler M, Ressler S, Campo-Fernandez B, Laich A, Jansen L, Widschwendter A, Viertler H-P, Bacher N, Morandell D, Muller-Holzner E, Durst M, Jansen-Durr P, Zwerschke W. Expression of the high-risk human papillomavirus type 18 and 45 E7 oncoproteins in cervical carcinoma biopsies. *J Gen Virol* 2005; 86: 3235-3241.

[24] Sano T, Oyama T, Kashiwabara K, Fukuda T, Nakajima T. Immunohistochemical overexpression of p16 protein associated with intact retinoblastoma protein expression in cervical cancer and cervical intraepithelial neoplasia. *Pathol Int* 1998; 48: 580-585.

[25] Sano T, Oyama T, Kashiwabara K, Fukuda T, Nakajima T. Expression status of p16 protein is associated with human papillomavirus oncogenic potential in cervical and genital lesions. *Am J Pathol* 1998; 153: 1741- 1748.

[26] Klaes R., Friedrich T., Spitkovsky D., Ridder R., Rudy W, Petry U, Dallenbach-Hellweg G, Schmidt D, von Knebel Doeberitz M. Overexpression of $p16^{INK4a}$ as a specific marker for dysplastic and neoplastic epithelial cells of the cervix uteri. *Int J Cancer* 2001; 92: 276-284.

[27] Milde-Langosch K, Riethdorf S, Kraus-Poppinghaus A, Riethdorf L, Loning T. Expression of cyclin-dependent kinase inhibitors $p16^{MTS1}$, $p21^{WAF1}$, and $p27^{KIP1}$ in HPV-positive and HPV-negative cervical adenocarcinomas.*Virchows Arch* 2001; 439: 55-61.

[28] Volgareva GM, Zavalishina LE, Frank GA, Andreeva YuYu, Petrov AN, Kisseljov FL, Spitkovsky DD. Expression of protein marker p16^{INK4a} in uterine cervical cancer. *Arkh Patol* 2002;64(1): 22-24. (In Russian).

[29] Klaes R, Benner A, Friedrich T, Ridder R, Herrington S, Jenkins D, Kurman RJ, Schmidt D, Stoler M, von Knebel Doeberitz M. P16^{INK4a} immunohistochemistry improves interobserver diagnosis of cervical intraepithelial neoplasia. *Am J Surg Pathol.* 2002; 26: 1389-1399.

[30] Volgareva GM, Zavalishina LE, Andreeva YY, Frank GA, Krutikova EI, Golovina DA, Bliev AY, Spitkovsky DD, Ermilova VD , Kisseljov FL. Protein p16^{INK4a} as a marker of dysplastic and neoplastic alterations in cervical epithelial cells. *BMC Cancer* [online]. 2004; Aug 31; 4(1):58. Available from: URL: http://www.pubmedcentral.gov/articlerender.fcgi?tool=pubmed&pubmedid=15339339.

[31] Negri G, Vittadello F, Romano F, Kasal A, Rivasi F, Girlando S, Mian C, Egarter-Vigl E. P16^{INK4a} expression and progression risk of low-grade intraepithelial neoplasia of the cervix uteri. *Virchovs Arch* 2004; 445: 616-620.

[32] Wang J-L, Zheng B-Y, Li X-D, Angstrom MS, Wallin K-L. Predictive significance of the alteration of p16^{INK4a}, p14^{ARF}, p53 and proliferating cell nuclear antigen expression in the progression of cervical cancer. *Clin Cancer Res* 2004; 10: 2407-2414.

[33] Qiao X, Bhuiya TA, Spitzer M. Differentiating high-grade cervical intraepithelial lesion from atrophy in postmenopausal women using Ki67, cyclin E, and p16 immunohistochemical analysis. *J Lower Genital Tract Disease* 2005; 9: 100-107.

[34] Murphy N, Ring M, Heffron CCBB, King B, Killalea AG, Hughes C, Martin CM, McGuinness E, Sheils O, O'Leary JJ. p16^{INK4a}, CDC6, and MCM5: predictive biomarkers in cervical preinvasive neoplasia and cervical cancer. *J Clin Pathol* 2005; 58: 525-534.

[35] Nieh S, Chen Su-Feng, Chu T-Y, Lai H-C, Fu E. Expression of p16^{INK4a} in Papanicolaou smears containing atypical squamous cells of undetermined significance from the uterine cervix. *Gynecol Oncol* 2003; 91: 201-208.

[36] Murphy N, Ring M, Killalea AG, Uhlmann V, O'Donovan M, Mulcahy F, Turner M, McGuinness E, Griffin M, Martin C, Sheils O, O'Leary JJ. p16^{INK4a} as a marker for cervical dyskaryosis: CIN and cGIN in cervical biopsies and ThinPrep^{TM} smears. *J Clin Pathol* 2003; 56: 56-63.

[37] Trunk MJ, Dallenbach-Hellweg G, Ridder R, Petry U, Ikenberg H, Schneider V, von Knebel Doeberitz M. Morphologic characteristics of p16^{INK4a}-positive cells in cervical cytology samples. *Acta Cytol* 2004; 48: 771-782.

[38] Dallenbach-Hellweg G, Trunk MJ, von Knebel Doeberitz M. Traditional and new molecular methods for early detection of cervical cancer. *Arkh Patol* (the Russian Journal of Pathology) 2004; N5: 35-39.

[39] Nieh S, Chen S-F, Chu T-Y, Lai H-C, Lin Y-S, Fu E, Gau C-H. Is p16^{INK4a} expression more useful than human papillomavirus test to determine the outcome of atypical squamous cells of undetermined significance-categorized Pap smear? A comparative analysis using abnormal cervical smears with follow-up biopsies. *Gynecol Oncol* 2005; 97: 35-40.

[40] Solomon D, Davey D, Kurman R, Moriarty A, O'Connor D, Prey M, Raab S, Sherman M, Wilbur D, Wright T Jr. The 2001 Bethesda System: terminology for reporting results of cervical cytology. *J Am Med Assoc* 2002; 287: 2114-2119.

[41] Kratzke RA, Greatens TM, Rubins JB, Maddaus MA, Niewoehner DE, Niehans GA, Geradts J. *Rb* and $p16^{INK4a}$ expression in resected non-small cell lung tumors. *Cancer Res* 1996; 56: 3415-3420.

[42] Milde-Langosch K, Ocon`E, Loning T. *P16/MTS1* inactivation in owarian carcinomas: high frequency of reduced protein expression associated with hyper-methylation or mutation in endometrioid and mucinous tumors. *Int J Cancer* 1998; 79:`61-65.

[43] Kawhivabara K, Oyama T, Sano T, Fukuda T, Nakajima T. Correlation between methylation status of the *p16/CDKN2* gene and the expression of p16 and Rb proteins in primary non-small cell lung cancers. *Int J Cancer (Pred Oncol)* 1998; 79: 215-220.

[44] Agoff SN, Lin P, Morihara J, Mao C, Kiviat NB, Koutsky LA. $p16^{INK4a}$ expression correlates with degree of cervical neoplasia: a comparison with Ki-67 expression and detection of high-risk HPV types. *Mod Pathol* 2003; 16: 665-673.

[45] Kanao H, Enomoto T, Ueda Y, Fujita M, Nakashima R, Ueno Y, Miyatake T, Yoshizaki T, Buzard GB, Kimura T, Yoshino K, Murata Y. Correlation between $p14^{ARF}$/ $p16^{INK4a}$ expression and HPV infection in uterine cervical cancer.*Cancer Letters* 2004; 213: 31-37.

[46] Wang J-L, Zheng B-Y, Li X-D, Nokelainen K, Angstrom T, Lindstrom MS, Wallin K-L. $p16^{INK4a}$ and $p14^{ARF}$ expression pattern by immunochemistry in human papillomavirus-related cervical neoplasia. *Mod Pathol* 2005; 18: 629-637.

[47] Lambert AP, Anschau F, Schmitt VM. $p16^{INK4a}$ expression in cervical premalignant and malignant lesions. *Exp Mol Pathol* 2005; Oct 27 (Abstract ahead of print).

[48] Lin Z-H, Shen X-H, Jin Z, Kim Y, Lee E, Kim H, Kim I. Human papillomavirus genotyping by oligonucleotide microarray and $p16^{INK4a}$ expression in uterine cervical intraepithelial neoplasm and invasive carcinoma in Korean women. *Pathol Int* 2005; 55: 491-496.

[49] Naeger LK, Goodwin EC, Hwang E-S, DeFikippis, Zhang H, DiMaio D.Bovine papillomavirus E2 protein activates a complex growth-inhibitory program in p53-negative HT-3 cervical carcinoma cells that includes repression of cyclin A and cdc25A phosphatase genes and accumulation of hypophosphorylated retinoblastoma protein.*Cell Growth &Differetiation* 1999; 10: 413-422.

[50] Samoylova EV, Shaikhaiev GO, Petrov SV, Kisseljova NP, Kisseljov FL. HPV infection in cervical-cancer cases in Russia. *Int J Cancer* 1995; 61: 337-341.

[51] Nguyen T.T., Nguyen CT, Gonzales FA, Nichols PW, Yu MC, Jones PA. Analysis of cyclin-dependent kinase inhibitor expression and methylation pattern in human prostate cancers. *Prostate* 2000; 43: 233-242.

[52] Darnell GA, Antalis TM, Rose BR, Suhrbier A. Silencing of integrated human papillomavirus type 18 oncogene transcription in cells expressing serpin B2. *J Virol* 2005; 79: 4246-4256.

[53] Di Vinci A, Perdelli L, Banelli B, Salvi S, Casciano I, Gelvi I, Allemanni G, Margallo E, Gatteschi B, Romani M. $p16^{INK4a}$ promoter methylation and protein expression in breast fibroadenoma and carcinoma. *Int J Cancer* 2004; 114: 414-421.

[54] Nilsson K, Landberg G. Subcellular location, modification and protein complex formation of the cdk-inhibitor p16 in Rb-functional and Rb- inactivated tumor cells. *Int. J. Cancer* 2006; 118: 1120-1125.

[55] Reinstein E, Scheffner M, Oren M, Ciehanover A, Schwartz A. Degradation of the E7 human papillomavirus oncoprotein by the ubiquitin-proteasome system: targeting via ubiquitination of the N-terminal residue.*Oncogene* 2000; 19: 5944-5950.

[56] Kanduc D. Translational regulation of human papillomavirus type 16 E7 mRNA by the peptide SEQIKA, shared by rabbit alpha(1)-globin and human cytokeratin 7. *J Virol* 2002; 76: 7040-7048.

In: New Research on Cervical Cancer
Editor: George Z. Rolland, pp. 149-174
ISBN 1-60021-300-6

Chapter 6

STRUCTURAL AND FUNCTIONAL GENOMICS AS A TOOL FOR THE UNDERSTANDING OF THE MOLECULAR BASIS OF UTERINE CERVICAL CANCER: ONCOGENOMICS

Guelaguetza Vazquez-Ortiz*, Mauricio Salcedo and Patricia Piña-Sanchez
Oncology Genomics Laboratory, Oncology Diseases Research Unit, Oncology Hospital, National Medical Center SigloXXI-IMSS, Mexico City, Mexico

ABSTRACT

Cervical cancer (CC) is the second cause of cancer deaths in women worldwide. High risk human papillomavirus (HPV) infection is the major initiating event in cervical carcinogenesis, of the two most common HPV types (HPV16 and 18), which are present in more than 60-70% of invasive CC. The progressive histopathologic changes that occur during cervical carcinogenesis can be divided in distinctive multiple stages, ranging from low to high grade lesions, which, nevertheless, still do not carry 100% risk of progression, indicating that some additional factors are involved in CC tumorigenesis. In the recent years, the discovery of a number of disease biomarkers, including $p16^{INK4a}$, through immunohistochemical and mRNA studies, has enhanced the diagnostic accuracy of both cervical cytology and histology. More recently, development of high-throughput technologies, such as single nucleotide polymorphism (SNP) analysis, comparative genomic hybridization (CGH) and gene expression profiling using SAGE and cDNA microarrays, has significantly increased the potential for biomarker discovery. Over the past few years our group has used this technology including matrix CGH, SAGE, cDNA

* Correspondence concerning this article should be addressed to: Unidad de Investigación Médica en Enfermedades Oncológicas, Centro Médico Nacional Siglo XXI-IMSS. Av. Cuauhtemoc 330, Col. Doctores. Delegación Cuauhtemoc, Mexico, DF. 06720. Phone: +55 56276900 Ext. 22706. Fax. +55 57610952. E-mail: *guelav@yahoo.com*, maosal89@yahoo.com

expression and tissue microarrays in CC samples at different stages from early to cancer and CC cell lines. Our findings indicate some differences in gene expression between cell lines and tissue samples, regardless of having the same HPV type. Also, genes overexpressed in other cancers are also present in CC. Moreover, some genes encoding proteins related to tumorigenesis are overexpressed in CC, as well as CC cell lines, regardless of the presence or absence of HPV and its particular types. In addition these techniques have facilitated an increased understanding of the pathogenesis for cervical cancer.

Keywords: HPV, cervical cancer, oncgenomics, CGH, microarrays, SAGE

Introduction

Cervical cancer (CC) is the second most common cancer among women worldwide and the first cause of death in Mexican women by neoplasm [1]. In cancer research, as well as in other major areas of modern biology, a revolutionary transition has begun. In general, cancer progression is not a single but a multistep process and includes many genomic structural abnormalities. Among them, genomic gains and losses, particularly deletion of tumour suppressor genes and amplification of oncogenes are associated with cancer progression and its malignant phenotype. Regarding carcinomas of the cervix, infection with HPV is known to play a crucial role in the immortalization of epithelial cells. CC is caused mainly by the infection of a high-risk HPV group of human papillomaviruses (HPVs). This group of HPVs (represented by HPV 16 and 18 types) has been detected in low grade squamous intraepithelial lesion (LSIL), high grade squamous intraepithelial lesion (HSIL) and invasive cancers. After high-risk HPV infection, two viral oncogenic proteins, E6 and E7, play a critical role in inducing cervical cancers by interacting with p53 and pRB, respectively, for the inactivation of these cellular regulatory proteins [2-3].

It has been reported that except for CC, most cancer development frequently results from p53 gene mutation. The p53 mutation is detected in more than 50% of cancer types, but little in cervical cancer cell types. In most CC however, the function of p53 is down-regulated by the E6 protein of HPV 16 whereby E6 binds to p53, resulting in the degradation of E6–p53 complexes through the ubiquitin pathway. The viral E6 protein is also required for the continuous growth of HPV-immortalized cells. In similar way, E7 of HPV is also associated with the inactivation of retinoblastoma tumor suppressor gene product [4].

The persistence of HPV infection in patients that do not develop SIL or CC [5], and the long latency of the transition from high grade SIL to carcinoma suggest that host factors are required for the malignant transformation of epithelial cells [6-7].

This progression or transition also has been shown to be associated with the accumulation of multiple genetic alterations including p16 expression, telomere shortening, telomerase expression, besides the already cited inactivation of p53 and pRb tumor suppressor genes. All these interactions results in the deregulation of important cellular functions, such as tumor suppression, apoptosis, cell cycle control, transcriptional regulation and immune evasion [8].

It is widely known that HPV during first steps of infection is present as a replicative autonomous plasmid, whereas in CC is commonly found as an integrated form. It remains unclear whether HPV integration is a random event; however, it shows a clear predilection for genomic fragile sites, like the MYC locus. In addition, HPV integration causes disruption of the E2 gene and this is followed by an overexpression of the E6 and E7 oncoproteins. E2 protein up-regulates E6/E7 transcription from episomal DNA but represses it in the case of integrated DNA. The activator function of the E2 protein seems to counteract the repressive chromatin structure formed over episomal DNA suggesting that integration could be an irreversible event that initiates genomic instability and cell immortalization [9].

Specifically, the induction of genomic instability by HPV seems to be particularly important for the establishment and development of an invasive tumour, since this increased genomic plasticity would generate cellular clones with enhanced transforming and invasive potential [10].

Structural Genomics in Uterine Cervical Cancer

It is accepted that further genetic events, whether induced by or independent of HPV infection, are required for progression to cervical cancer. In this scenario, HPV E7 and E6 expressing cells allows cell structural alterations such as translocations and deletions. Although cytogenetic studies on CC have identified a number of non-random karyotypic changes involving chromosomes 1, 3, 5 and 17, the search of specific alterations is partially known due to heterogeneity in this tumour. In other words, the conventional cytogenetic analyses have not provided definite clues on genomic alterations in this neoplasia [11-12].

Comparative genomic hybridization (CGH) serves as a screening test for DNA copy-number changes in tumour genomes, to avoid the problem of misidentification of chromosomes and to allow entire tumour genome for gains and losses in a single experiment. This method is based on co-hybridization of differentially labelled genomic tumour DNA and normal DNA to normal metaphase chromosome preparation [13].

In cervical lesions, CGH has been applied to study all the different stages of this tumor; detecting specific patterns of chromosomal imbalances involving loss of 2q33, 3p, 4, 5q, 6q, 11q and 18q, and gain of 1q, 3q, 5p and 8q, that arises at early stages during cervical carcinoma development. These results suggest that the common gain of chromosome 3q is one of the most important genetic alterations that could define the transition from a pre-malignant lesion to an invasive carcinoma [14-15]

In order to obtain a CC chromosomal alterations profile, 334 CC cases from Progenetix database (www.progenetix.com) were analyzed. Progenetix is a public access and repository database where we are actively contributing. This analysis indicate that all chromosomes present genomic alterations, however; it is interesting to observe that the most significant alterations are gains in 1q, 3q, 5p, 6p and 8q, and losses in 2q, 3p, 4 and 6q (Figure 1). Since lack of information about HPV status in the reported cases of the Progenetix database, at present, it is not possible to identify specific chromosomal imbalances related to HPV presence. Recent reports indicate that HPV integration sites are randomly distributed over the whole genome [16], meaning that a specific genomic alteration in CC due to HPV presence could be a rare event.

Some of these imbalances have been already related to specific clinical behaviours, such as losses of chromosome 11p ($P < 0.0001$) and 18q ($P < 0.01$) which were associated with poor prognosis in CC without lymph node metastasis. Little is known about the identity of specific genes that might be the targets of regional chromosomal imbalances [17].

Matrix-based CGH or array CGH widely available in different platforms (UCSF, Agilent, Affymetrix, VYSIS, etc.), overcomes this problem increasing the sensitivity for the detection of DNA copy number changes at specific loci. This is through the use of well defined genomic DNA fragments whose mapping location is known, and are arrayed onto a solid surface thereby achieving a resolution of copy number imbalances up to the single gene level [18-20].

In order to refine the patterns of chromosomal imbalances present in CC, and also to identify specific genes that might be targets of copy number changes at single gene level; we have applied microarray CGH (GENOSENSOR VYSIS) platform and more recently the UCSF platform, (paper in preparation) on different cervical lesions including HSIL, CC, as well as uterine cervix carcinoma derived cell lines. This results identify that the most common DNA gains were located at the Retinol binding proteins 1 and 2 (RBP1-RBP2) (3q21-q22) genes, the sub-telomeric clone of 5ptel C84C11/T3 D5S23 a satellite marker at 5p15.2 and the DAB2 gene (5p13) in 58.8% of the samples. The most common losses were found at the FHIT gene (3p14.2)(see Figure 1) in 47% of the samples, followed by deletions at D8S504 marker (8p23.3), CTDP1- SHGC- 145820 (18qtel), KIT (4q11-q12), D1S427-FAF1 (1p32.3), D9S325 (9qtel), EIF4E (eukaryotic translation initiation factor 4E, 4q24), RB1 (13q14), and DXS7132 (Xq12) present in 5/17 (29.4%) of the samples. It is clear that chromosomal gains are more frequent than losses in cervical cancer. In general, the frequency of genetic alterations in CC augments with increasing degrees of dysplasia, from 19% in LSIL and HSIL to 85% in invasive cancer [21].

Detection of the TERC gene amplification has been recently proposed as a potential marker for the evaluation of cervical carcinoma progression [22]; however, we detected an amplification of this clone in less than 10% of the samples analyzed by CGH arrays. Following this, FISH analyses have detected a higher prevalence of nuclei with a diploid pattern than those with a tetraploid pattern, even in the high-grade lesions. Furthermore, the percentage of nuclei with more than two copies of 3q, including the tetraploid cells ranged between 3.3 to 50% of the HSIL. Dellas et al., used in situ hybridization to analyze the prevalence of 3q amplifications in cervical cancer tissue arrays, detecting low level amplifications in the majority of the studied tumors [23]. These results suggest that these low copy number gains might not be adequately detected by chromosome or even array CGH, due to the contamination with normal cells and/or the presence of a high number of diploid or tetraploid cells in the sample.

RBP1 gene encodes for a carrier protein involved in the transport of retinol (vitamin A alcohol) from the liver storage site to peripheral tissue. Vitamin A is a fat-soluble vitamin necessary for growth, reproduction, differentiation of epithelial tissues, and vision. This gene harbours four exons encoding 24, 59, 33, and 16 amino acid residues, respectively. The second intervening sequence occupies 19 kb of the 21 kb of the gene (NM_002899 Accesion number at http://smd.stanford.edu/cgi-bin/source/sourceResult). This protein is also involved in proliferation and differentiation of epidermal tissues probably interacting with HOX homeotic genes [24]. In this context, we recently identify that some of the HOX genes are up-regulated in CC [25], thus, we hypothesized that at least RBP1 proteins could be related in CC with HOX gene expression.

As previously described, C-MYC proto-oncogene is widely known to be involved in many essential biologic functions like regulation of normal and neoplastic cell kinetics [26] and its overexpression may play a role in the multistep carcinogenesis of many kinds of neoplasias. Very recently, by means of microRNA it has been demonstrated that C-MYC gene could be up-regulated [27], and its overexpression is commonly observed in altered WNT pathway [28]. In addition, it has been extensively demonstrated the importance of the role of C-MYC (overexpression and amplification) in the development of CC.

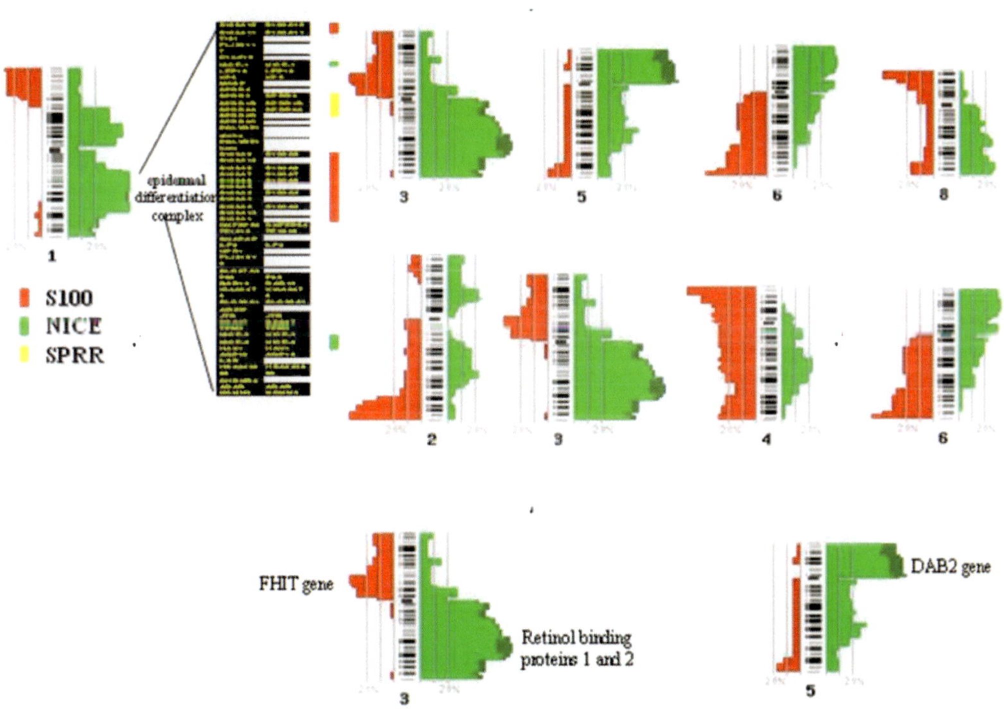

Figure 1. Ideograms showing significant alterations in CC samples by CGH experiments. The figure shows chromosomes 3, 5, 6 and 8 gains (green area) and losses in chromosomes 2, 3, 4 and 6 (red area). The long arm of chromosome 1 is showing the Epidermal Differentiation Complex (EDC), this complex is conformed by S100 genes, NICE and SPRR genes. FHIT gene is located at chromosome 3, which appears to be lost as well as RBP1 and 2. Chromosome 5 shows DAB2 gain.

In CGH studies, it is frequently observed the gain of copy changes in 8q24 (C-MYC gene locus). These findings have been validated by applying Southern blot experiments in CC samples and cDNA microarrays analysis, RNA-RNA in situ hybridization and also immunohistochemistry assays, obtaining the same result about C-MYC alteration. Based on this, we can demonstrate that in this gene, a direct relation between gene amplification and gene overexpression (transcripts and protein) exist (Figure 2). These results support that C-

MYC oncogene is one of the most typical gene alterations involved in cervical carcinogenesis. Meaning that alterations on this gene are associated with: microRNAs [29], gain of copy number, gene upregulation [30], and HPV integration (due to its close integration site to C-MYC locus) [16].

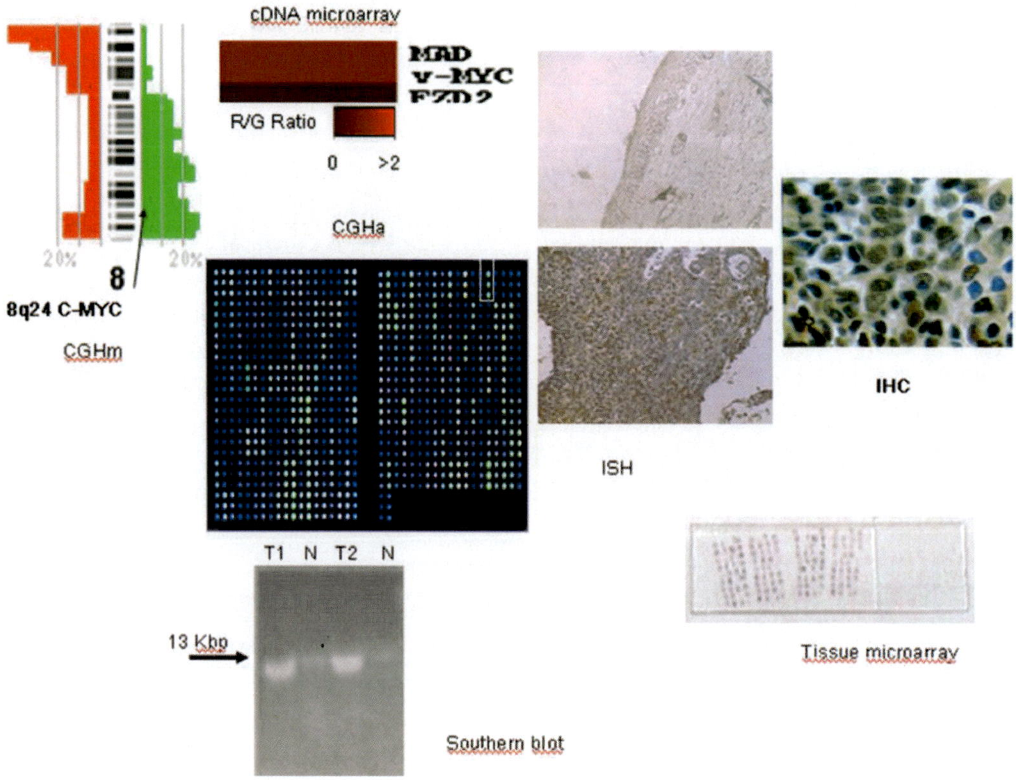

Figure 2. Correlation between genetic alteration of C-MYC and its transcript and protein over-expression.

SINGLE NUCLEOTIDE POLYMORPHISMS IN CERVICAL CANCER

As previously reviewed, infection with high risk HPV is a necessary but not a sufficient cause of CC and it has been assumed that additional factors are involved in the persistence and progression of HPV infection. One of these factors could be the immune response of the host [31-33].

The genetic differences that influence the primary immune response may determine those who are at highest risk for progression to CC. Most research efforts have focused on the association of CC risk with MHC complex, specially class II MHC alleles [34-36] However, in this chapter we will review another genetic polymorphisms recently studied in the literature.

It is a fact that a polygenic disease like cancer is attributable in part to polymorphisms of multiple interacting genes. This phenotypic variation may also reflect environmental variations, as well as gene-by-enviromental interactions that may be complex and unpredictable [37].

Single Nucleotide Polymorphisms (SNPs) are the most common form of polymorphism in the human genome, in the current dbSNP database release, there are more than 10 million. These are highly abundant and can be used as markers; many SNPs also have functional consequences if they occur in the coding or regulatory regions of a gene [38].

Association studies, can detect differences between the SNP patterns of the controls and cases, thereby indicating which pattern is most likely associated with the disease-causing gene. Until now, CC population-based case-control studies have been partial, in the attempt to associate one or a few "candidate genes" with disease.

SNP profiling offers an alternative method of molecular profiling in cancer. To date, a whole genome SNP profile of CC has not been performed. However, through traditional genotyping approaches several SNPs have been associated with increase of cervical cancer. The new Affymetrix 500K mapping array is the first product to utilize the product of the International HapMap Project. This system can assay up to 50,000 SNPs in a single experiment. By using the Affymetrix 100K array, the researchers have demonstrated the power of this technology through significant discoveries in diseases such as cancer. Other commercial platforms for SNPs study are Perlegen Wafers, Molecular inversion probes (ParAllele, Bioscience), Whole Genome Genotyping Bead Array (Illumina).

Despite advances in large scale genotyping technologies, scepticism persist regarding the use of SNP genotyping and genetic association studies. The major concern in SNPs studies is the high rate of false positives. An association between a phenotype and a polymorphism can occurs as a result of randomness in the population and case control which can be increased when many SNPs or phenotypes are tested. This can be overcome by testing a large enough case-control population [39-40].

Bearing this in mind, a number of SNPs have been implicated in cervical cancer, many with conflicting data, and thus should be viewed with caution. A number of these SNPs are reviewed below.

Tumor Necrosis Factor (TNFα) is a potent pro-inflammatory cytokine, which induces cell death of certain tumor cell lines. Under certain conditions it can stimulate cell proliferation and also induce cell differentiation and is the major mediator of inflammation in the mucosa and first barrier against epitheliotropic viruses like HPV [41]. Some SNP in TNFα gene seems to be biologically important, a G to A transition at position -308 of the TNFα gene increase in vitro transcription by 6-9-folds [42]. This SNP is associated to susceptibility for several types of cancer [43]. TNFα -308 low secretor phenotype (GG) is associated with precursor lesions of cervix while compared to women with normal cytology [44]. The transition G to A at position -238 is associated with various diseases, including endometrial carcinoma, but controversial results have been shown in SIL and CC [45]. The TNFα locus also contains a five microsatellite compound by CA/GT dinucleotide repeat, and the number of TNFα repeats correlated with TNFα secretion [46]. In precursor lesions of CC, TNFα-11 alone cannot be considered as a predisposition factor, however when is analyzed with other risk factor like HPV viral type and HLA-DQ6, the risk is 15-folds greater than control women. It is not still clear whether TNFα-11 allele is associated with high or low secretion of the TNFα. These polymorphisms are biologically important and could be associated with a more intense inflammatory activity which plays a role in cancer progression as well as viral infections.

Glutathione S-Transferases (GSTs) are multifunctional phase II enzymes that metabolise and detoxify a broad range of xenobiotics and carcinogens. GSTs conjugate gluthatione to various potentially carcinogenic compounds to form thioethers. This reaction could be the first step in the detoxification process, facilitating the excretion of a variety of carcinogens, reactive oxygen species, and chemotherapeutic agents, with a diversity of substrate specificities [47-49]. Several polymorphisms have been identified (http://www.ncbi.nlm.nih.gov/SNP/) in this gene; in Asian population GSTM1 and GSTT1 deletion genotype have a high frequency [50-51]. However it has been suggested that GSTM1 null allele may result from unequal crossing-over, this and others variants have been investigated as risk factors for the predisposition to different cancers [52-54]. A few studies in CC suggest that GSMT1 and GSTT1 null genotypes were more common among cases than controls, but these were not significantly associated with an increased risk of CC development. However, null genotype is associated to CC after adjustment for smoking and HPV infection. GSTP1 present a polymorphism (GA or GG) in codon 105 in which VAL replaces ILE, this allele display a significantly lower enzyme activity and less effective capability of detoxification [55]. Ma et al., found a significant combined effect of smoking and GSTP1 gene on CC, smokers with GSTP1 AA had a risk of CC 3-folds higher than non-smokers with GSTP1 GG [56].

Interleukin 10 (IL-10) is a T-helper type 2 cytokine which has a suppressive effect on cell-mediated immunity it also inhibits the synthesis of a great number of cytokines, including IFN-gamma, IL2, IL3, TNF and GM-CSF. An increased IL-10 expression was reported in certain tumors, such as non-small cell lung cancer, renal cell, ovarian, colon, and skin cancers. Polymorphism -1082 in its gene promoter correlates with differential amounts of its production [57]. Fifty SNPs have been reported in NCBI database until now for this gene. In CC and SIL an increased secretion of IL-10 has been reported; however its association with polymorphism -1082 is controversial [58], due to population differences and other associated cofactors.

FAS. Is a receptor for TNFSF6/FASL and participate in the apoptosis induction, and it mediates the recruitment of the adapter molecule FADD and caspase-8 to form the death–inducing signalling complex (DISC). This complex activates the proteolytic caspase-8 activity, which initiates the subsequent cascade of caspases mediating apoptosis. SNP -670 of FAS (A/G) gene promoter influences the expression by different transcriptional efficiency of this gene [59]. This SNP has been examined in women affected by CC showing that G allele (low transcription) increased the risk for CC compared with A allele in Japanese and Chinese population, however, in Polish women this association has not been found [60].

Tumor suppressor gene (TP53) is the most studied tumor suppressor gene. Many functions are attributable to p53, like transcriptional activation, DNA repair, regulation angiogenesis, induction growth arrest, apoptosis, senescence and differentiation. This determines a central role for TP53 as a master regulator of tumor suppression [61-62]. NCBI database report 227 polymorphisms in TP53, one of them is located in the codon Arg72Pro, which has been extensively studied (mainly in CC) for cancer susceptibility. Controversial results indicate that TP53Arg72 may represent an important risk factor for HPV associated cancer development [63]. Differences in biochemical and biological activities of these polymorphic proteins have been studied. Storey et al. (1998), shown that the protein harbouring p53Arg72 is more sensitive to degradation by E6/HPV16 and 18, than p53Pro72 [64]. Respect to transcriptional activity p53Pro is a more efficient transcriptional activator than p53Arg72; however, p53Arg72 may induce apoptosis more efficiently than p53Pro72 [65]. On the other hand, in normal population this SNP present differences in geographical distribution (http://www-p53.iarc.fr/p53resources.html). Our preliminary studies are showing that in healthy women the p53Arg72 homozygous is the most frequently SNP found, and could be taken as a risk factor *per se* in Mexican population; however these results must be further studied.

The reasons for discrepancies or poor reproducibility of the results about polymorphism associated to risk for CC could be diverse. First, it is a fact that distribution of SNPs between ethnic human populations is highly diverse and variable, which has been affected by population dynamic, mutations, recombination, and selection. The goal of HapMap project is to identify SNPs, particularly haplotypes between different populations. In this context, a SNP could represent a risk factor in a population or ethnic group, but not in another one, probably due to another risk factors like environmental. Thus, we must know the distribution of polymorphisms and haplotypes between normal populations and disease populations. Second, in contrast to monogenic diseases, cancer diseases are polygenic, meaning that variation in the presence/absence of the disease is attributable, in part, to polymorphism of multiple interacting genes, excepting the inherited cancers as hereditary medullary thyroid carcinoma, multiple endocrine neoplasias, familiar breast and ovarian cancers, Li-Fraumeni syndrome, familial retinoblastoma.

Even when CC is the second common cancer among women worldwide, hall-markers and SNP studies have been limited. This scenario invites to do efforts to identify and characterize the combination of genetic variants relevant in this neoplasm.

High-throughput approaches to identify these genetics variants are required for large-scale genome-wide. Other factors affecting the statistical power in the detection of genetic association of polymorphism and CC should be considered, such as sample size, adequate selection of cases and controls, ethnic diversity, etc. [66-67]. The isolated statistical significance does not guarantee a genetic association, and lack of formal statistical significance does not exclude the possibility of an association [68].

Functional Genomics Sage: A First Review of the Transcriptome Analysis of the Human Normal Cervix

A brief review of the current understanding of the genetic and genomic alterations associated with CC will set the actual state of this neoplasia. One of the most interesting challenges in the molecular and cell biology is to quantify the transcripts present in a cell or in a population of cells in order to determine the cellular transcriptome (expressed genes) in those systems.

It has been mentioned that the identification of a number of genes expressed can provide a theoretical basis for accurately counting the number of expressed genes and the total number of genes in a given cell type. This is for a better understanding of the mechanism(s) which governs the expression of thousands of genes at very low levels.

At present, there are several techniques used to detect transcripts, since almost individual techniques as reverse transcriptase in polymerase chain reaction (RT-PCR), until high-throughput methodologies as cDNA microarrays. However, the most meticulous, systematic and interesting technology for transcriptome analysis is the Serial Analysis of gene expression (SAGE). To date, there are several variants of this strategy such as Long SAGE (L-SAGE), microSAGE, SAGE Adaptation to Downsized Extracts (SADE) [69-70] and very recently miRAGE [71].

In general, as SAGE methodology is not dependent on pre-existing databases of expressed genes, it provides an unbiased view of gene expression profiles within the mRNA populations. SAGE allows the simultaneous quantitative and qualitative analysis of thousands of gene transcripts based on three principles: first, 14mers are sufficient to uniquely identify 95% of cell transcripts; second, cloning of these 14 bp tags serially with the insertion of a restriction enzyme recognition sequence as an anchor, the throughput is considerably increased, and third, the expression level of a transcript is directly proportional to the number of times a specific tag is observed in the final count [72].

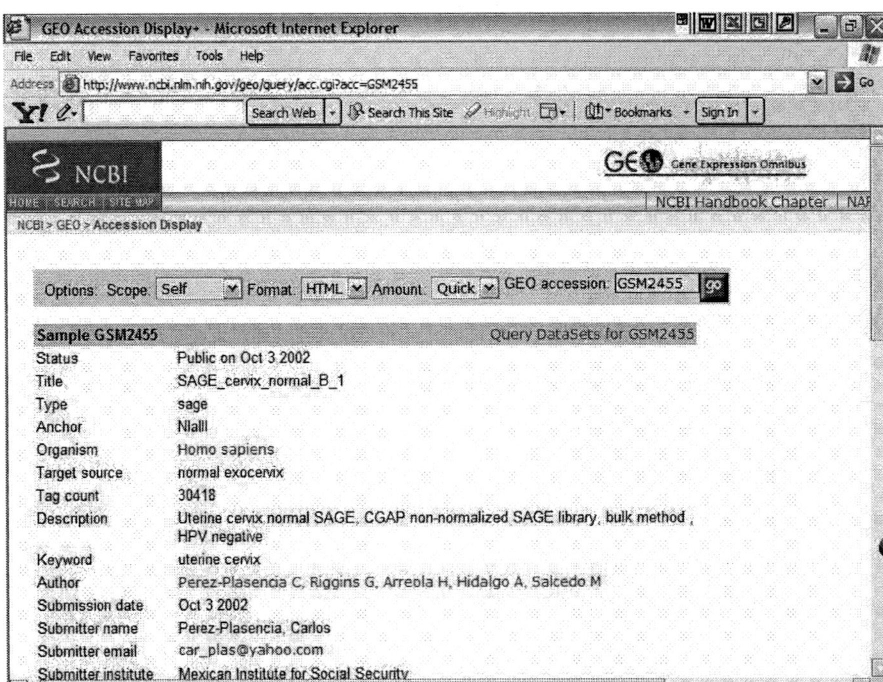

Figure 3. Normal Cervix SAGE Library.

Some advantages of this platform are: 1) the information generated is digital in format; 2) the data obtained can be compared with data generated with other laboratory or with data available in public database, and 3) the information generated is virtually "immortal" which is constantly updated and subjected to reinterpretation. The most important disvantage is that SAGE is not ideally suited for the comparison of multiple samples in a relatively short time. At present, the SAGEmap database consist of over 5 million transcript tags representing more than 100 libraries from different tissues and cell lines [SAGEmap NCBI [http://www.ncbi.nih.gov/SAGE] [73].

In a collaborative effort with the National Cancer Institute's initiative named Cancer Genome Anatomy Project (CGAP; Dr. Gregory Riggins), we obtained the first analysis of global gene expression in primary normal exocervical epithelium followed by a database analysis in order to relate each tag to its corresponding gene (Figure 3). The SAGE-cervix library yielded 30,418 sequenced tags, which were used to generate a table representing those genes expressed in normal human cervix without any infectious disease and providing an estimate of the genes normally expressed by the normal uterine cervix. For a complete list of the expressed genes in this library, please visit the SAGEmap website http://www.ncbi.nlm.nih.gov/SAGE. This catalogue of expressed genes represents the first attempt to generate a comprehensive and profound analysis of the cervical epithelium expression profile. The wealth of information obtained allows detection of genes involved in normal epithelium physiology, as well as possible target genes of HPV infection. In general, tag frequency in a typical SAGE experiment follows a normal distribution, our library followed this kind of distribution [74]. In this context, Kuznetzov et al., reported that all observed large-scale gene expression data sets in yeast, mouse, and human cells follow a Pareto-like distribution model skewed by many low-abundance transcripts [75].

Tags with a frequency of 1 were not considered for quantitative purposes, because these are likely to represent artefacts of sequencing or of the SAGE procedure according previous reports. The most frequently represented tag in the current report had a frequency of 515 (16,930 tags per million TPM). An estimate of such data indicates that this gene tag corresponding to S100A8 gene, has an expression level of ~5,150 copies per cell, similar numbers of tags to what is observed in digital Northern's of other top expressed tags in SAGE libraries [76].

Among the most frequently expressed tags in our library (Table 1), some of them corresponded to ubiquitously expressed transcripts such as GRIN2C, FTH1, GNS, RPLP2, and RPL21. The presence of this type of transcripts is a common result in SAGE experiments with an expected heterogeneity in their expression levels [77], indicating a possible role as novel housekeeping genes. A number of genes related to calcium homeostasis were identified and this set of genes included S100A8, S100A9, and SPRR3, which also belong to a complex of genes that are subject to coordinate regulation during keratinocyte differentiation. Interestingly, the studies in normal pancreas and pancreatic cancers among the first tissues to be studied by shown that the most genes differentially expressed in these kinds of tissues were also the S100A gene [78].

The S100 family share spatial and temporal expression and interrelated functions with other two gene families: cornified envelope precursor proteins (involucrin [SPRRs]) and the intermediate filament associated proteins. All these families belong to a genetic complex named the epidermal differentiation complex (EDC) which is located on the 1q21 chromosome (see Figure 1). It is worth to note that by CGH analysis the chromosome 1q is commonly gained, suggesting that this genomic complex is crucial in the carcinogenesis of the uterine cervix [79]. Approximately 30 genes belonging to the EDC are clustered together in a 200 Mb region, from which there are 20 genes expressed the in cervical SAGE library. These data support the idea of a strong relationship between cervical epithelium and calcium influxes with endocrine glands activity.

Table 1. Top expressed genes in SAGE normal cervical library

TAG sequence	No of Tags	TPM	UniGene ID	Cluster name
TACCTGCAGA	515	16930	Hs.416073	S100A8, S100 calgranulin A
TAGGTTGTCT	356	11703	Hs.374596	TPT1 tumor protein, translationally-controlled 1
TTTCCTGCTC	276	9073	Hs.139322	SPRR3 Small proline-rich protein 3
GAGGGAGTTT	201	6607	Hs.523463	RPL27A ribosomal protein L27a
GTGACCACGG	188	6180	Hs.436980	GRIN2C Glutamate receptor, N-methyl D-aspartate 2C
GTGGCCACGG	184	6049	Hs.112405	S100A9 S100 calcium binding protein A9 (calgranulin B)
GCATAATAGG	168	5523	Hs.381123	RPL21 Ribosomal protein L21
TCAGATCTTT	161	5292	Hs.446628	RPS4X ribosomal protein S4, X-linked
GTTGTGGTTA	155	5095	Hs.99785	Homo sapiens cDNA: FLJ21245 fis, clone COL01184
GGATTTGGCC	151	4964	Hs.437594	RPLP2 Ribosomal protein, large P2
TTGGGGTTTC	143	4701	Hs.448738	FTH1 Ferritin, heavy polypeptide 1
TTGGTCCTCT	138	4536	Hs.381172	RPL41 ribosomal protein L41
TGCACGTTTT	130	4273	Hs.265174	RPL32 ribosomal protein L32
ACAAAGCATT	128	4208	Hs.369982	IGFBP5 insulin-like growth factor binding protein 5
AGGGCTTCCA	122	4010	Hs.401929	OL-64 visceral adipose-specific SERPIN
CCACTGCACT	114	3747	Hs.107003	CCNB1IP1 Cyclin B1 interacting protein 1
GGCAAGCCCC	107	3517	Hs.148340	RPL10A ribosomal protein L10a
CTGGGTTAAT	105	3451	Hs.334534	GNS glucosamine (N-acetyl)-6-sulfatase
TGCACTTCAA	103	3386	Hs.62886	SPARCL1 SPARC-like 1 (mast9, hevin)

aTPM: Tags per million; [(Tag frequency)(1000,000) /Total No of sequenced tags].

In order to obtain better knowledge of the functional categories of global gene expression profile from SAGE cervix data, the Fatigo Data mining website http://fatigo.bioinfo.cnio.es was employed [80].

Figure 4 shows the distribution of expressed genes by functional categories defined by the Gene Ontology Consortium. As seen, the most frequent individual transcripts (more than 60%) correspond to genes involved in maintenance and basic metabolism. On the other hand, genes corresponding to other processes such as cell growth regulation, morphogenesis, cell differentiation, or death were as not frequently expressed as the maintenance ones. In a similar way, the SAGE normal colon, colon cancer, normal breast and breast carcinoma libraries were also analyzed. As expected the results show a quite similar distribution between libraries even when there are normal and cancer tissues. This finding indicates that independently of the cell type and status, most of the cellular processes should have a similar profile maintaining specific gene expression.

The overwhelming information derived from this kind of analysis justifies the effort and provides a better knowledge of cervical biology and physiology. In a near future, it could also provide an insight of cervical physiology or genomic changes during HPV infection and in other pathologies affecting cervical tissue.

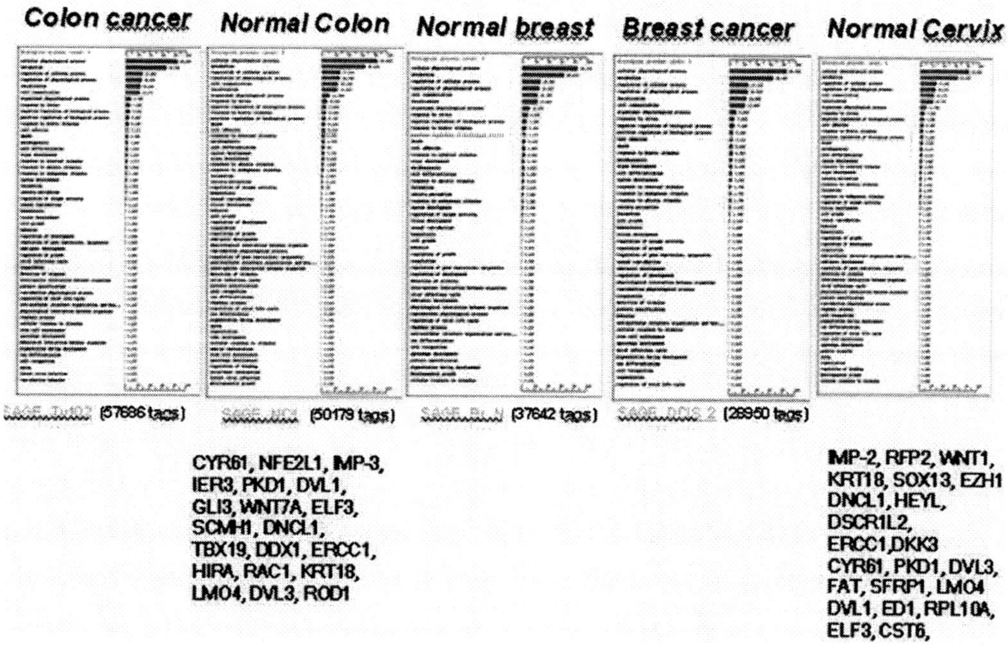

Figure 4. Distribution of expressed genes by functional categories defined by the Gene Ontology Consortium. The analysis of the distribution of normal colon, colon carcinoma, normal breast, breast carcinoma and normal cervix SAGE libraries show similarities.

Gene Expression Profiling in Cervical Cancer

Traditional methods of differential cloning have been employed successfully to isolate unique genes associated with disease. Nevertheless, these techniques have limited use in the study of multifactorial diseases such as CC. As previously mentioned, new high-throughput technologies for gene analysis have the potential to allow an unbiased search for novel unexpected alterations specific to disease stages.

Complementary DNA (cDNA) microarrays, with their ability to determine the expression pattern of thousands of genes simultaneously and to obtain molecular signatures of the state of activity of a cell, are better suited to such studies. It is generally recognized that expression of several genes is coordinated both spatially and temporally and this coordination changes during development and progression of cancer. Analysis of these data set using commercially available software, allows genes to be grouped according to molecular function and biological processes. This facilitates an increased understanding of the pathogenesis of different cancers by identifying potential pathways implicated in disease development. Differentially expressed genes identified comparing normal with malignant cells, in this manner may also represent molecular targets for future drug discovery [81-82].

Initially, microarrays were individually spotted with either oligonucleotides or cDNAs and required reference and test DNA samples that were labelled with different fluorescent dyes. While the fluorescent ratios of the two samples could be compared, absolute mRNA quatitation was difficult. Following this, a number of commercially available, whole genome microarrays were introduced.

These methods were first applied to tissue culture and animal models of HPV transformation and only recently to tissue samples from women with invasive cervical cancer. Now the general interest has begun to focus on identification of specific biomarkers that may help predict outcome or response to treatment, or which may be potential targets for drug discovery in the future (as gene therapy).

The first steps in gene expression profiling for CC study were performed using differential display. By using this technique a novel cDNA fragment named C4.8 was discovered from comparing tumorigenic versus non-tumorigenic HPV16 immortalized keratinoctyes expression [83]. Following the studies about HPV transformation in keratinocytes, it was described that E6 and E7 from HPV16, down-regulates the expression of interferon responsive genes and insulin like growth factor binding protein [84] and also up-regulates those NFkappaB responsive genes [85]. Besides, whole HPV16 genome integration effect was identified; a set of 85 genes mainly IFN responsive genes show changes in their expression levels after HPV16 integration. This expression pattern subsequently matched to another result obtained from HPV33 integration which also overexpress NFkappaB, however, the novel result obtained from this experiment is that MAPK pathway is under-expressed after HPV integration [86].

In one of the largest studies realized in this direction, genes commonly involved in cell proliferation or associated with the extracellular matrix were found to be up-regulated in squamous intraepithelial lesions and cancer [87]. Quantification of the most significant expression changes indicated a progressive increase from LSIL to HSIL to invasive cancer. Also, in a wide expression analysis in women from Hong Kong SPP1 (Osteopontin), CDKN2A (p16), RPL39L, Clorf1, MAL, p11, ARS and NICE-1 were found to be up-regulated [88].

Another more specific study identifies those genes that were over-expressed only in adenocarcinomas and under-regulated in squamous carcinoma. These genes were CEACAM5, TACSTD1, S100P and MSLN. Interestingly, the genes involved in epidermal differentiation complex such as S100A9 and ANXA8 were up-regulated in the squamous type, suggesting that these genes are histotype associated [89]. A different study using microarrays to determine expression patterns of normal exfoliated cervical cells and normal tissue, conclude that the exfoliated ones expression partially represents the expression of the tissue. This means that exfoliated cells are complex enough to provide potential differentiation between disease and normal tissue in order to identify applicable biomarkers [90].

Following the biomarker discovery context, our group has used 8400 unique genes cDNA arrays to examine the expression profiles of six cell lines derived from human cervical cancer, HPV positive tumor samples and normal HPV negative epithelium tissues [91-92]. Hierarchical clustering between normal cells, HPV16 and HPV18 infected cells identified different expression patterns depending of the HPV type present in the sample however; all cells share the same expression in some genes, meaning that these, could represent the minimum cluster of genes that the cell needs to function properly (Figure 5). The Gene Ontology analysis (GO) of the differentially regulated genes in cervical cancer revealed that, most of the genes were assigned to 10 major cellular processes, showing as key functions of various cellular activities involved in cervical cancer development. The GO analysis organizes the regulated genes into three separated ontologies, comprising biological process, cellular component, and molecular function. The GO show a set of well-defined terms and relationships through which the role of a particular gene, gene product or gene-product group in the pathogenesis could be inferred.

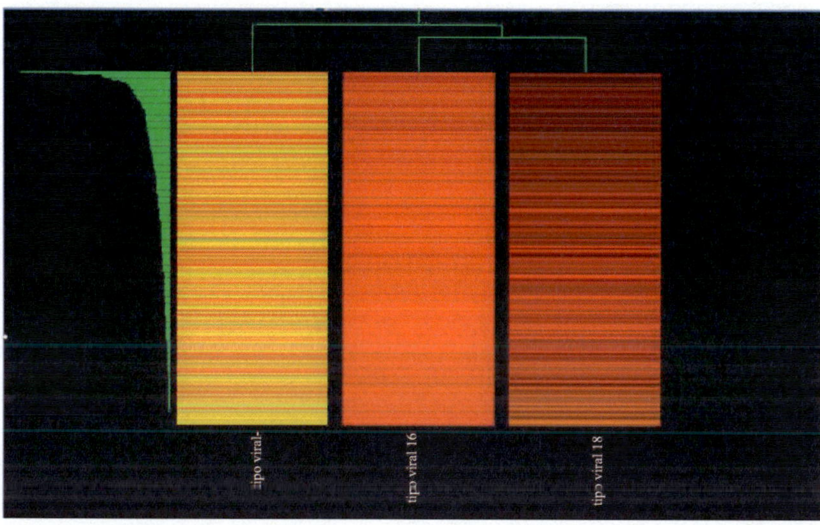

Figure 5. Cluster of normal cervix, HPV16, and HPV18 infected cells. The cluster analysis of normal, HPV16 and HPV18 cells demonstrate that genes (in red) are shared in all samples. Genes represented in yellow are genes that are only expressed in normal cells, while, genes represented by black lines are only present HPV18 cells. This means that each type of sample presents a characteristic pattern of expression that could be determined by the HPV type present.

Genes which are associated with synthesis and cellular metabolism are commonly referred in the differential gene expression analysis in tumor tissues, as compared to normal counterparts. We also observed almost a complete downregulation of genes coding for proteins involved in apoptosis in cervical cancer specimens suggesting a great importance of these gene products for the development of cervical cancer cells. In contrast, the expression of the survivin gene was instead up-regulated which also correlates with previous published results. The consistency in survivin alteration between these studies could be regarded as a validation of the assay [93] (Figure 6). In addition, the expression of some oncogenes such as feline sarcoma (Snyder-Theilen) viral, and GRO3 were also upregulated, suggesting that these gene products not previously described in CC might be involved in its progression (see Figure 6).

It is noteworthy that a proliferative marker, PAI1 presented an increased expression in the studied specimens. This is compatible with the previous finding, that cells expressing PAI1 increased as a function of increasing cervical lesion grade, possibly as a proliferation marker of cervical cancers [94-95]. There are only a few genes that share DNA amplifications and also mRNA overexpression. In previously matrix CGH studies realized by our group PAI1 gene presents an amplification and a markedly overexpression by means of cDNA arrays. A whole protein expression profile both in normal and tumoral cells, evidenced by two dimensional gel electrophoresis and peptide mass fingerprinting analysis surprisingly identified PAI1 protein level up-regulated (paper in preparation) meaning that this gene could be used as a potential molecular marker for the disease at different levels.

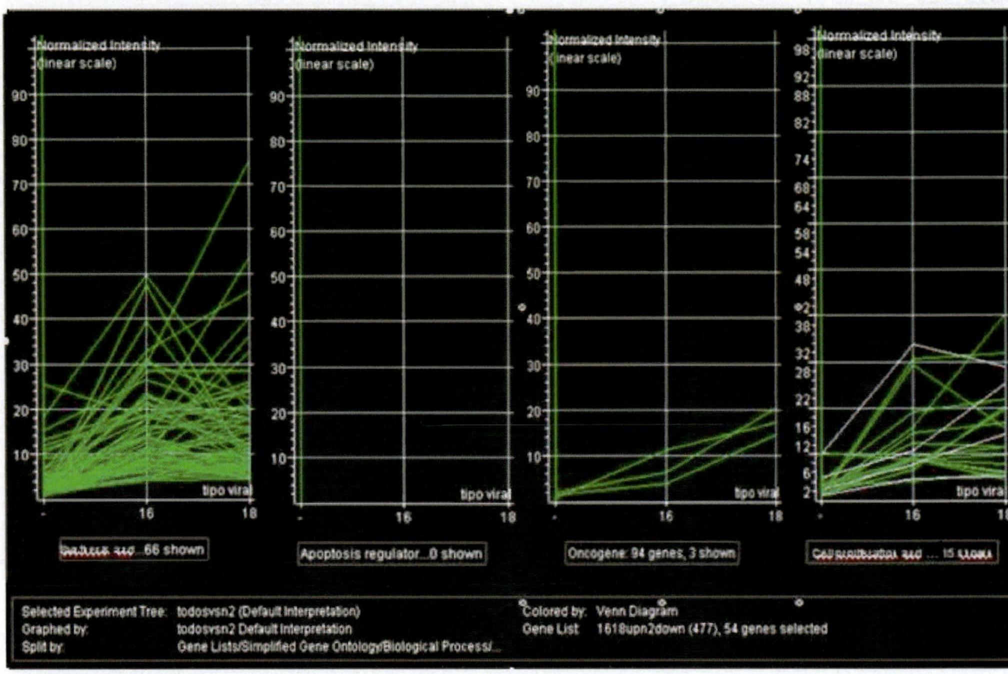

Figure 6. Gene Ontology Analysis of normal, HPV16, and HPV18 infected cells. The X axis shows the type of sample and the Y axis the folds of overexpression, in each studied cluster. The panel of the left demonstrate that genes belonging to "Synthesis and cellular metabolism" cluster, present a clear up-regulation in HPV positive cells ranging from a 6 to 70 fold of over-expression. The apoptosis cluster show that almost all the apoptosis cluster studied genes present a basal expression, while the oncogene cluster only present two transcripts that show a clear significant over-expression. The cell adhesion bunch present overexpression.

Interestingly, the pathway belonging to response to oxidative stress was completely up-regulated. On the other hand, regulation of extracellular matrix expression related genes is a key to tissue remodelling in normal and pathologic processes that lead to tissue carcinogenesis. Interestingly, almost all the genes in this cellular process were highly up-regulated. Among this genes were TIMP1, Integrins alpha 1 and 4, cadherin 2 and 11, Cathepsins F, B L2, MMP 9, 10 11 and 12 (see Figure 6). The transcript and protein overexpression of three of these genes were validated, resulting in a progressive expression through different stages of cervical carcinogenesis [96]. Other differentially regulated genes in cervical cancer belong to the cell growth and maintenance group, however, this group presents less significative difference.

The overexpression of p16^{INK4a} a Cdk inhibitor, has been demonstrated in a number of microarray studies using cervical cytology and histology specimens and also primary culture of cervical cells [97]. These results have been validated by using Real time RT-PCR, flow cytometry and immunohistochemistry. The up-regulation of p16^{INK4a} in cervical lesions is believed to be a consequence of functional inactivation of pRb by high risk HPV E7 protein. The absence of this protein staining in normal cervical epithelium, inflammatory lesions and low grade dysplasias associated with low risk HPV types, means that it may help to identify HSIL and CC in biopsy and cytology specimens, thus reducing false positive and negative results in cancer screening [98]. The degree of staining correlates significantly with the degree of dysplasia, with immunostaining showing a 100% sensitivity and 95% specificity for the detection of HSIL.

Vascular endothelial growth factor (VEGF) is a cytokine that plays a central role in angiogenesis. VEGF protein and mRNA expression have been shown to be increased in HSIL and CC compared to its normal copunterpart, by gene expression profiling, RT-PCR, Immunohistochemistry and *in situ* hybridization assays [99].

In addition to the genes previously described, many thousands of other differentially expressed genes have been identified by microarray analysis. In certain cases, the function of these genes has not been elucidated, whereas in others, their significance in disease pathogenesis remains to be determined. Differentially expressed genes, identified by this technique, may become targets of new drug discovery endeavours, and patterns of expression may aid in the determination of prognosis for individual patients, facilitating individual or personalized treatments.

MicroRNA Profiles in Cancer Cells

MicroRNAs (miRNA) are a recently discovered family of short nonprotein-coding RNAs with diverse functions, including regulation of cellular differentiation, proliferation and apoptosis. To date 629 human miRNA have been identified. These small RNA are highly conserved, approximately 21 mer molecules that regulate expression of genes by binding to the 3' untranslated regions (3'-UTR) of specific mRNAs, repressing their translation and may represent an alternative epigenetic mechanism of gene silencing [100]. Therefore, it is not surprising that studies implicating miRNA in cancer are being published, since cancers ultimately arise from disrupted gene expression. However, the interaction between miRNAs and specific oncogenes and cell cycle regulatory genes is not fully understood [101]. Recently, several miRNAs in HPV infected cells have been identified, thus it is important to identify which miRNA are modified during CC carcinogenesis since HPV infection, and which are the secondary events caused by the infection. Nevertheless, recent discoveries identified viral miRNAs such as in Herpes virus, Polyoma virus and SV40; this new area could generate information about viral miRNAs that could explain some of the mechanisms of the carcinogenesis. The potential implications of miRNA in cancer are enormous, if expression profiling of panels of human miRNAs can be used to correctly classify cancers [71]. In the last 2 years a significant number of publications in this area, however miRNA research is still in its infancy. More work is required to fully understand the role of these small RNAs in the regulation of oncogenic and tumor suppressor pathways, but it is evident its huge potential for therapeutic targeting using silencing technology.

Conclusion

Cervical cancer is the second most common female malignancy worldwide and the first cause of dead by neoplasm in Mexican female population. Unlike many other cancers, CC has a well defined pre-malignant phase that could be detected by cervical cytology screening. The progressive histologic and cytologic changes that occur during the multistep process of cervical carcinogenesis can be divided in several stages as LSIL, HSIL and invasive tumor. The natural history of these cervical precursor lesions is difficult to study because they are usually biopsied or otherwise treated as soon as detected. However, it is clear that HSIL lesions are more likely to regress that to progress to invasive disease. The recognition of the consistent and strong association of HPV infection with development of cervical cancer has identified this virus as the main etiological factor for this type of cancer. However, currently HPV is viewed as a necessary but not sufficient factor for CC development meaning that cell factor are also required for cervical carcinogenesis. To date, molecular profiling techniques have identified a number of biomarkers for cervical cancer and pre-cancer, including some very interesting SNPs in several genes, besides the overexpression of $p16^{INK4a}$, VEGF, TERT in tumor tissues. Although, the cost and complexity of the numerous molecular profiling strategies discussed in this chapter mean that their use in the management of individual patients is likely to be limited; their strength lies in their ability to identify additional biomarkers, which may further facilitate early diagnosis, predict prognosis and treatment response, and may become targets for future drug development. Molecular profiling techniques are likely to aid the rapid identification of novel biomarkers that may be targets for the development of new therapies. In addition, the tissue profiling from cases demonstrating both sensitivity and resistance to chemotherapy and radiotherapy may help delineate genes that can predict an individual tumor response to a given treatment.

Acknowledgements

We want to thank for the support provided from Dr Carles Ciutat (Universidad de Barcelona), Dr. H. Mayani (IMSS), Dr. JA Garcia (KECK, Graduate Institute, CA, USA), Dr. M. Lazos (HGM, SS), Dr. A Mantilla (HO, IMSS), Dr. E. Garrido, (CINVESTAV, IPN), Dra. B. Gonzalez-Yebra (U. de Gto., León Mexico), Dr. C. Pérez and Dra. L. Taja (INCAN, SS), Dr R. Lopez (IIB UNAM), Dr. Michael Baudis (Progenetix), Dr. G. Riggins (Duke University), Dr. M. Jose and Dra. T. Govezensky (IIB, UNAM), Dr. F. Cruz-Talonia (CENACLID, SS), Dr. I. Petersen (Charite Hospital, Berlin, Germany), Dra. DM Hernandez (HO, IMSS), Gynecology Service of the Oncology Hospital CMN, Siglo XXI-IMSS, Oncology Genomics Laboratory, CONACyT (M-34686, Fondos sectoriales 7114), Coordinación de Investigación en Salud and FOFOI-IMSS and Dirección General de Estudios de Posgrado-UNAM.

REFERENCES

[1] Salmeron J, Lazcano-Ponce E, Lorincz A, Hernandez M, Hernandez P, Leyva A, Uribe M, Manzanares H, Antunez A, Carmona E, Ronnett BM, Sherman ME, Bishai D, Ferris D, Flores Y, Yunes E, Shah KV: Comparison of HPV-based assays with Papanicolaou smears for cervical cancer screening in Morelos State, Mexico. *Cancer Causes Control* 2003; 14(6):505-512.

[2] Bosch FX, Durst M, Schwarz E, Boukamp P, Fusenig NE, Zur HH: The early genes E6 and E7 of cancer associated human papilloma viruses as targets of tumor suppression? *Behring Inst Mitt* 1991;(89):108-121.

[3] von Knebel DM, Rittmuller C, Zur HH, Durst M: Inhibition of tumorigenicity of cervical cancer cells in nude mice by HPV E6-E7 anti-sense RNA. *Int J Cancer* 1992; 51(5):831-834.

[4] Zur HH: Papillomaviruses causing cancer: evasion from host-cell control in early events in carcinogenesis. *J Natl Cancer Inst* 2000; 92(9):690-698.

[5] Hildesheim A, Schiffman MH, Gravitt PE, Glass AG, Greer CE, Zhang T, Scott DR, Rush BB, Lawler P, Sherman ME, .: Persistence of type-specific human papillomavirus infection among cytologically normal women. *J Infect* Dis 1994; 169(2):235-240.

[6] Zur HH: Disrupted dichotomous intracellular control of human papillomavirus infection in cancer of the cervix. *Lancet* 1994; 343(8903):955-957.

[7] Heselmeyer K, Schrock E, du MS, Blegen H, Shah K, Steinbeck R, Auer G, Ried T: Gain of chromosome 3q defines the transition from severe dysplasia to invasive carcinoma of the uterine cervix. *Proc Natl Acad Sci U S A* 1996; 93(1):479-484.

[8] Munger K, Howley PM: Human papillomavirus immortalization and transformation functions. *Virus Res* 2002; 89(2):213-228.

[9] Ried T, Heselmeyer-Haddad K, Blegen H, Schrock E, Auer G: Genomic changes defining the genesis, progression, and malignancy potential in solid human tumors: a phenotype/genotype correlation. *Genes Chromosomes Cancer* 1999; 25(3):195-204.

[10] Cahill DP, Kinzler KW, Vogelstein B, Lengauer C: Genetic instability and darwinian selection in tumours. *Trends Cell Biol* 1999; 9(12):M57-M60.

[11] Atkin NB, Baker MC: Small metacentric marker chromosomes in unbanded archival material from carcinomas of the cervix uteri. *Cytobios* 1991; 65(262-263):179-185.

[12] Rao PH, rias-Pulido H, Lu XY, Harris CP, Vargas H, Zhang FF, Narayan G, Schneider A, Terry MB, Murty VV: Chromosomal amplifications, 3q gain and deletions of 2q33-q37 are the frequent genetic changes in cervical carcinoma. *BMC Cancer* 2004; 4:5.

[13] Heselmeyer K, Schrock E, du MS, Blegen H, Shah K, Steinbeck R, Auer G, Ried T: Gain of chromosome 3q defines the transition from severe dysplasia to invasive carcinoma of the uterine cervix. *Proc Natl Acad Sci U S A* 1996; 93(1):479-484.

[14] Heselmeyer K, Schrock E, du MS, Blegen H, Shah K, Steinbeck R, Auer G, Ried T: Gain of chromosome 3q defines the transition from severe dysplasia to invasive carcinoma of the uterine cervix. *Proc Natl Acad Sci U S A* 1996; 93(1):479-484.

[15] Rao PH, rias-Pulido H, Lu XY, Harris CP, Vargas H, Zhang FF, Narayan G, Schneider A, Terry MB, Murty VV: Chromosomal amplifications, 3q gain and deletions of 2q33-q37 are the frequent genetic changes in cervical carcinoma. *BMC Cancer* 2004; 4:5.

[16] Wentzensen N, Vinokurova S, von Knebel DM: Systematic review of genomic integration sites of human papillomavirus genomes in epithelial dysplasia and invasive cancer of the female lower genital tract. *Cancer Res* 2004; 64(11):3878-3884.
[17] Hidalgo A, Schewe C, Petersen S, Salcedo M, Gariglio P, Schluns K, Dietel M, Petersen I: Human papilloma virus status and chromosomal imbalances in primary cervical carcinomas and tumour cell lines. *Eur J Cancer* 2000; 36(4):542-548.
[18] Solinas-Toldo S, Lampel S, Stilgenbauer S, Nickolenko J, Benner A, Dohner H, Cremer T, Lichter P: Matrix-based comparative genomic hybridization: biochips to screen for genomic imbalances. *Genes Chromosomes Cancer* 1997; 20(4):399-407.
[19] Pinkel D, Segraves R, Sudar D, Clark S, Poole I, Kowbel D, Collins C, Kuo WL, Chen C, Zhai Y, Dairkee SH, Ljung BM, Gray JW, Albertson DG: High resolution analysis of DNA copy number variation using comparative genomic hybridization to microarrays. *Nat Genet* 1998; 20(2):207-211.
[20] Pollack JR, Perou CM, Alizadeh AA, Eisen MB, Pergamenschikov A, Williams CF, Jeffrey SS, Botstein D, Brown PO: Genome-wide analysis of DNA copy-number changes using cDNA microarrays. *Nat Genet* 1999; 23(1):41-46.
[21] Hidalgo A, Monroy A, Arana RM, Taja L, Vazquez G, Salcedo M: Chromosomal imbalances in four new uterine cervix carcinoma derived cell lines. *BMC Cancer* 2003; 3:8.
[22] Heselmeyer-Haddad K, Janz V, Castle PE, Chaudhri N, White N, Wilber K, Morrison LE, Auer G, Burroughs FH, Sherman ME, Ried T: Detection of genomic amplification of the human telomerase gene (TERC) in cytologic specimens as a genetic test for the diagnosis of cervical dysplasia. *Am J Pathol* 2003; 163(4):1405-1416.
[23] Dellas A, Torhorst J, Jiang F, Proffitt J, Schultheiss E, Holzgreve W, Sauter G, Mihatsch MJ, Moch H: Prognostic value of genomic alterations in invasive cervical squamous cell carcinoma of clinical stage IB detected by comparative genomic hybridization. *Cancer Res* 1999; 59(14):3475-3479.
[24] Thompson A, Quinn MF, Grimwade D, O'Neill CM, Ahmed MR, Grimes S, McMullin MF, Cotter F, Lappin TR: Global down-regulation of HOX gene expression in PML-RARalpha + acute promyelocytic leukemia identified by small-array real-time PCR. *Blood* 2003; 101(4):1558-1565.
[25] Lopez R, Garrido E, Pina P, Hidalgo A, Lazos M, Ochoa R, Salcedo M: HOXB homeobox gene expression in cervical carcinoma. *Int J Gynecol Cancer* 2006; 16(1):329-335.
[26] Adhikary S, Eilers M: Transcriptional regulation and transformation by Myc proteins. *Nat Rev Mol Cell Biol* 2005; 6(8):635-645.
[27] O'Donnell KA, Wentzel EA, Zeller KI, Dang CV, Mendell JT: c-Myc-regulated microRNAs modulate E2F1 expression. *Nature* 2005; 435(7043):839-843.
[28] Urakami S, Shiina H, Enokida H, Kawakami T, Tokizane T, Ogishima T, Tanaka Y, Li LC, Ribeiro-Filho LA, Terashima M, Kikuno N, Adachi H, Yoneda T, Kishi H, Shigeno K, Konety BR, Igawa M, Dahiya R: Epigenetic inactivation of Wnt inhibitory factor-1 plays an important role in bladder cancer through aberrant canonical Wnt/beta-catenin signaling pathway. *Clin Cancer Res* 2006; 12(2):383-391.

[29] Liu CG, Calin GA, Meloon B, Gamliel N, Sevignani C, Ferracin M, Dumitru CD, Shimizu M, Zupo S, Dono M, Alder H, Bullrich F, Negrini M, Croce CM: An oligonucleotide microchip for genome-wide microRNA profiling in human and mouse tissues. *Proc Natl Acad Sci U S A* 2004; 101(26):9740-9744.

[30] Salcedo M, Taja L, Utrera D, Chavez P, Hidalgo A, Perez C, Benitez L, Castaneda C, Delgado R, Gariglio P: Changes in retinoblastoma gene expression during cervical cancer progression. *Int J Exp Pathol* 2002; 83(6):275-286.

[31] Walboomers JM, Jacobs MV, Manos MM, Bosch FX, Kummer JA, Shah KV, Snijders PJ, Peto J, Meijer CJ, Munoz N: Human papillomavirus is a necessary cause of invasive cervical cancer worldwide. *J Pathol* 1999; 189(1):12-19.

[32] Mayrand MH, Coutlee F, Hankins C, Lapointe N, Forest P, de LM, Roger M: Detection of human papillomavirus type 16 DNA in consecutive genital samples does not always represent persistent infection as determined by molecular variant analysis. *J Clin Microbiol* 2000; 38(9):3388-3393.

[33] Brummer O, Hollwitz B, Bohmer G, Kuhnle H, Petry KU: Human papillomavirus-type persistence patterns predict the clinical outcome of cervical intraepithelial neoplasia. *Gynecol Oncol* 2006.

[34] Maciag PC, Schlecht NF, Souza PS, Franco EL, Villa LL, Petzl-Erler ML: Major histocompatibility complex class II polymorphisms and risk of cervical cancer and human papillomavirus infection in Brazilian women. *Cancer Epidemiol Biomarkers Prev* 2000; 9(11):1183-1191.

[35] Ghaderi M, Nikitina ZL, Wallin K, Wiklund F, Hallmans G, Lenner P, Dillner J, Sanjeevi CB: Tumor necrosis factor A and MHC class I chain related gene A (MIC-A) polymorphisms in Swedish patients with cervical cancer. *Hum Immunol* 2001; 62(10):1153-1158.

[36] Matsumoto K, Yasugi T, Nakagawa S, Okubo M, Hirata R, Maeda H, Yoshikawa H, Taketani Y: Human papillomavirus type 16 E6 variants and HLA class II alleles among Japanese women with cervical cancer. *Int J Cancer* 2003; 106(6):919-922.

[37] Kirk BW, Feinsod M, Favis R, Kliman RM, Barany F: Single nucleotide polymorphism seeking long term association with complex disease. *Nucleic Acids Res* 2002; 30(15):3295-3311.

[38] Gray IC, Campbell DA, Spurr NK: Single nucleotide polymorphisms as tools in human genetics. *Hum Mol Genet* 2000; 9(16):2403-2408.

[39] Stephens M, Sloan JS, Robertson PD, Scheet P, Nickerson DA: Automating sequence-based detection and genotyping of SNPs from diploid samples. *Nat Genet* 2006; 38(3):375-381.

[40] Zehbe I, Tachezy R, Mytilineos J, Voglino G, Mikyskova I, Delius H, Marongiu A, Gissmann L, Wilander E, Tommasino M: Human papillomavirus 16 E6 polymorphisms in cervical lesions from different European populations and their correlation with human leukocyte antigen class II haplotypes. *Int J Cancer* 2001; 94(5):711-716.

[41] Basile JR, Zacny V, Munger K: The cytokines tumor necrosis factor-alpha (TNF-alpha) and TNF-related apoptosis-inducing ligand differentially modulate proliferation and apoptotic pathways in human keratinocytes expressing the human papillomavirus-16 E7 oncoprotein. *J Biol Chem* 2001; 276(25):22522-22528.

[42] Kroeger KM, Carville KS, Abraham LJ: The -308 tumor necrosis factor-alpha promoter polymorphism effects transcription. *Mol Immunol* 1997; 34(5):391-399.

[43] Ho SY, Wang YJ, Chen HL, Chen CH, Chang CJ, Wang PJ, Chen HH, Guo HR: Increased risk of developing hepatocellular carcinoma associated with carriage of the TNF2 allele of the -308 tumor necrosis factor-alpha promoter gene. *Cancer Causes Control* 2004; 15(7):657-663.

[44] Duarte I, Santos A, Sousa H, Catarino R, Pinto D, Matos A, Pereira D, Moutinho J, Canedo P, Machado JC, Medeiros R: G-308A TNF-alpha polymorphism is associated with an increased risk of invasive cervical cancer. *Biochem Biophys Res Commun* 2005; 334(2):588-592.

[45] Ju W, Kang S, Kim JW, Park NH, Song YS, Kang SB, Lee HP: Promoter polymorphism in the matrix metalloproteinase-1 and risk of cervical cancer in Korean women. *Cancer Lett* 2005; 217(2):191-196.

[46] Crouau-Roy B, Briant L, Bouissou C, Stravropoulos C, Pociot F, Cambon-Thomsen A, Clayton J: Tumor necrosis factor microsatellites in four European populations. *Hum Immunol* 1993; 38(3):213-216.

[47] Mannervik B: Novel polymorphisms in the glutathione transferase superfamily. *Pharmacogenetics* 2003; 13(3):127-128.

[48] Mannervik B, Board PG, Hayes JD, Listowsky I, Pearson WR: Nomenclature for mammalian soluble glutathione transferases. *Methods Enzymol* 2005; 401:1-8.

[49] Rebbeck TR: Molecular epidemiology of the human glutathione S-transferase genotypes GSTM1 and GSTT1 in cancer susceptibility. *Cancer Epidemiol Biomarkers Prev* 1997; 6(9):733-743.

[50] Lemos MC, Cabrita FJ, Silva HA, Vivan M, Placido F, Regateiro FJ: Genetic polymorphism of CYP2D6, GSTM1 and NAT2 and susceptibility to haematological neoplasias. *Carcinogenesis* 1999; 20(7):1225-1229.

[51] Schlade-Bartusiak K, Sasiadek M, Kozlowska J: The influence of GSTM1 and GSTT1 genotypes on the induction of sister chromatid exchanges and chromosome aberrations by 1,2:3,4-diepoxybutane. *Mutat Res* 2000; 465(1-2):69-75.

[52] Zhong S, Wyllie AH, Barnes D, Wolf CR, Spurr NK: Relationship between the GSTM1 genetic polymorphism and susceptibility to bladder, breast and colon cancer. *Carcinogenesis* 1993; 14(9):1821-1824.

[53] Anwar WA, bdel-Rahman SZ, el-Zein RA, Mostafa HM, Au WW: Genetic polymorphism of GSTM1, CYP2E1 and CYP2D6 in Egyptian bladder cancer patients. *Carcinogenesis* 1996; 17(9):1923-1929.

[54] Lee E, Huang Y, Zhao B, Seow-Choen F, Balakrishnan A, Chan SH: Genetic polymorphism of conjugating enzymes and cancer risk: GSTM1, GSTT1, NAT1 and NAT2. *J Toxicol Sci* 1998; 23 Suppl 2:140-142.

[55] Teixeira JP, Gaspar J, Silva S, Torres J, Silva SN, Azevedo MC, Neves P, Laffon B, Mendez J, Goncalves C, Mayan O, Farmer PB, Rueff J: Occupational exposure to styrene: modulation of cytogenetic damage and levels of urinary metabolites of styrene by polymorphisms in genes CYP2E1, EPHX1, GSTM1, GSTT1 and GSTP1. *Toxicology* 2004; 195(2-3):231-242.

[56] Ma Q, Lin G, Qin Y, Lu D, Golka K, Geller F, Chen J, Shen J: GSTP1 A1578G (Ile105Val) polymorphism in benzidine-exposed workers: an association with cytological grading of exfoliated urothelial cells. *Pharmacogenetics* 2003; 13(7):409-415.

[57] Turner DM, Williams DM, Sankaran D, Lazarus M, Sinnott PJ, Hutchinson IV: An investigation of polymorphism in the interleukin-10 gene promoter. *Eur J Immunogenet* 1997; 24(1):1-8.

[58] Roh JW, Kim MH, Seo SS, Kim SH, Kim JW, Park NH, Song YS, Park SY, Kang SB, Lee HP: Interleukin-10 promoter polymorphisms and cervical cancer risk in Korean women. *Cancer Lett* 2002; 184(1):57-63.

[59] Huang QR, Morris D, Manolios N: Identification and characterization of polymorphisms in the promoter region of the human Apo-1/Fas (CD95) gene. *Mol Immunol* 1997; 34(8-9):577-582.

[60] Dybikowska A, Sliwinski W, Emerich J, Podhajska AJ: Evaluation of Fas gene promoter polymorphism in cervical cancer patients. *Int J Mol Med* 2004; 14(3):475-478.

[61] Nakamura Y: Isolation of p53-target genes and their functional analysis. *Cancer Sci* 2004; 95(1):7-11.

[62] Zhao R, Gish K, Murphy M, Yin Y, Notterman D, Hoffman WH, Tom E, Mack DH, Levine AJ: Analysis of p53-regulated gene expression patterns using oligonucleotide arrays. *Genes Dev* 2000; 14(8):981-993.

[63] Jee SH, Won SY, Yun JE, Lee JE, Park JS, Ji SS: Polymorphism p53 codon-72 and invasive cervical cancer: a meta-analysis. *Int J Gynaecol Obstet* 2004; 85(3):301-308.

[64] Storey A, Thomas M, Kalita A, Harwood C, Gardiol D, Mantovani F, Breuer J, Leigh IM, Matlashewski G, Banks L: Role of a p53 polymorphism in the development of human papillomavirus-associated cancer. *Nature* 1998; 393(6682):229-234.

[65] Thomas M, Kalita A, Labrecque S, Pim D, Banks L, Matlashewski G: Two polymorphic variants of wild-type p53 differ biochemically and biologically. *Mol Cell Biol* 1999; 19(2):1092-1100.

[66] Gordon D, Finch SJ: Factors affecting statistical power in the detection of genetic association. *J Clin Invest* 2005; 115(6):1408-1418.

[67] Cardon LR, Bell JI: Association study designs for complex diseases. *Nat Rev Genet* 2001; 2(2):91-99.

[68] Ioannidis JP, Ntzani EE, Trikalinos TA, Contopoulos-Ioannidis DG: Replication validity of genetic association studies. *Nat Genet* 2001; 29(3):306-309.

[69] Velculescu VE, Vogelstein B, Kinzler KW: Analysing uncharted transcriptomes with SAGE. *Trends Genet* 2000; 16(10):423-425.

[70] Cheval L, Virlon B, Billon E, Aude JC, Elalouf JM, Doucet A: Large-scale analysis of gene expression: methods and application to the kidney. *J Nephrol* 2002; 15 Suppl 5:S170-S183.

[71] Cummins JM, He Y, Leary RJ, Pagliarini R, Diaz LA, Jr., Sjoblom T, Barad O, Bentwich Z, Szafranska AE, Labourier E, Raymond CK, Roberts BS, Juhl H, Kinzler KW, Vogelstein B, Velculescu VE: The colorectal microRNAome. *Proc Natl Acad Sci USA* 2006; 103(10):3687-3692.

[72] Dinel S, Bolduc C, Belleau P, Boivin A, Yoshioka M, Calvo E, Piedboeuf B, Snyder EE, Labrie F, St-Amand J: Reproducibility, bioinformatic analysis and power of the SAGE method to evaluate changes in transcriptome. *Nucleic Acids Res* 2005; 33(3):e26.

[73] Lash AE, Tolstoshev CM, Wagner L, Schuler GD, Strausberg RL, Riggins GJ, Altschul SF: SAGEmap: a public gene expression resource. *Genome Res* 2000; 10(7):1051-1060.

[74] Ruijter JM, van Kampen AH, Baas F: Statistical evaluation of SAGE libraries: consequences for experimental design. *Physiol Genomics* 2002; 11(2):37-44.

[75] Kuznetsov VA, Knott GD, Bonner RF: General statistics of stochastic process of gene expression in eukaryotic cells. *Genetics* 2002; 161(3):1321-1332.

[76] Perez-Plasencia C, Riggins G, Vazquez-Ortiz G, Moreno J, Arreola H, Hidalgo A, Pina-Sanchez P, Salcedo M: Characterization of the global profile of genes expressed in cervical epithelium by Serial Analysis of Gene Expression (SAGE). *BMC Genomics* 2005; 6:130.

[77] Jansen BJ, van RF, de JG, Zeeuwen PL, Schalkwijk J: Serial analysis of gene expression in differentiated cultures of human epidermal keratinocytes. *J Invest Dermatol* 2001; 116(1):12-22.

[78] Rosty C, Ueki T, Argani P, Jansen M, Yeo CJ, Cameron JL, Hruban RH, Goggins M: Overexpression of S100A4 in pancreatic ductal adenocarcinomas is associated with poor differentiation and DNA hypomethylation. *Am J Pathol* 2002; 160(1):45-50.

[79] Hidalgo A, Baudis M, Petersen I, Arreola H, Pina P, Vazquez-Ortiz G, Hernandez D, Gonzalez J, Lazos M, Lopez R, Perez C, Garcia J, Vazquez K, Alatorre B, Salcedo M: Microarray comparative genomic hybridization detection of chromosomal imbalances in uterine cervix carcinoma. *BMC Cancer* 2005; 5:77.

[80] Al-Shahrour F, az-Uriarte R, Dopazo J: FatiGO: a web tool for finding significant associations of Gene Ontology terms with groups of genes. *Bioinformatics* 2004; 20(4):578-580.

[81] Wooster R: Cancer classification with DNA microarrays is less more? *Trends Genet* 2000; 16(8):327-329.

[82] Kikuchi T, Daigo Y, Katagiri T, Tsunoda T, Okada K, Kakiuchi S, Zembutsu H, Furukawa Y, Kawamura M, Kobayashi K, Imai K, Nakamura Y: Expression profiles of non-small cell lung cancers on cDNA microarrays: identification of genes for prediction of lymph-node metastasis and sensitivity to anti-cancer drugs. *Oncogene* 2003; 22(14):2192-2205.

[83] Nees M, van WE, Bakos E, Schneider A, Durst M: Identification of novel molecular markers which correlate with HPV-induced tumor progression. *Oncogene* 1998; 16(19):2447-2458.

[84] Berger AJ, Baege A, Guillemette T, Deeds J, Meyer R, Disbrow G, Schlegel R, Schlegel R: Insulin-like growth factor-binding protein 3 expression increases during immortalization of cervical keratinocytes by human papillomavirus type 16 E6 and E7 proteins. *Am J Pathol* 2002; 161(2):603-610.

[85] Nees M, Geoghegan JM, Hyman T, Frank S, Miller L, Woodworth CD: Papillomavirus type 16 oncogenes downregulate expression of interferon-responsive genes and upregulate proliferation-associated and NF-kappaB-responsive genes in cervical keratinocytes. *J Virol* 2001; 75(9):4283-4296.

[86] Ruutu M, Peitsaro P, Johansson B, Syrjanen S: Transcriptional profiling of a human papillomavirus 33-positive squamous epithelial cell line which acquired a selective growth advantage after viral integration. *Int J Cancer* 2002; 100(3):318-326.

[87] Chen Y, Miller C, Mosher R, Zhao X, Deeds J, Morrissey M, Bryant B, Yang D, Meyer R, Cronin F, Gostout BS, Smith-McCune K, Schlegel R: Identification of cervical cancer markers by cDNA and tissue microarrays. *Cancer Res* 2003; 63(8):1927-1935.

[88] Wong YF, Cheung TH, Tsao GS, Lo KW, Yim SF, Wang VW, Heung MM, Chan SC, Chan LK, Ho TW, Wong KW, Li C, Guo Y, Chung TK, Smith DI: Genome-wide gene expression profiling of cervical cancer in Hong Kong women by oligonucleotide microarray. *Int J Cancer* 2006; 118(10):2461-2469.

[89] Chao A, Wang TH, Lee YS, Hsueh S, Chao AS, Chang TC, Kung WH, Huang SL, Chao FY, Wei ML, Lai CH: Molecular characterization of adenocarcinoma and squamous carcinoma of the uterine cervix using microarray analysis of gene expression. *Int J Cancer* 2006.

[90] Steinau M, Lee DR, Rajeevan MS, Vernon SD, Ruffin MT, Unger ER: Gene expression profile of cervical tissue compared to exfoliated cells: impact on biomarker discovery. *BMC Genomics* 2005; 6(1):64.

[91] Vazquez-Ortiz G, Ciudad CJ, Pina P, Vazquez K, Hidalgo A, Alatorre B, Garcia JA, Salamanca F, Peralta-Rodriguez R, Rangel A, Salcedo M: Gene identification by cDNA arrays in HPV-positive cervical cancer. *Arch Med Res* 2005; 36(5):448-458.

[92] Vazquez-Ortiz G, Pina-Sanchez P, Hidalgo A, Lazos M, Moreno J, Alvarado I, Cruz F, Hernandez DM, Perez-Plascencia C, Salcedo M: [Global expression analysis in uterine cervical cancer: metabolic pathways and altered genes]. *Rev Invest Clin* 2005; 57(3):434-441.

[93] Borbely AA, Murvai M, Konya J, Beck Z, Gergely L, Li F, Veress G: Effects of human papillomavirus type 16 oncoproteins on survivin gene expression. *J Gen Virol* 2006; 87(Pt 2):287-294.

[94] neri-Navarro A, ias-Lopez G, Oceguera-Villanueva A, Del Toro-Arreola S, Bravo-Cuellar A, Perez-Montfort R, Orbach-Arbouys S: Urokinase-type plasminogen activator and plasminogen activator inhibitors (PAI-1 and PAI-2) in extracts of invasive cervical carcinoma and precursor lesions. *Eur J Cancer* 1998; 34(4):566-569.

[95] Horn LC, Pippig S, Raptis G, Fischer U, Kohler U, Hentschel B, Martin R: Clinical relevance of urokinase-type plasminogen activator and its inhibitor type 1 (PAI-1) in squamous cell carcinoma of the uterine cervix. *Aust N Z J Obstet Gynaecol* 2002; 42(4):383-386.

[96] Vazquez-Ortiz G, Pina-Sanchez P, Vazquez K, Duenas A, Taja L, Mendoza P, Garcia JA, Salcedo M: Overexpression of cathepsin F, matrix metalloproteinases 11 and 12 in cervical cancer. *BMC Cancer* 2005; 5(1):68.

[97] Hudelist G, Czerwenka K, Singer C, Pischinger K, Kubista E, Manavi M: cDNA array analysis of cytobrush-collected normal and malignant cervical epithelial cells: a feasibility study. *Cancer Genet Cytogenet* 2005; 158(1):35-42.

[98] Klaes R, Friedrich T, Spitkovsky D, Ridder R, Rudy W, Petry U, lenbach-Hellweg G, Schmidt D, von Knebel DM: Overexpression of p16(INK4A) as a specific marker for dysplastic and neoplastic epithelial cells of the cervix uteri. *Int J Cancer* 2001; 92(2):276-284.

[99] Kanda K, Ueda M, Futakuchi H, Yamaguchi H, Mori K, Terai Y, Ueki M: Transcriptional expression of the genes implicated in angiogenesis and tumor invasion in cervical carcinomas. *Gynecol Oncol* 2005; 98(3):453-461.

[100] Cullen BR: Derivation and function of small interfering RNAs and microRNAs. *Virus Res* 2004; 102(1):3-9.

[101] Calin GA, Sevignani C, Dumitru CD, Hyslop T, Noch E, Yendamuri S, Shimizu M, Rattan S, Bullrich F, Negrini M, Croce CM: Human microRNA genes are frequently located at fragile sites and genomic regions involved in cancers. *Proc Natl Acad Sci USA* 2004; 101(9):2999-3004.

In: New Research on Cervical Cancer
Editor: George Z. Rolland, pp. 175-188
ISBN 1-60021-300-6

Chapter 7

HISTONE DEACETYLASE INHIBITORS INDUCE GROWTH INHIBITION, CELL CYCLE ARREST AND APOPTOSIS IN HUMAN CERVICAL CANCER CELLS

***Noriyuki Takai*[1,*]*, H. Phillip Koeffler*[2]*, Hisashi Narahara*[1]**
[1]Department of Obstetrics and Gynecology, Oita University Faculty of Medicine, Oita, Japan;
[2]Division of Hematology/Oncology, Cedars-Sinai Medical Center/UCLA School of Medicine, Los Angeles, USA.

ABSTRACT

Objectives: We investigated the effect of a variety of histone deacetylase inhibitors (HDACIs) [suberoyl anilide bishydroxamine, valproic acid, trichostatin A, and sodium butyrate] on three cervical cancer cell lines.
Methods: Cervical cancer cells were treated with various concentrations of HDACIs, and their effects on cell growth, cell cycle, apoptosis, and related measurements were investigated.
Results: The 3-(4,5-dimethylthiazol-2-yl)-2,5-diphenyltetrazolium bromide assays showed that all cervical cancer cell lines were sensitive to the growth inhibitory effects of HDACIs. Cell cycle analysis indicated that their exposure to HDACIs decreased the proportion of cells in the S-phase and increased the proportion in the G0/G1 phases of the cell cycle. Induction of apoptosis was confirmed by annexin V staining of externalized phosphatidylserine and loss of the transmembrane potential of mitochondria. This induction occurred in concert with altered expression of genes related to cell

* Correspondence concerning this article should be addressed to Noriyuki Takai, M.D., Ph.D., Department of Obstetrics and Gynecology, Oita University Faculty of Medicine, 1-1 Idaigaoka, Hasama-machi, Oita 879-5593, Japan. Tel: 81-97-586-5922; Fax: 81-97-549-5087; E-mail: takai@med.oita-u.ac.jp.

growth, malignant phenotype, and apoptosis. Furthermore, HDACIs treatment of these cell lines increased acetylation of H3 and H4 histone tails.
Conclusion: These results raise the possibility that HDACIs may prove particularly effective in the treatment of cervical cancers.

Keywords: cell cycle, apoptosis, acetylation, cervical cancer.

INTRODUCTION

One of the most important mechanisms in chromatin remodeling is the post-translational modification of the N-terminal tails of histones by acetylation, which contributes to a 'histone code' determining the activity of target genes [1]. Transcriptionally silent chromatin is composed of nucleosomes in which the histones have low levels of acetylation on the lysine residues of their amino-terminal tails. Acetylation of histone proteins neutralizes the positive charge on lysine residues and disrupts nucleosome structure, allowing unfolding of the associated DNA with subsequent access by transcription factors, resulting in changes in gene expression.

Acetylation of core nucleosomal histones is regulated by the opposing activities of histone acetyltransferases (HATs) and histone deacetylases (HDACs). HDACs catalyze the removal of acetyl groups on the amino-terminal lysine residues of core nucleosomal histones, and this activity is generally associated with transcriptional repression. Aberrant recruitment of HDAC activity has been associated with the development of certain human cancers [2]. Transcription factors such as Mad-1, BCL-6, and ETO have also been shown to assemble HDAC-dependent transcriptional repressor complexes [3-5].

HDAC inhibitors (HDACIs) such as trichostatin A (TSA) and sodium butyrate (NaB) can inhibit cancer cell growth *in vitro* [6] and *in vivo* [7], revert oncogene-transformed cell morphology [8], induce apoptosis [9], and enhance cell differentiation [10]. Several classes of HDACIs have been identified, including: (a) short-chain fatty acids [e.g., butyrates and valproic acid (VPA)]; (b) organic hydroxamic acids [e.g., TSA and suberoyl anilide bishydroxamine (SAHA)]; (c) cyclic tetrapeptides [e.g., trapoxin]; and (d) benzamides [e.g., MS-275] [11]. The structure of SAHA is related to that of TSA, a natural product isolated from *Streptomyces hygroscopicus* that was initially used as an antifungal antibiotic [11]. Phenylbutyrate has been used as a single agent in the treatment of ß-thalassemia, toxoplasmosis, and malaria.

The inhibition of HDACs by SAHA occurs through a direct interaction with the catalytic site of the enzyme, as shown by X-ray crystallography studies [12]. The result of HDAC inhibition is believed not to have a generalized effect on the genome but rather only effects the transcription of a small subset of the genome. Differential display analysis of transformed lymphoid cell lines revealed that the expression of only 2-5 % of transcribed genes is changed significantly after treatment with TSA [13].

SAHA is a potentially new therapeutic approach to cancer treatment and phase I clinical trials for the treatment of a variety of solid and hematological tumors have been finished [14], and VPA is an established drug in the long-term therapy of epilepsy. Some HDACIs (e.g.

TSA and trapoxin) are of limited therapeutic use because of poor bioavailability in vivo as well as toxic side-effects at high doses. NaB and phenylbutyrate are degraded rapidly after i.v. administration and therefore require high doses exceeding 400 mg/kg/day [15]. Furthermore, these compounds are not specific for HDACs because they also inhibit phosphorylation and methylation of proteins, as well as DNA methylation [16].

We have performed a study designed to define the biologic and therapeutic effects HDACIs in treating cervical cancer. We focused particularly on SAHA and VPA, which are recognized as the least toxic HDACIs. We examined whether these compounds were able to mediate inhibition of cell growth, cell cycle arrest, apoptosis, and expression of genes related to the malignant phenotype in cervical cancer cell lines.

MATERIALS AND METHODS

Cell Lines

The CaSKi, ME-180, and SiHa human cervical cancer cell lines were obtained from the American Type Culture Collection (Manassas, VA). These cells were maintained as monolayers at 37°C in 5% CO_2/air in Dulbecco's Modified Eagle Medium (DMEM) (Gibco, Rockville, MD) containing 10% heat-inactivated fetal bovine serum (FBS) (Omega, Tarzana, CA).

Chemicals

SAHA was obtained from Alexis (Lausen, Switzerland). VPA, TSA, and NaB were obtained from Sigma (St. Louis, MO). The diluent used as a control in the experiments was phosphate-buffered saline (PBS).

MTT Assays

3-(4,5-Dimethylthiazol-2-yl)-2,5-diphenyltetrazolium bromide (MTT; Sigma, St. Louis, MO) was dissolved in PBS (5 mg/mL) and was used to measure cellular proliferation. Cells (1×10^3) were incubated with 100 μL of culture medium for 48 h in 96-well plates, and 10 μL of MTT solution was added. After 4 h of incubation, solubilization solution (50 μL of 20% SDS) was added, and cells were then incubated at 37°C for 16 hrs. In this assay, MTT is cleaved to an orange formazan dye by metabolically active cells. The dye was directly quantified using an enzyme-linked immunoabsorbent assay reader at 540 nm. All experiments were done independently at least three times in triplicate per experimental point.

Cell Cycle Analysis by Flow Cytometry

The cell cycle was analyzed by flow cytometry after 2 days of culturing either with or without HDACIs, as described [17,18]. Cervical cancer cells (5×10^4) were exposed to HDACIs in six-well, flat-bottomed plates for 48 hrs. Total cells, both cells in the suspension and adherent cells, were collected, washed, and suspended in cold PBS. Cells were fixed in chilled 75% methanol and stained with propidium iodine (PI). Analysis was performed immediately after staining using the CELLFit program (Becton Dickinson, San Jose, CA), whereby the S-phase was calculated using an RFit model. All experiments were done independently at least three times in triplicate per experimental point.

Measurement of Apoptosis (*flow-cytometric analysis with the annexin V/PI assay*)

An early step in the process of cell death (apoptosis and necrosis) is the redistribution of phosphatidylserine (PS) from the inner leaflet to the outer leaflet of the plasma membrane due to the loss of membrane asymmetry [19]. The externalized PS can be readily visualized by incubating intact cells with a fluorescent derivative of the protein annexin-V, a phospholipid-binding protein. PI, a fluorochrome, is used to label DNA. Unlike necrotic cells, apoptotic cells do not lose their cell membrane integrity and are thus impermeable for dyes such as PI. Therefore, the combination of annexin-V and PI staining permits the simultaneous quantification of vital, apoptotic, and necrotic cells.

Cells were plated and grown overnight until they reached 80% confluence, and then treated with HDACIs. After 48 hrs, detached cells in the medium were collected, and the remaining adherent cells were harvested by trypsinization. The cells (1×10^5) were washed with PBS and resuspended in 250 μL of binding buffer (annexinV-FITC kit; Becton Dickinson) containing 10 μL of 20 μg/mL PI and 5 μL of annexin V-FITC, which binds to phosphatidylserine translocated to the exterior of the cell membrane early in the apoptosis pathway as well as during necrosis. After incubation for 10 min at room temperature in a light-protected area, the samples were analyzed on a FACSCalibur flow cytometer (Becton Dickinson). FITC and PI emissions were detected in the FL-1 and FL-2 channels, respectively. For each sample, data from 30,000 cells were recorded in list mode on logarithmic scales. Subsequent analysis was done with CellQuest software (Becton Dickinson). We could discriminate intact cells (annexin–/PI–) from apoptotic cells (annexin+/PI–) and necrotic cells (annexin+/PI+) after treatment with HDACIs. All experiments were done independently at least three times in triplicate per experimental point.

Mitochondrial Transmembrane Potential

The electron gradient across the mitochondrial membrane space during normal respiration is called the mitochondrial transmembrane potential (MTP). Disruption of the MTP is one of the earliest intracellular events following the induction of apoptosis. The

MitoCapture Apoptosis Detection Kit (Biovision Research Products, Palo Alto, CA) provides a simple, fluorescent-based method for distinguishing between healthy and apoptotic cells by detecting the changes in MTP.

Cells were prepared for FACS as described above and stained using the Mitocapture Apoptosis Detection kit obtained from Biovision with a fluorescent lipophilic cationic reagent that assesses mitochondrial membrane permeability, according to the manufacturer's recommendation. Briefly, cells were incubated with the MitoCapture reagent at 37 °C in a 5% CO_2 incubator for 15 min. This assay uses an intramitochondrial dye, which forms aggregates in healthy cells, leading to increased 575 fluorescence (PI channel, FL2) and indicating a normal MTP. In apoptotic cells, however, the dye is excluded from the mitochondria, leading to a loss of 575 fluorescence (aggregate) and an increase in 525 fluorescence (FITC channel, FL1) (monomer). Data were converted to density plots using System 2 software. In some experiments, FACS data were confirmed by fluorescent microscopy using a wide band pass filter. Cells with intact mitochondria exhibited focal red cytosolic fluorescence, whereas cells with permeabilized mitochondria exhibited diffuse green cytosolic fluorescence. Cells lacking red fluorescence and having green fluorescence were scored positive. All experiments were done independently at least three times in triplicate per experimental point.

Western Blot Analysis

Cells were washed twice in PBS, suspended in lysis buffer [50 mM Tris (pH 8.0), 150 mM NaCl, 0.1% SDS, 0.5% sodium deoxycholate, 1% NP40, phenylmethylsulfonyl fluoride at 100 µg/mL, aprotinin at 2 µg/mL, pepstatin at 1 µg/mL, and leupeptin at 10 µg/mL], and placed on ice for 30 min. After centrifugation at 15,000 × *g* for 15 min at 4°C, the suspension was collected. Protein concentrations were quantified using the Bio-Rad protein Assay Dye Reagent Concentrate (Bio-Rad Laboratories, Hercules, CA) according to the manufacturer's recommendation. Whole cell lysates (40 µg) were resolved by SDS-PAGE in a 4-15% gel, transferred to a polyvinylidene difluoride membrane (Immobilon; Amersham, Arlington Heights, IL), and probed sequentially with antibodies against acetylated H3 (1:1,000, Upstate, Lake Placid, NY), acetylated H4 (1:1,000, Upstate), $p21^{WAF1}$ (Ab-1, 1:1,000, Oncogene, San Diego, CA), $p27^{KIP1}$ (C-19, 1:1,000, Santa Cruz Biotechnology, Santa Cruz, CA), cyclin A (clone 25, 1:1,000, BD Pharmingen, San Jose, CA), E-cadherin (G-10, 1:1,000, Santa Cruz Biotechnology), bcl-2 (100, 1:1,000, Santa Cruz Biotechnology), and anti-GAPDH mAb (Research Diagnostics, Flanders, NJ). The blots were developed using the enhanced chemiluminescent (ECL) kit (Amersham).

Statistical Analysis

All numerical data were expressed as means ± SD. Significance was determined by conducting a paired Student's *t*-test.

RESULTS

Effects of HDACIs on the Proliferation and Viability of Cervical Cancer Cell Lines in vitro

We examined the antitumor effects of HDACIs on three cervical cancer cell lines *in vitro*, using an MTT assay with an exposure of 2 days to the HDACIs. CaSKi, ME-180, and SiHa cervical cancer cells showed significant sensitivity to HDACIs, as can be seen in Figure 1. The effective dose of the HDACIs that inhibited 50 % growth (ED_{50}) of the cervical cancer cell lines is shown in Table 1 and ranged between 1.0 x 10^{-6} M and 5.1 x 10^{-6} M for SAHA; between 3.2 x 10^{-4} M and 7.8 x 10^{-4} M for VPA; between 2.7 x 10^{-4} M and 9.3 x 10^{-4} M for NaB and between 4.3 x 10^{-8} M and 9.8 x 10^{-8} M for TSA. The CaSKi cells were the most sensitive to the inhibitory effects of HDACIs (CaSKi> ME-180> SiHa) (Table 1).

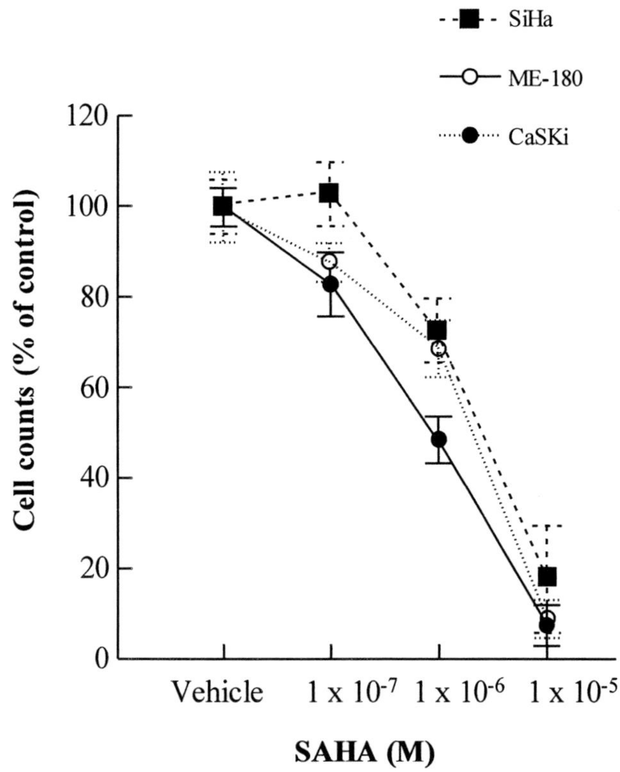

Figure 1. Effect of SAHA on the growth of human cervical cancer cell lines in vitro. CaSKi, ME-180, and SiHa cervical cancer cells were treated with either SAHA at various concentrations (1×10^{-7} - 1×10^{-5} M) or the dilutant (control) for 48 hrs, and growth (% of control) was measured using 3-(4,5-dimethylthiazol-2-yl)-2,5-diphenyltetrazolium bromide assay. Results represent means ± SD of three independent experiments with triplicate dishes.

Table 1. Inhibition of proliferation (ED_{50}) of cervical cancer cell lines by HDACIs

	SAHA	VPA	NaB	TSA
CaSKi cells	1.0×10^{-6} M	3.2×10^{-4} M	2.7×10^{-4} M	4.3×10^{-8} M
ME-180 cells	4.5×10^{-6} M	6.3×10^{-4} M	4.8×10^{-4} M	8.1×10^{-8} M
SiHa cells	5.1×10^{-6} M	7.8×10^{-4} M	9.3×10^{-4} M	9.8×10^{-8} M

The numbers indicate the concentration of HDACIs that induced 50% growth inhibition (ED_{50}) in each cervical cancer cell line. The ED_{50} was determined by plotting the inhibition of growth of the cervical cancer cells in the presence of increasing concentrations of each HDACI [SAHA, 1 x 10^{-7} M to 1 x 10^{-5} M, (see Figure 1); VPA, 1 x 10^{-4} M to 5 x 10^{-3} M; NaB, 1 x 10^{-4} to 5 x 10^{-3} M; TSA, 1 x 10^{-8} to 3 x 10^{-7} M). HDACIs, histone deacetylase inhibitors; SAHA, suberoyl anilide bishydroxamine; VPA, valproic acid; NaB, sodium butyrate; TSA, trichostatin A.

Cell-Cycle Analysis of Cervical Cancer Cells after Exposure to HDACIs

Cervical cancer cells cultured for 2 days in the presence of HDACIs showed an accumulation in the G0/G1 phase of the cell cycle, with a concomitant decrease in the proportion of those in the S phase (Table 2). For example, a total of 40.6 ± 8.1% of the untreated CaSKi cells, compared with 71.4 ± 10.6% of cells cultured with 3×10^{-6} M of SAHA, were in the G0/G1 phase. A total of 31.5 ± 4.5% of the CaSKi untreated cells, compared with 9.1 ± 3.0% of cells cultured with 3×10^{-6} M of SAHA were in the S phase (Fig. 2). This was representative of all the cell lines tested.

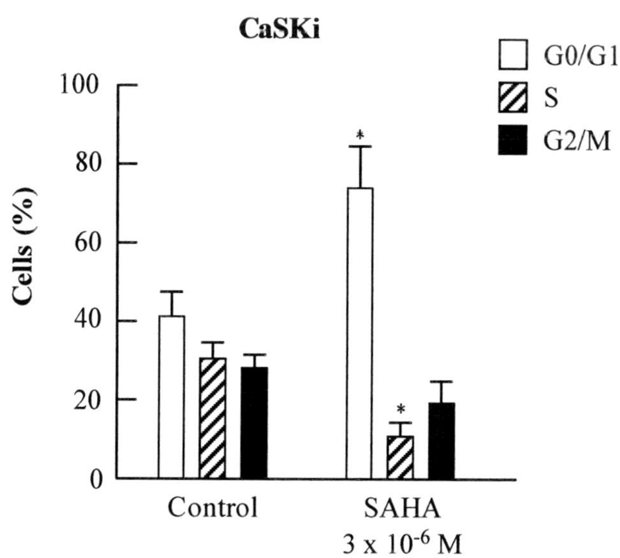

Figure 2. Cell-cycle analysis of CaSKi cells by flow cytometry. CaSKi cells were cultured with SAHA for 48 hrs, harvested, and stained with PI. Control cells were treated with vehicle alone. Cell-cycle analysis was performed by flow cytometry (see Materials and Methods). Results represent means ± SD of three independent experiments. *$p<0.05$ vs. the control group (Student t-test).

Table 2. Cell cycle changes mediated by HDACIs in three cervical cancer cell lines

		Vehicle	SAHA 3×10^{-6} M	VPA 1×10^{-3} M	NaB 1×10^{-3} M	TSA 1×10^{-7} M
	G0/G1 (%)	40.6 ± 8.1	71.4 ± 10.6	65.0 ± 7.8	69.5 ± 12.7	73.5 ± 10.9
CaSKi cells	S (%)	31.5 ± 4.5	9.1 ± 3.0	10.1 ± 2.7	11.0 ± 5.2	8.1 ± 2.8
	G2/M (%)	28.8 ± 3.1	19.5 ± 5.2	25.0 ± 9.2	20.1 ± 9.2	18.5 ± 5.7
	G0/G1 (%)	52.9 ± 11.2	74.0 ± 9.7	69.4 ± 15.7	69.2 ± 7.9	75.4 ± 9.1
ME-180 cells	S (%)	25.4 ± 5.6	11.0 ± 3.7	9.5 ± 7.6	13.9 ± 3.8	9.9 ± 5.2
	G2/M (%)	22.7 ± 6.1	15.1 ± 6.5	21.4 ± 6.9	17.0 ± 5.0	15.0 ± 2.7
	G0/G1 (%)	41.2 ± 7.8	61.5 ± 9.9	55.7 ± 9.7	59.9 ± 11.3	60.4 ± 8.1
SiHa cells	S (%)	35.4 ± 5.7	14.9 ± 5.8	23.8 ± 6.0	21.0 ± 3.8	13.0 ± 6.5
	G2/M (%)	23.4 ± 4.9	24.4 ± 7.1	20.9 ± 3.9	19.8 ± 5.1	26.6 ± 5.7

Cervical cancer cells were plated in triplicate wells and grown in the presence or absence (control) of the HDACIs for 2 days at the indicated concentration and cell cycle distribution was measured. Means ± SD.

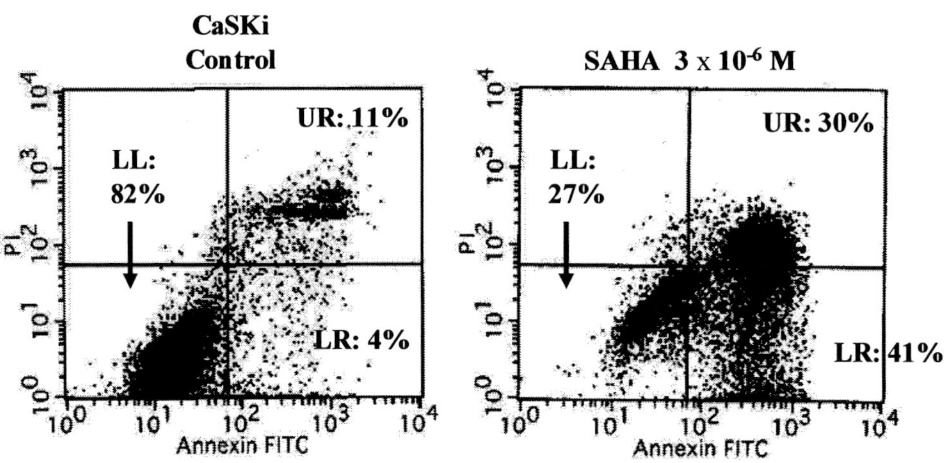

Figure 3. Cell death measured by annexin-V and PI staining detected by flow cytometry. CaSKi cells were treated with 3×10^{-6} M of SAHA for 48 hrs. Cells were then stained with annexin-V and PI. The positive cells were detected by flow cytometry. The viable cells were negative for both annexin-V and PI staining (the lower left quadrant of the cytograms, LL), apoptotic cells were positive for annexin-V staining but negative for PI staining (the lower right quadrant, LR), and necrotic cells were positive for both annexin-V and PI staining (the upper right quadrant, UR). Each experiment was repeated three times. Two typical flow cytometry results are shown. Histograms for untreated (A) and treated cells (B) at 48 hrs are shown.

Apoptotic Changes in HDACIs-Treated Cervical Cancer Cells

To assess the capability of cervical cancer cells to undergo apoptosis in response to drug exposure and to help distinguish between different types of cell death, we double-stained HDACIs-treated cells with annexin V and PI and analyzed the results using flow cytometry. Annexin V binding combined with PI labeling was performed for the distinction of early apoptotic (annexin V+/PI–) and necrotic (annexin V+/PI+) cells. At increasing doses of HDACIs, we also detected a simultaneous increase in both the annexin V+/PI– fraction (early apoptotic) and annexin V+/PI+ (regarded as necrotic) subpopulations (Fig. 3). For example, after incubations with 3 × 10^{-6} M of SAHA for 48 hrs, 41.4 ± 10.9% of CaSKi cells were annexin V+/PI–, and 29.9 ± 9.1% annexin V+/PI+. Untreated CaSKi cells were 3.9% annexin V+/PI–, and about 11% annexin V+/PI+. A typical cyto-diagram obtained by flow cytometry and CellQuest software is shown in Fig. 3, and the results (mean ± SD in triplicate) of all of the cell lines are shown in Table 3.

Table 3. Cell death measured by annexin-V and PI staining detected by flow cytometry in cervical cancer cells

		Vehicle	SAHA 3 × 10^{-6} M	VPA 1 × 10^{-3} M	NaB 1 × 10^{-3} M	TSA 1 × 10^{-7} M
CaSKi cells	Viable (LL) (%)	82.4 ± 11.8	27.3 ± 7.0	19.8 ± 5.5	33.3 ± 9.5	19.7 ± 2.3
	Apoptosis (LR) (%)	3.9 ± 1.1	41.4 ± 10.9	56.0 ± 12.2	46.4 ± 16.0	60.3 ± 15.3
	Necrosis (UR) (%)	11.0 ± 6.7	29.9 ± 9.1	24.2 ± 7.9	20.2 ± 9.1	20.1 ± 5.7
ME-180 cells	Viable (LL) (%)	90.4 ± 14.2	25.0 ± 3.5	23.9 ± 5.7	39.2 ± 11.1	20.7 ± 8.2
	Apoptosis (LR) (%)	5.0 ± 2.1	53.3 ± 14.0	45.0 ± 9.7	38.8 ± 8.7	42.4 ± 7.5
	Necrosis (UR) (%)	4.6 ± 1.0	22.0 ± 9.0	30.7 ± 6.0	22.0 ± 5.4	36.9 ± 5.8
SiHa cells	Viable (LL) (%)	88.2 ± 20.0	20.7 ± 7.6	31.5 ± 5.7	27.4 ± 7.7	19.7 ± 5.2
	Apoptosis (LR) (%)	5.4 ± 4.1	48.2 ± 7.4	49.8 ± 10.1	40.5 ± 12.5	44.2 ± 9.2
	Necrosis (UR) (%)	6.5 ± 5.2	31.1 ± 4.8	18.7 ± 6.7	32.0 ± 11.9	36.1 ± 7.5

For further information, see Figure 3. Each experiment was repeated three times. Means ± SD.

Loss of MTP in Response to HDACIs

Loss of MTP has been shown to occur prior to nuclear condensation and caspase activation and is linked to cytochrome *c* release in many, but not all, apoptotic cells [20,21]. Using MitoCapture staining and flow cytometry, we analyzed the MTP in three cervical cancer cell lines treated with HDACIs. Intracellular fluorescence was assayed by FACS after loading cells with an intramitochondrial dye. High fluorescence at 575 nm (FL2) corresponds to the aggregated form of the dye and is proportional to an intact MTP, whereas loss of MTP leads to a loss of 575 fluorescence and an increase in fluorescence at 525 nm (FL1) (monomeric form of the dye). As seen in Fig. 4, untreated cells exhibit high 575 fluorescence, indicating normal MTP. Treatment of cells with SAHA results in loss of 575 fluorescence and an increase in fluorescence at 525, indicating loss of MTP (Table 4).

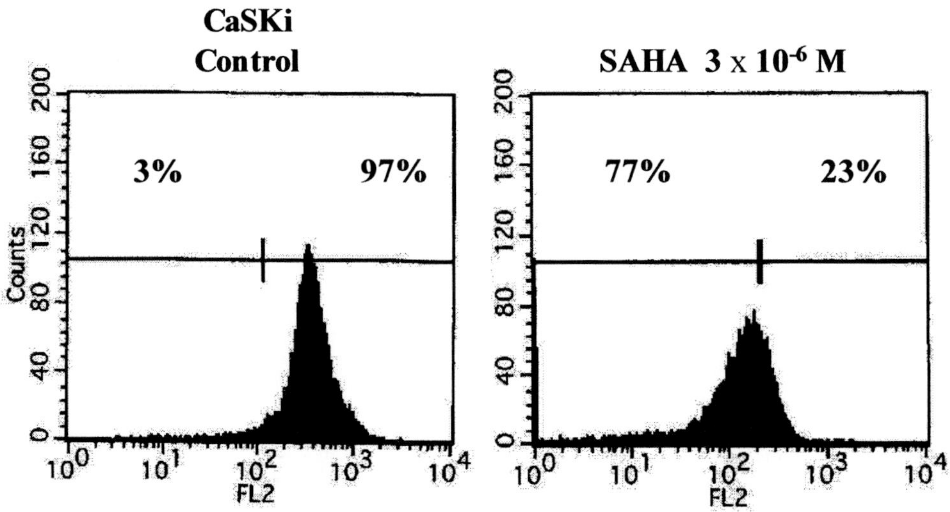

Figure 4. Effect of SAHA treatment on MTP analyzed using the MitoCapture assay. CaSKi cells were treated with SAHA for 48 hrs and harvested for flow cytometry. Each histogram profiles the number of cells relative to their fluorescent intensity. In healthy cells, intramitochondrial dye forms aggregates, leading to increased FL2 fluorescence. In apoptotic cells, the dye is not included in the mitochondria, resulting in a loss of FL2 fluorescence.

Table 4. Apoptotic cells measured by MTP in cervical cancer cells

		Vehicle	SAHA 3×10^{-6} M	VPA 1×10^{-3} M	NaB 1×10^{-3} M	TSA 1×10^{-7} M
CaSKi cells	Viable (%)	97.1 ± 1.1	23.2 ± 2.7	30.4 ± 4.6	31.1 ± 9.1	20.4 ± 3.9
	Apoptosis (%)	2.9 ± 0.5	76.8 ± 5.1	69.6 ± 7.7	68.9 ± 12.5	79.6 ± 9.1
ME-180 cells	Viable (%)	97.0 ± 0.5	26.1 ± 5.1	31.8 ± 5.3	33.3 ± 5.0	23.6 ± 7.8
	Apoptosis (%)	3.0 ± 0.9	73.9 ± 10.2	68.2 ± 8.1	66.7 ± 8.9	76.4 ± 12.5
SiHa cells	Viable (%)	98.2 ± 0.2	30.7 ± 5.7	35.0 ± 2.7	39.2 ± 7.0	24.9 ± 8.0
	Apoptosis (%)	1.8 ± 0.2	69.3 ± 9.9	65.0 ± 7.6	60.8 ± 11.8	75.1 ± 19.1

For further information, see Figure 4. Each experiment was repeated three times. Means ± SD.

Effect of HDACIs on the Acetylation of Histones

Treatment of three cervical cancer cell lines with all HDACIs dramatically increased the levels of acetylated histone H3 and H4. Representative data are shown in Figure 5A.

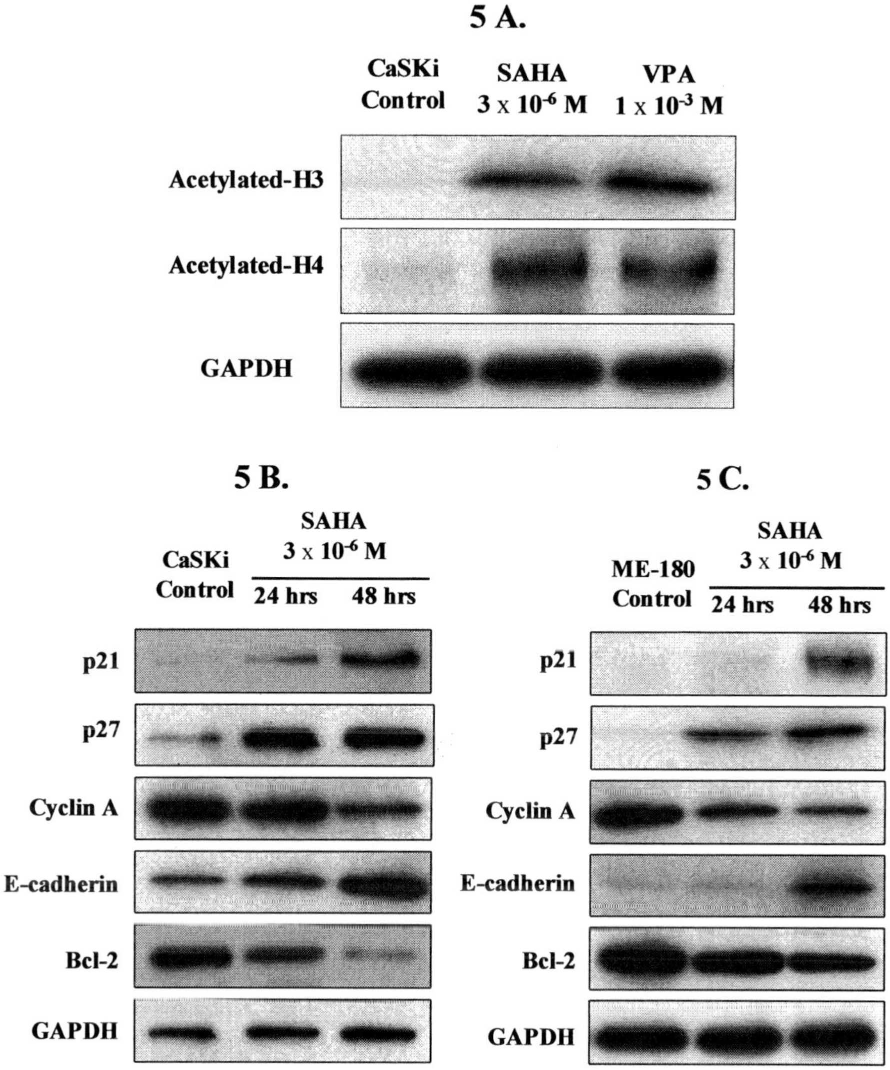

Figure 5. Cell cycle- and apoptosis-related protein expression in CaSKi cells (A, B) and ME-180 cells (C), as measured by Western blot analysis. CaSKi cells and ME-180 cells were treated with 3×10^{-6} M SAHA and 1×10^{-3} M VPA, and cell lysates were harvested after 24 and 48 hrs. Western blot analysis was performed with a series of antibodies. Figure 5A: acetylated histone H3, acetylated histone H4; Figure 5B and 5C: $p21^{WAF1}$, $p27^{KIP1}$, cyclin A, E-cadherin, and bcl-2. Control cells were treated with vehicle alone. The amount of protein was normalized by comparison to GAPDH levels.

Effect of HDACIs on the Expression of Cell-Cycle and Apoptosis-RELATED Proteins as well as E-Cadherin

$p21^{WAF1}$ and $p27^{KIP1}$ are cyclin-dependent kinase inhibitors that bind to cyclin-dependent kinase complexes and decrease kinase activity, and they may act as key regulators of the G0/G1 accumulation (reviewed in [17,18]). We examined the effect of HDACIs on the expression of $p21^{WAF1}$ and $p27^{KIP1}$ in three cervical cancer cell lines by Western blot analysis

(CaSKi treated with SAHA, Fig. 5B; ME-180 treated with SAHA, 5C; other data not shown). HDACIs markedly upregulated the level of $p21^{WAF1}$ and $p27^{KIP1}$ proteins, which were expressed at negligible levels in the three untreated cervical cancer cell lines. Conversely, SAHA (3×10^{-6} M) decreased cyclin A levels by 50% and decreased bcl-2 amounts by 20% in the CaSKi cells (Fig. 5B). SAHA lowered the expression of cyclin A by 25%, and decreased bcl-2 expression by 50% in the ME-180 cells (Fig. 5C).

E-cadherin binds to β-catenin and can act as a tumor suppressor gene; its promoter has CpG islands that are frequently methylated in selected cancers. HDACIs markedly increased the expression level of E-cadherin in three cervical cancer cell lines (Figs. 5B, 5C).

CONCLUSION

Epigenetic mechanisms, such as DNA methylation and histone deacetylation, may play a role in the proliferation of human cancer cells. HDACIs can prevent proliferation and induce differentiation in numerous transformed cell types, including neuroblastomas, erythroleukemia, acute myelogenous leukemia, and carcinomas of the skin, breast, prostate, bladder, lung, colon, endometrium, and ovary [22]. The effect of HDACIs on human cervical cancers, however, has never been fully examined. This stimulated us to examine the effect of HDACIs on cervical cancer cell lines for the first time.

We have demonstrated that HDACIs are highly effective in suppressing the growth of human cervical cancer cells. These events are associated with the accumulation of acetylated H3 and H4 histone proteins. The prominent arrest of cancer cells in the G0/G1 phase of the cell cycle is likely to account for these effects. $p21^{WAF1}$ and $p27^{KIP1}$ are cyclin-dependent kinase inhibitors that have important roles in blocking the cell cycle in the G_1 phase [23]. Protein levels of both $p21^{WAF1}$ and $p27^{KIP1}$ increased following treatment of cervical cancer cells with HDACIs, supporting their contribution as a possible mechanism by which these agents inhibit cervical cancer growth.

Our results show that HDACIs decreases cyclin A levels, and this appears to occur at the transcription level. Therefore, HDACIs cause decreased expression of cyclin A and increased expression of $p21^{WAF1}$, which probably combine to modulate the activity of the downstream pRb/E2F axis, triggering cell cycle arrest [24].

Also, we found that treatment with HDACIs dramatically and significantly increased the number of apoptotic cells in cervical cancer cell lines. This effect was associated with a decrease in the levels of the anti-apoptotic protein bcl-2.

The E-cadherin gene is involved in cell-cell adhesion, and loss of function has been associated with enhanced metastatic growth of tumor cells [25]. Inactivation of this gene by hypermethylation has been observed in breast carcinoma cells and in primary breast tumors [26]. In our opinion transcription of E-cadherin is upregulated in endometrial and ovarian cancer cells treated with HDACIs, suggesting a gain of tumor suppressor function in response to inhibition of histone deacetylase.

In summary, this is the first report showing that HDACIs exhibit antiproliferative activity and potently induces apoptosis in human cervical cancer cells. These events are accompanied by induction of $p21^{WAF1}$and $p27^{KIP1}$ and down-regulation of several anti-apoptosis and cell cycle-related proteins, bcl-2, cyclin A, and E-cadherin. The present findings raise the possibility that HDACIs may prove particularly effective in the treatment of cervical cancers.

ACKNOWLEDGMENTS

The study was supported by a Grant-in-Aid (No. 16790961 to Noriyuki Takai) for Scientific Research from the Ministry of Education, Culture, Sports, Science, and Technology, Japan.

REFERENCES

[1] Strahl BD, Allis CD. The language of covalent histone modifications. *Nature* 2000;403:41–45.
[2] Verdin E, Dequiedt F, Kasler HG. Class II histone deacetylases: versatile regulators. *Trends Genet* 2003;19:286-293.
[3] Laherty CD, Yang WM, Sun JM, Davie JR, Seto E, Eisenman RN. Histone deacetylases associated with the mSin3 corepressor mediate mad transcriptional repression. *Cell* 1997;89:349–356.
[4] Dhordain P, Lin RJ, Quief S, Lantoine D, Kerckaert JP, Evans RM, Albagli O. The LAZ3(BCL-6) oncoprotein recruits a SMRT/mSIN3A/histone deacetylase containing complex to mediate transcriptional repression. *Nucleic Acids Res* 1998;26:4645–4651.
[5] Gelmetti V, Zhang J, Fanelli M, Minucci S, Pelicci PG, Lazar MA. Aberrant recruitment of the nuclear receptor corepressor-histone deacetylase complex by the acute myeloid leukemia fusion partner ETO. *Mol Cell Biol* 1998;18:7185–7191.
[6] Yoshida M, Kijima M, Akita M, Beppu T. Potent and specific inhibition of mammalian histone deacetylase both in vivo and in vitro by trichostatin A. *J Biol Chem* 1990;265:17174–17179.
[7] Yoshida M, Hoshikawa Y, Koseki K, Mori K, Beppu T. Structural specificity for biological activity of trichostatin A, a specific inhibitor of mammalian cell cycle with potent differentiation-inducing activity in Friend leukemia cells. *J Antibiot* 1990;43:1101–1106.
[8] Yoshida M, Horinouchi S, Beppu T. Trichostatin A and trapoxin: novel chemical probes for the role of histone acetylation in chromatin structure and function. *Bioessays* 1995;17:423–430.
[9] Marks PA, Richon VM, Rifkind RA. Histone deacetylase inhibitors: inducers of differentiation or apoptosis of transformed cells. *J Natl Cancer Inst* 2000;92:1210–1216.
[10] Zhou Q, Melkoumian ZK, Lucktong A, Moniwa M, Davie JR, Strobl JS. Rapid induction of histone hyperacetylation and cellular differentiation in human breast tumor cell lines following degradation of histone deacetylase-1. *J Biol Chem* 2000;27:35256–35263.

[11] De Ruijter AJ, van Gennip AH, Caron HN, Kemp S, van Kuilenburg AB. Histone deacetylases (HDACs): characterization of the classical HDAC family. *Biochem J* 2003;370:737-749.

[12] Finnin MS, Donigian JR, Cohen A, Richon VM, Rifkind RA, Marks PA, Breslow R, Pavletich NP. Structures of a histone deacetylase homologue bound to the TSA and SAHA inhibitors. *Nature* 1999;401:188-193.

[13] Van Lint C, Emiliani S, Verdin E. The expression of a small fraction of cellular genes is changed in response to histone hyperacetylation. *Gene Expr* 1996;5:245-253.

[14] O'Connor OA, Heaney ML, Schwartz L, Richardson S, Willin R, MacGregor-Cortelli B, Curly T, Moskowitz C, Portlock C, Horwitz S, Zelenetz AD, Frankel S, Richon VM, Marks P, Kelly WK. Clinical experience with intravenous and oral formulations of the novel histone deacetylase inhibitor suberoylanilide hydroxamic acid in patients with advanced hematologic malignancies. *J Clin Oncol* 2006;24:166-73.

[15] Warrel RP Jr, He LZ, Richon VM, Calleja E, Pandolfi PP. Therapeutic targeting of transcription in acute promyelocytic leukemia by use of an inhibitor of histone deacetylase. *J Natl Cancer Inst* 1998;90:1621-1625.

[16] Newmark HL, Young CW. Butyrate and phenylacetate as differentiating agents: practical problems and opportunities. *J Cell Biochem Suppl* 1995;22:247-253.

[17] Takai N, Desmond JC, Kumagai T, Gui D, Said JW, Whittaker S, Koeffler HP. Histone deacetylase inhibitors have a profound anti-growth activity in endometrial cancer cells. *Clin Cancer Res* 2004;10:1141-1149.

[18] Takai N, Kawamata N, Gui D, Said JW, Miyakawa I, Koeffler HP. Human ovarian carcinoma cells: histone deacetylase inhibitors exhibit antiproliferative activity and potently induce apoptosis. *Cancer* 2004;101:2760-2770.

[19] Rimon G, Bazenet CE, Philpott KL, Rubin LL. Increased surface phosphatidylserine is an early marker of neuronal apoptosis. *J Neurosci Res* 1997;48:563-570.

[20] Chen Y, Kramer DL, Diegelman P, Vujcic S, Porter CW. Apoptotic signaling in polyamine analogue-treated SK-MEL-28 human melanoma cells. *Cancer Res* 2001;61:6437-6444.

[21] Sandberg EM, Sayeski PP. Jak2 tyrosine kinase mediates oxidative stress-induced apoptosis in vascular smooth muscle cells. *J Biol Chem* 2004;279:34547-34552.

[22] Richon VM, Sandhoff TW, Rifkind RA, Marks PA. Histone deacetylase inhibitor selectively induces $p21^{WAF1}$ expression and gene-associated histone acetylation. *Proc Natl Acad Sci USA* 2000;97:10014-10019.

[23] Johnson DG, Walker CL. Cyclins and cell cycle checkpoints. *Ann Rev Pharm Toxicol* 1999;39:295-312.

[24] Freytag SO. Enforced expression of the c-myc oncogene inhibits cell differentiation by precluding entry into a distinct predifferentiation state in G_0/G_1. *Mol Cell Biol* 1988;8:1614-1624.

[25] Takeichi M. Cadherin cell adhesion receptors as a morphogenetic regulator. *Science* 1991;251:1451–1455.

[26] Graff JR, Herman JG, Lapidus RL, Chopra H, Xu R, Jarrard DF, Isaacs WB, Pitha PM, Davidson NE, Baylin SB. E-cadherin expression is silenced by DNA hypermethylation in human breast and prostate carcinomas. *Cancer Res* 1995;55:5195–5199.

In: New Research on Cervical Cancer
Editor: George Z. Rolland, pp. 189-216
ISBN 1-60021-300-6

Chapter 8

CHINESE WOMEN AND CANCER AS CONTAGIOUS: SCREENING IMPLICATIONS

Eleanor Anne Holroyd*
School of Nursing and Midwifery, Royal Melbourne Institute of Technology, Bundoora, Melbourne, Australia

ABSTRACT

This chapter will draw on empirical work conducted in South East Asia that depict a contemporary picture of women's health behaviors, beliefs and attitudes about cervical screening and cancer. Compared with other regions, South Asia has a relatively high rate of cervical cancer, much of this morbidity should be avoidable with cervical screening, but uptake rates remain low. This chapter will be approached from a socio- cultural basis and then aligned to inform the provision of appropriate preventive health strategies.

A particular focus will be on marginalized women, isolated by circumstances of poverty, migration and race; this will include domestic workers and new migrants. The discussion will draw how socio -cultural beliefs pose barriers to medically based health preventative behaviors and the intersection of these themes. Socio-cultural issues of fatalism, embarrassment, modesty, and cancer as a contagion will be elaborated upon. In addition, the structural reality of long working hours, workplace stigmatization, illegal status and financial impoverishment will be examined in respect to how these influence screening attendance patterns. Lay-professional interactions that eclipse negotiating engendered relationships will also provide a lenses from which to interpret women's' perceptions of pain, embarrassment, fertility, associations with promiscuity and other risk factors.

The conclusion will highlight the importance of mainstreaming gender, society and culture into the more traditional and medicals health care education and service provision systems that exist in SE Asia.

Keywords: Chinese, cervical cancer, screening, beliefs.

* Correspondence concerning this article should be addressed to Eleanor Anne Holroyd

INTRODUCTION

Culture prescribes appropriate behavior within a reality that assures individuals a place in their social network, provides a purpose in life, (Kleinman, 1980) and promotes well-being. Thus health beliefs and practices must be understood within the sociocultural contexts in which they have meaning. Within a culture, women share knowledge and beliefs assumed to influence participation in health screening and early detection behaviors (Facione & Katapodi, 2000) suggesting that health care services need to be provided in a structure that is responsive to cultural requirements. A woman's culture and prior socialization experiences will have a direct bearing on how she responds to the meaning of cancer (Mo, 1992).

Health-related behaviors are influenced by culturally associated ideas about the body, family systems, about lay and professional interactions, health information available and the nature of social support (Masi, et al 1993). Health beliefs can influence health behavior in culturally specific ways, which can interfere with a women's ability to utilize services (Van der Stuyft et al, 1989). Asian women, in particular new immigrants, have been documented to under-utilize health-care systems, use popular and folk healthcare sectors and to wait to seek medical help until they have depleted all other sources, reflecting their lack of knowledge of services, paucity of economic resources and a shortage of time (Bernal & Meleis 1995). Issues of class, transition, gender and immigration together with role and identity tensions between host country and those of the country of origin all contribute to the propesntiy to engage in or not to engage in health related behaviours.

An evaluation of cultural and structural barriers to undertaking health-preventative behaviors such as cervical screening needs to be contextualised in terms of history, norms and values which enable certain women to accept or reject one particular approach to health, disease and illness over another (Kleinman 1980). Different cultures experience specific structural constraints to healthcare utilisation which often are overlooked and include a lack of knowledge of service availability and language barriers encountered when attending public health services. Evidence from a number of South East Asian countries suggests that a multifactorial approach needs to be used in order to r increasing screening attendance, including consideration of cultural and socio- economic factors. Yet despite the acknowledgment of these factors in predicting screening patterns, little is known about how these factors promote or hinder screening attendance for Asian women (Straughan & Seow, 1998).

Cultural Influences on South East Asian Women's Health Beliefs and Behaviours

Fot Asian women feelings of invulnerability to reproductive cancer represent a strong contrast to the over-stated vulnerability often expressed in studies of women from other cultural groups (Facione et al., 1997; Rajaram & Rashidi, 1998; Thompson et al., 1997). Studies of recently immigrated Chinese women report an association with the need for preventative health behaviors with white women rather than themselves, and the belief that if women reduced their level of stress and their tendencies to be bad-tempered they could prevent breast cancer (Hoeman et al., 1996).

A related issue reported in a number of studies is that many Chinese believe that talking about health related problems can cause these problems to happen (Facione et al., in press; Kagawa-Singer, 1997; Mo, 1992). Perceived susceptibility to reproductive cancer has been reported to be lower in Chinese-Americans in contrast to Caucasian Americans (Facione et al., 2000; Hoeman et al., 1996; Lu, 1995. Furthermore, culturally defined gender roles for women are of importance, because they dictate the kinds of support, both emotional and finanacial a woman may have available to encourage her to attend for screening (Bilimoria & Morrow, 1995; Kagawa-Singer, 1995; McDonald, Thorne, & Pearson, 1999; Morgan, Park, Cortes, 1995; Rajaram & Rashidi, 1998).

Specific Chinese cultural barriers to screening behaviors include avoidance of social assertiveness and the association of cervical screening procedures with immodesty and sexually inappropriate behaviors (Marin & Marin, 1991; Mo, 1992). Cervical screening is a self-directed activity that requires women to have a strong self-belief in their ability to exercise personal control over life events with fatalism a substantial barrier to Asian women participating in screening tests since they believe that there is very little they can do to change their life destiny (Straughan & Seow, 1998). Mo (1992) has reported a fatalistic view and notions of pre- destination in Chinese-American populations, a finding also reported among Chinese populations residing in the Asian region (Dibble et al., 1997; Hoeman et al., 1996; Lu, 1995; Salazar, 1996; Seow et al., 1995).

In the Philippines health beliefs have been primarily influenced by Malaysian culture and further influenced by Indian, Spanish, Chinese, Mexican and American belief systems. Filipinos associate disease with the life course processes and with both natural and supernatural elements. The key elements of Filipino health practices being that of flushing the body and a balance of heat and cold. These practices serve to protect the boundaries of the body and so offset threats by natural and supernatural forces (McKenzie & Chrisman 1977). Heat and cold regulation of the body plays a large part in Filipino health-related behaviors with heat and massage being commonly used to treat such disorders. For Filipino women there is the belief that exposure to cold brought about by late night showering or evening air can make one susceptible to colds, bronchitis, pneumonia or shivers and have the effect of destroying ones health and beauty (Constable, 1997). Bodily protection involves safeguarding the body from supernatural elements. Maintaining social relationships, mental health, and ensuring personal success are considered supernatural matters in that they are controlled by fatalistic elements with the ability to sleep seen as a sign of mental wellness. Upon immigration, the Filipino folk remedies that endure tend to be those that are cheaper, trusted and considered successful, as well as those that can be used in conjunction with the formal medicinal systems of the host country (McKenzie & Chrisman 1977, National Demographic Health Survey (NDHS,1998).

Immigrant Women Workers in South East Asia

Immigrant domestic helpers are commonly used for household labour in the more developed of the South East Asian nations, working and erratic hours (Feldman, Sapienza, & Kane, 1999) and are comparatively poorly paid. These women tend to be socially stigmatized and marginalized, have limited access to health and social resources with heightened potential for mental health concerns due to isolation and abuse as well as chronic illnesses. They have demanding roles, which include responsibility for the care of children and households while having to accommodate new values, norms and languages. Adding to these strains, many of these women have left behind families and young children in their counties of origin who are financially dependent on their incomes.

In Hong Kong in early 2001 there were 200,000 female domestic helpers. Filipino domestic workers began working in Hong Kong homes during the early 1970s, originally employed by English speaking expatriate families. A minimum wage has existed since 1985 with a legally binding two-year employment contract established between employer and domestic helper. The employment contract stipulates the regulation conditions which include a minimum salary set at $US464/ month, a minimum standard of lodging to be provided or payment towards lodging needed and holiday pay and travel allowance back to the Philippines every two year. In addition, all expenses on food, electricity and health care must either be provided or subsidized. In 1996 a domestic helpers salary was less than half of that of Hong Kong's median salary (being $HK 9500/month in 1996) (Hong Kong General Household Survey, 1996) and does not go far to meet the cost of living. Foreign domestic helpers have made significant contributions to Hong Kong's economy although they have received little recognition for their contribution. Throughout the 1980s and 1990s the number of foreign domestic workers in Hong Kong grew and hostility toward them increased. During this period the English and Chinese newspapers featured antagonistic letters and editorials regarding domestic helpers' use of public spaces on Sundays (Bagely, Madrid and Bolitho, 1997). In addition, to the lowering of the statutory minimum wage, domestic workers were also criticized for not being grateful for the privilege of working in Hong Kong (Constable 1997).

Immigrant domestic workers were found to be less likely than locals to use health care services and were more likely to perceive a poorer health status, even greater than those faced by the uninsured and the poor (Weitzman & Berry, 1992). For Filipino immigrant women dwelling in the US "extreme modesty" associated with undressing and having a stranger touch ones body has been cited as a considerable barrier to accessing reproductive healthcare services (Stern 1985). A survey of 218 Filipino immigrants, aged 50 years older, residing in Los Angeles and found that 48% of women reported receipt of a cervical smear within the past 2 years yet only 14% of women were adherent to the guidelines for regular screening intervals. The study went on to report that Filipino-American associated modesty with reproductive cancer screening (Maxwell, Bastani, Umme and Warda, 2000).

Constable (1997) in a recent ethnographic account of the lives of Filipino domestic workers in Hong Kong contended that unlike Chinese workers in the past, these women were not differentiated from their employers simply by economic class and status but they are also marginalised by their ethnic and national identity and status as temporary workers.

Immigrants tend to occupy a marginal position in a host country by virtue of language, socialisation, education and differences in cultural belief systems. Filipino domestic workers are doubly marginalized by virtue of their gender and social position.

Thus in order to provide adequate and culturally sensitive health care, health policy makers and health providers need to understand the reproductive health-related behaviors and beliefs among specific ethnic groups residing within their society.

Socio-Structural Barriers to Cervical Screening Attendance in South East Asia

Social barriers to Chinese women attending for reproductive cancer screening tend to be associated with income, education, and immigration status rather than solely the result of culturally dictated behaviors and culturally shared beliefs. Poverty is well documented to be a confounding variable in many health seeking behaviors (Facione & Dodd, 1995; Facione & Giancarlo, 1998; Freeman & Wasfie, 1989; Katz et al., 1993; Lauver et al., 1995) whereas education, whether formal or informal, influences the breadth of ideas available to a cultural group (Navon, 1999).

In Hong Kong cervical cancer is the ninth cause of death and the fifth most common cause of new cancer (HK Cancer Registry, 2002). Hong Kong has a moderately high rate of cervical cancer (Adab and Hedley, 1997) with an incidence of 12.7 cases per 100 000 women (Hong Kong Cancer Registrar, 2002), yet a proportion associated morbidity and morality should be preventable through cervical screening (Marcus & Crane, 1998; Adab & Hedley, 1997). In Hong Kong, there is no organized cervical screening programme and surveys indicate uptake rates of 55-60% (FPA, 1999; Adab & McGee, 2001).

The uptake of preventive health behaviours has also been found to be associated with culturally located beliefs about one's age, being married and the expectation of procreativity in both Hong Kong Chinese and US dwelling Chinese citizens (Hoeman et al., 1996; Twinn et al., 1999). Hoeman et al. (1996) reported a lack of social assertiveness in respect to information seeking, particularly in regard to reproductive health matters, to be another cultural barrier to health screening behaviours in Chinese women.

Socio economic influences in cancer incidence and mortality in ethnic populations include poverty, educational level and access to diagnostic and medical treatment facilities. These factors are further influenced by acceptability, attitudes and beliefs about cancer, social stigma, lifestyle differences in personal customs or habits, reproductive habits, and sexual practices in the population (Kagawa-Singer, 1995). The gender of the practitioner has consistently emerged in previous studies of South East Asian women as a factor influencing uptake rates (Fylan, 1998; Johnston et al., 1996; Pritchard et al., 1995; Temple-Smith et al., 1995). Indeed, female practitioners have been noted to reduce embarrassment during the procedure amongst a range of ethnic groups which include Chinese, Indian and Vietnamese women (Naish et al., 1994; Yu & Rymer, 1998, Fylan 1998). In summary the social and organizational barriers to women attending for cervical cancer screening are complex including income and education levels, immigration status, gender role accommodation together with cultural notions of fatalism and social stigma.

Chinese Women and Cervical Screening Beliefs

A recent Hong Kong(HK) based study (Holroyd et al 2001; Twinn et al, 2000) investigated beliefs and barriers to screening attendance from the perspective of women and medical practitioners through a combination of postal questionnaire and focus group interviews. The mean age of the 47 screened focus group attendees was 43.2 years with the range distribution between 26 years and 55 years. A total of 94% of the attendees had been living in HK for the past 7 years and 96 % were married with 46% having two children and 26% having three children. A total of 41% of the women had a monthly household income of below $HK15000 compared to a median monthly household income of HK$17,500 in Hong Kong in 1996 (Census & Statistics Dept 2001). The mean age of the unscreened attendees was 48.7 years (ranging between 36 to 60 years). All the unscreened women were married and their ages ranged from 27-60 years. All but three of these women had more then one child. These high numbers of women who were married with children in both screened and unscreened groups reflect Hong Kong's population distribution of the cohort of women of similar age.

Although some women described screening, as a means of self-protection, frequently screening was not self-initiated instead it was generally prompted by marriage and childbirth. In many Asian cultures the expectation of obedience to a spouse is in conflict with another cultural expectation to remain healthy in order to serve the needs of the family. Women who deal with these conflicting cultural expectations and the anxieties of potential cervical cancer need direct interventions to help them arrive at a personally acceptable solution. This requires a community-based, culturally sensitive care delivery system that partners with women's organization and support agencies.

Several married women reported that they had someone with whom they could share their most intimate concerns, in particular to discuss their health concerns this affirming that culturally expected gender roles dictate the support women have for early cancer detection behavior (Facione & Gaincarlo, 1998; Frank-Stromborg, Wassner, & Nelson, 1998; Kagawa-Singer, 1995; Kagawa-Singer, 1997; Mo, 1992; Salazar, 1996). Of note is that Chinese women have been shown to hide their participation in cancer screening from their male partners or not to seek help for symptoms because their husbands did not want a male doctor to perform such examinations (Mo, 1992). Chinese women have been reported to behave less autonomously about health-related decisions than their counterparts in western countries (Hoeman et al., 1996; Kagawa-Singer, 1995; Kagawa-Singer, 1997; Mo, 1992; Salazar, 1996), who share decisions about their body with their husband and partner. Chinese women tend to use information from family members and friends as well as the information that they receive from the media and the medical community when they make decisions about cancer screening (Baldwin, 1996; Facione el al., 2000; Facione & Giancarlo, 1998; Rajaram & Rashidi, 1998; Skinner et al., 1998; Thompson et al., 1997).

Asian women with young children report to seek cervical screening to stay healthy so that they could continue to be available for their children. Thus frequently for women from South East Asian countries making personal health decisions is influenced by having a confidant to discuss health issues with, being married and having younger children (indicating the presence of emotional support), and having a regular doctor (indicating support form the healthcare system). For Chinese women, when dealing with health conditions that are tied to one's life cycle, the influence of ones family appears to be significant (Straughan and Seow, 1998).

For the women from Holroyd et al's study reported above personal contact with friends or relatives who had experience of cervical or other types of cancer acted as a promoter to attend for screening. Family or peer stories of cancer were cited by several women to influence them to see their doctors for cervical screening. Consequently, the decision about whether to see a doctor for cancer screening may be influenced by others experiences as opposed to self initiation. The following illustration provides an example:

> My friends tell me that regular screening, whether any problems are identified or not, could give the family an account of my health condition. Otherwise, it would be too late when the disease shows up.

The Importance of Female Practitioners

Generally female cervical smear-takers were preferred over males as seen in the following testimony:

> If I choose to go for cervical screening I would definitely go to a female doctor, I currently have a female GP she is very patient and a good listener, it would be easier, less embarrassing, many Hong Kong women prefer female doctors.

In general Asian women prefer a female physician to carry out breast and pelvic examinations and provide advice about attending for future smears (Facione et al, 2000). Having a female perform the examination was explicitly seen by some women to mitigate such concerns as embarrassment and immodesty. Testimony about the embarrassment associated with being examined by a male doctor is found in the following:

> And it's more embarrassing with a male doctor than a female doctor. I will be less afraid to ask a female doctor sensitive questions. I won't dare to ask a male doctor.

Marriage, Promiscuity, and Disharmony as Potential Risks

The Chinese women interviewed in the reported study voiced the risks associated with cervical cancer to include promiscuity, young age of marriage, youth or old age and poor personal hygiene of their husbands or themselves as well as the use of tampons. The most frequently perceived risk was that of having had a promiscuous life. These are exemplified in the following testimony:

Don't be promiscuous, and don't start having sexual intercourse at an early age. If you're healthy, you should be alright. Do not have casual sex. If you are promiscuous you can easily get it from other people.

The women reported that they felt that preventive health behavior should be deferred until a women was 40 years of age or older or until they are married and could at least legitimately request reproductive care. It is of note here that despite the previous claim of needing to wait until marriage that all of women were married and by cultural implications legitimately sexually active yet had not chosen to attend screening. All of the screened women reported attending regularly after marriage reflecting an association of the commencement of cervical screening with marriage. The justification of marriage to participate in screening poses two possible explanations; one which legitimizes requests for reproductive health care as opposed to waiting for symptoms. Secondly, it is possible that the notion of it being socially unacceptable to attend for cervical screening is public rhetoric aimed at women who have been or are sexually active suggesting the importance of "right" and "proper" behavior for Chinese women (Wolf, 1968).

A cultural tendency to wait for symptoms so implying a lack of knowledge of the importance of risk is well exemplified in the following telephone testimony:

But the main reason that I don't go is that I am not sick and I have no time so why go?

Some women went on to report the importance of balance and moderation in their lives as a preventive strategy for cancer. A similar finding is reflected in the international literature that being associated with offsetting illness by methods that maintain balance among the body humors (Mo, 1992). These methods of maintaining balance included food choices, the use of herbs, mental exercises, and the avoidance of stress. Older screened women only used traditional healing methods and sought health services when a cancer illness had not responded to other efforts at symptom management.

Unscreened Chinese women placed a significant reliance on signs and symptoms related to the disease to prompt attendance in comparison to screened women who saw screening attendance behavior as linked to preventive health. Unscreened women appeared to associate attendance for health care with sickness thus delaying attendance, rather than the prevention of disease, which is essential to reduction in morbidity and mortality rates from cervical cancer. Similar cultural and social barriers to screening attendance such as the decision to delay treatment tend to o include lack of symptom appraisal and lack of symptom knowledge; Boffetta & Parkin, 1995; Coates et al., 1992; Facione & Dodd, 1995; Lauver & Chang, 1991), low personal risk estimation (Facione & Giancarlo, 1998; Hiatt et al., 1996;), and misattribution of possible threat (Burgess et al., 1988; Coates et al., 1992; Facione et al., 1997; Mandelblatt et al., 1995).

"I'm so Busy"

Chinese women interviewed identified a range of social factors acting as barriers to attendance such as: working full-time, a lack of childcare, having busy lives, and the associated costs. An understanding of personal interpretation of gender roles and relationships and the influence of past peer or family history posing barriers to attending regularly was linked to these factors. The following testimony provides an illustration of these perceived barriers:

> I can't go to the Health Care clinic. It's so troublesome that I am required to attend the private practice. Besides making an appointment, I need to take a day off in order to go for it, particularly because I'm working during the day. This is troublesome.

And

> My kid's still young. I think if someone can take care of my kid while I go for the Pap smear, I'd feel more relaxed. .... The doctor said why did you bring your son with you. I said there's no one to take care of him so I brought him with me. And the doctor replied, find someone to do it next time.

The cost of the screening procedure was consistently identified as factors influencing women's; attendance patterns by both the screened and unscreened focus groups and well as unscreened women from the telephone interviews. In Hong Kong commonly the charge for cervical screening ranges between $HK100-300 (average income), with one third of women surveyed attending providers (government services) who did not charge. For example;

> I think one should pay for medical services but the charges shouldn't too high.

"Really Embarrassed"

Women described their embarrassment associated with cervical screening. Screened women, however, appeared to manage these feelings and attended regularly for screening whereas embarrassment appeared to contribute to the denial of need amongst unscreened women, a finding also reported in Twinn and Cheng (2000). Notions of embarrassment are well exemplified in the following quote by a screened woman.

> I started going when my son was a few years old. Each time was a big struggle. I was really shy and felt really embarrassed. I felt deprived of any confidence every time I went and the feeling when I came out of the place was very hard to describe.

This testimony suggests the importance of culturally based modesty and reluctance to seek medical consultation regarding non-symptomatic concerns about the body. Chinese women's self – perceived modesty find further links in their emphasis on the importance of a female smear-taker. Physical examination of intimate body parts by a non-family member combined with a sense of modesty about the body in general is barrier for Asian women attending for reproductive screening services (Dibble et al., 1997; Hoeman et al., 1996; Kagawa-singer, 1997; Lu, 1995; Mo B, 1992; Salazar, 1996).

Chinese women's notions of modesty extended to include a concern for maintaining expectations of "correct" female behavior and further reflects the attitudes of her male sexual partner. Chinese values with respect to modesty and sexuality, especially in unmarried women, have been shown to partially account for Chinese women's lack of attention to reproductive health (Mo, 1992). In addition, among traditional Cantonese-Chinese, *ham suup* is used as a derogatory term to denote a person who is overly concerned with talking about her body or who even expresses curiosity or is knowledgeable about the body (Mo, 1992). This concept is well illustrated in the following testimony from an unscreened focus group attendee:

> I find it quite embarrassing for others when I want to talk about my body, having your most private parts exposed, if I am not asked to do it I won't do it.

Similar perceptions relating to embarrassment and modesty are shown in the following:

> I would feel very bad and scared undressing and exposing my most private part to a doctor even more if the doctor was a man.

"It's so painful"

A further barrier influencing re-attendance rates for screened women was cited to be that of previous unpleasant experience associated with the procedure particularly pain and discomfort whether physical or emotional. This is well exemplified in the following testimony from a screened woman:

> During my last smear I felt so much pain, I was shaking all over and very hot. I wanted do to tell him to stop but I could not.

Similarly one unscreened woman reported in the telephone interview:

> I am very scared of the pain, all my friends tell me so, the doctors are sloppy and will not care about the pain, it is your pain.

It is possible that some women might experience pain partly as a somatisation of an emotional reaction to the screening procedure. The author's earlier work (Holroyd, Twinn, Shiu, 2001) in a Hong Kong Chinese population based study of 242 women of which 56.% were screened and 67.4% were unscreened found that 67.4% of women reported pain or the perception of pain to be almost universally associated with the procedure. In addition, many of the women cited an association between embarrassment, pain and the gender of the smear taker, which appeared important cultural and organizational factors influencing levels of shyness and discomfort (Seow et al, 1995, Yu & Rymer, 1998, Larsen & Olesen, 1998, Fylan, 1998; Ward et al., 1993).

Filipino Migrant Domestic Workers and Cervical Screening Beliefs

Hong Kong Filipino domestic workers may well be at risk for reproductive health problems for a variety of reasons, including the stressors associated with migration and the immigration process, adaptation to their new society, changes in their social support system, changes in socioeconomic status and level, and physical stressors including new pathogens (Aroian, 1990; Lipson & Meleis, 1989; Hatter-Pollara & Meleis, 1995).

Table 1. Socio-demographic Characteristics (N=98)

Item	Frequency (%)
Occupation	
Full-time domestic helper	95 (98%)
Other	2 (2%)
Missing data	1(1%)
Income (Hong Kong Dollars*)	
< $4,000	90 (92%)
$4,001-5,000	4 (4%)
$5,001-6,000	1 (1%)
> $6001	2 (2%)
Missing data	1 (1%)
Education level	
Secondary (high school)	33 (34%)
Vocational/secretarial (post-secondary)	23 (24%)
Tertiary (University)	42 (42%)
Marital status	
Never married	7(7%)
Married	80 (82%)
Separated	6 (6%)
Widowed	5 (5%)
Number of children	
None	9 (9%)
One	20 (21%)
Two	26 (27%)
Three or more	41 (43%)
Missing data	2 (2%)
Regular source of medical care	
General practitioner in the Philippines	43 (44%)
General practitioner in Hong Kong	25 (26%)
General practitioner in the Philippines and Hong Kong	2 (2%)
Specialist	5 (5%)
Other	3 (3%)
None	18 (18%)
Missing data	2 (2%)
Prior Pap smear	
Yes	46 (47%)
No, never	52 (53%)
Sexually active	
Yes	86 (88%)
No	4 (4%)
Prefer not to say	6 (6%)
Missing data	2 (2%)

Table 1. (Continued))

Item	Frequency (%)
Number of sexual partners	
None	4 (4%)
1 only	88 (90%)
2-3	2 (2%)
More than 10	1 (1%)
Missing data	3 (3%)
Family planning methods (more than one method used)	
Oral contraceptives	43 (444%)
Intrauterine contraceptive device	9 (9%)
Barrier method	13 (13%)
Rhythm method	4 (4%)
Sterilization	2 (2%)
Liqafed	9 (9%)
Depo-Provera injection	2 (2%)
Withdrawal	23 (23%)
None	11 (11%)
Missing data	2 (2%)
Hysterectomy	
Yes	5 (5%)
No	91 (93%)
Unsure	1 (1%)
Missing data	1 (1%)
Family or friends with cervical cancer	
Yes	20 (20%)
No	77 (79%)
Unsure	1 (1%)
Previously heard about Pap smears	
Yes	76 (78%)
No	22 (22%)
Smoking status	
Current smoker	1 (1%)
Ex-smoker	3 (3%)
Non-smoker	86 (88%)
Missing data	8 (8%)

* $7.80 Hong Kong = $1.00 US

The following reports a survey (Holroyd et al, 2003) of 98 female Filipino domestic helpers residing in Hong Kong who were given a questionnaire on their cervical screening and cancer health attitudes, beliefs, knowledge and attitudes, included *were:* smear history, knowledge, health beliefs and attitudes about cervical smears, and socio-demographic data. The women were between 24-54 years old (mean=37.9, SD=7.7), with an average of 3 pregnancies reported (SD=1.6, range=0-7). The majority of these women were employed as full-time domestic helpers (97%), earning less than $500.00 US/month (92%), married

(82%), with children (91%), non-smokers (88%), and had at least a secondary level of education (100%), with 66% of these women having completed post secondary education.

In respect to health practices and healthcare most of the women reported being sexually active (90%), with 44% taking an oral contraceptive. In all 70% reported having a regular source of medical care with 45% of the women reporting using a regular medical care in the Philippines. The majority of the women had previously heard about cervical smears (78%). However, more than half of these women (53%) reported never having a cervical smear taken (see Table 1). There were no significant differences in socio-demographic variables between women who had a prior cervical smear and those who never had one.

Cervical Smear History and Healthcare Behavior

Many women reported that having a cervical smear was not needed (20%, n=20), were unaware of the test (23%, n=23) or that they had no time have a Pap smear done (27%, n=26). Among women who previously had a cervical smear (N=47), approximately 40% (n=19) could not remember when their last cervical smear was taken. Only 32% (n=15) of these women recalled having a cervical smear within the last 2 years. However, the majority had been informed of a normal result (83%, n=39). The majority of the women had heard about cervical smears from health care professionals (77%, n=37) and had a cervical smear following the advice given by their physician or nurse (64%, n=30). Among the women having a prior cervical smear, most were taken at either a private specialists' clinic (47%, n=22) or at a government hospital (34%, n=16). Most of the women who had a cervical smear done were feeling healthy (79%, n=37) with only 40% (n= 19) basing their decision on their own initiative. (Table 2)

Knowledge About Cervical Smears and Cervical Cancer

Responses to statements assessing knowledge about cervical smears and cervical cancer can be found in Table 3. The majority of the women (77%) thought that cervical smears detect cancer of the uterus, and disagreed that cervical smear should begin from the first time of sexual intercourse (63%). Approximately one-third of the women thought that having a cervical smear every 3 years is often enough, that there is a risk of infection following a cervical smear (30%), and that not having regular cervical smears would not increase their risk of cervical cancer. Knowledge mean scores were good (mean=50.49, SD= 2.9), with possible scores ranging from 18-72. A t-test to compare mean knowledge scores about Pap Smears and Cervical Cancer between the women who previously had a Pap smear with those who never had a Pap smear, were significantly different (t=2.796, df=95, p=0.006). Women who had a prior Pap smear had significantly more knowledge about Pap smears and cervical cancer (mean=51.34, SD=2.5) than those who never had a Pap smear (mean=49.72, SD=3.2).

Table 2. Pap Smear History and Healthcare Behavior

Item	Frequency (%)
All subjects, N=98	
Reasons for avoiding Pap smear tests (more than one answer given)	
Embarrassment	12 (12%)
Fear of result	6 (6%)
Don't know where to go	6 (6%)
No time to go	26 (27%)
Consider test unnecessary	20 (20%)
Too expensive	4 (4%)
Unaware of test	23 (23%)
Missing data	12 (12%)
Women who had a prior Pap smear, N=47	
Last Pap smear	
<1 Year	13 (28%)
1-2 years	2 (4%)
2-3 years	5 (11%)
3-5 years	3 (6%)
5 + years	5 (11%)
can't remember	19 (40%)
Result of last Pap smear	
Informed, normal	39 (83%)
Not informed, presumed normal	6 (13%)
Informed abnormal	1 (1%)
Missing data	1 (1%)
How heard of Pap smear	
Mass media	1 (1%)
Healthcare professional	37 (77%)
Friends or relatives	7 (15%)
Other	1 (1%)
Missing data	1 (1%)
Inspiration to have Pap smear done	
Advised by MD/RN	30 (64%)
Advised by friend/relative	6 (30%)
Mass media	1 (1%)
Knows person with cervical cancer	1 (1%)
Brought by friend/relative	2 (4%)
Received letter to have Pap smear	1 (1%)
Missing data	6 (13%)
Location of last Pap smear	
Maternal/child health clinic	2 (4%)
General practitioner's clinic	3 (6%)
Private specialist's clinic	22 (47%)
Government hospital	16 (34%)
Other	2 (4%)
Missing data	2 (4%)

Table 2. (Continued)

Item	Frequency (%)
All subjects, N=98	
Reason for having last Pap smear	
Healthy	
Part of visit to MD	6 (13%)
On own initiative	19 (40%)
Other reason	12 (26%)
Had bleeding, vaginal discharge, or other symptom	8 (17%)
Missing data	2 (4%)

Health Beliefs and Attitudes Towards Having a Cervical Smear

Responses to statement regarding health beliefs and attitudes towards cervical cancer screening can be found in Table 4. A total of 91 women (93%) agreed that cancer was a serious disease with 86 (88%) and 95 (97%) retrospectively agreeing that having cancer would affect family, work and social life. Women were clearly believed that cervical smears helped to prevent cancer (91%) yet only 72 (74%) women believed that cancer could be cured if detected early. More than one-third of all the women thought that cervical smears would cause embarrassment (38%) and are expensive (40%). Nearly half (47%) of the women associated cervical smears with pain. The health beliefs and attitudes mean score was 59.79(SD= 4.2), with possible scores ranging from 14-70. A significant positive correlation between knowledge about cervical smears and cervical cancer, and health beliefs and attitudes towards cervical smears was found ($r=0.23$, $p=0.05$).

The socio–demographic and health characteristics identify the high rate of women using the Philippine health services as their provider suggesting a substantial gap in regular health screening given that the current employment contract stipulates a two-week holiday to the Philippines every two years and that many helpers do not elect to take this. During this holiday it is highly possible that health care in neglected in place of more pressing family obligations. It is of further note that while the majority of women were sexually active and used oral contraceptives despite Catholicism being reported in up to 90% of the Philippine population (NDHS, 1998). The high education level found together with high level of sexual activity and that less than 50% of helpers reported having had a prior cervical smear suggest a lack of information, awareness or accessibility of such services for these women.

Given that the majority of women (n= 52) had not had a smear and were within a reproductive age range with a sizeable majority of both attendees and non-attendees having had sexual intercourse this group so constituted a risk category for cervical cancer. This low incidence of both cervical screening and reported low rates of breast self-examination reported a previous study (Holroyd et al, 2001) adds support to the health risks that these immigrant domestic helpers face. Clearly there exists the perception that cervical smears are not needed, which may be linked to lack of awareness of eligibility, cost and availability of the test.

Table 3. Knowledge about Pap Smears and Cervical Cancer: Responses

Statement	**Agree**	**Disagree**	**Missing Data**
	N(%)	N(%)	N(%)
I'm too young/old to begin having Pap smears.	22 (22%)	**70 (72%)**	6 (6%)
Pap smears have to be done regularly to be effective.	**86 (88%)**	8 (8%)	4 (4%)
Pap smears are not necessary once a woman has reached menopause.	13 (13%)	**80 (82%)**	5 (5%)
Pap smears can detect abnormal cell changes in the cervix before cancer.	**88 (90%)**	5 (5%)	5 (5%)
Healthy women do not need to have a regular Pap smear.	7 (7%)	**87 (89%)**	4 (4%)
Women should begin having Pap smears from the time of first sexual intercourse.	**29 (30%)**	62 (63%)	7 (7%)
Having Pap smears at regular intervals could save my life.	**88 (90%)**	6 (6%)	4 (4%)
I only have to have a Pap smear if my doctor tells me I need one.	16 (16%)	**78 (80%)**	4 (4%)
Having a Pap smear every 3 years is often enough.	42 (43%)	**51 (52%)**	5 (5%)
If I hadn't had sex for ages, I wouldn't need to have a Pap smear.	9 (9%)	**83 (85%)**	6 (6%)
Pap smears help to prevent cervical cancer.	**89 (91%)**	5 (5%)	4 (4%)
There is no risk of infection following a Pap smear.	**64 (65%)**	29 (30%)	5 (5%)
The Pap smear is extremely reliable in the early detection of cervical cancer.	**88 (90%)**	6 (6%)	4 (4%)
Pap smears do not detect cancer of the uterus.	**17 (17%)**	75 (77%)	6 (6%)
Cervical cancer can be cured if detected early.	**93 (95%)**	1 (1%)	4 (4%)
Having many different sexual partners, increases the risk of women having changes in the cervix or of getting cancer.	**88 (90%)**	8 (8%)	2 (2%)
Not having regular Pap smears, increases the risk of women having changes in the cervix or of getting cancer.	**60 (61%)**	36 (37%)	2 (2%)
Having a previous abnormal Pap smear finding, increases the risk of women having changes in the cervix or of getting cancer.	**76 (78%)**	18 (18%)	4 (4%)

Table 4. Health Beliefs and Attitudes towards Having a Pap Smear: Responses.

Statement	Agree	Disagree	Unsure	Missing Data
	N(%)	N(%)	N(%)	N(%)
Cancer is a serious disease.	**91 (93%)**	2 (2%)	2 (2%)	3 (3%)
If I had cancer, it would affect my family.	**86 (88%)**	2 (2%)	7(7%)	3 (3%)
If I had cancer, it would affect my working and social life.	**95 (97%)**	0	0	3 (3%)
You can do something to avoid falling ill with cancer.	**79 (81%)**	3 (3%)	12 (12%)	4 (4%)
I sometimes worry about the possibility of getting cancer.	**89 (91%)**	0	6 (6%)	3 (3%)
I am just as likely to get cancer as any other woman my age.	**76 (78%)**	10 (10%)	9 (9%)	3 (3%)
I would be able to tell if I have cancer without going to the doctor.	10 (10%)	**68 (69%)**	17 (17%)	3 (3%0
If I did have cancer, I would rather not know that I had it.	9 (9%)	**84 (86%)**	1 (1%)	4 (4%)
Cancer cannot be cured even if it is detected early.	16 (16%)	**72 (74%)**	7 (7%)	3 (3%)
Having a Pap smear is likely to cause pain.	46 (47%)	**45 (46%)**	0	7 (7%)
Having a Pap smear is likely to cause embarrassment.	37 (38%)	**55 (56%)**	0	6 (6%)
The cost of a Pap smear is expensive.	39 (40%)	**53 (54%)**	0	6 (6%)
The Pap smear is effective in detecting cervical cancer early.	**86 (89%)**	1 (1%)	5 (5%)	6 (6%)
The Pap smear is a safe procedure.	**82 (84%)**	2 (2%)	8 (8%)	6 (6%)

Responses in **bold**, indicate a more favorable attitude towards having a Pap smear.

These results reflects the lack of knowledge about preventative services available for reproductive health issues for marginalised women in Hong Kong (Holroyd et al, 2001). However, it is of note, that the education levels of this group was more than three times that reported in the general population of women residing in the Philippines. Such a finding may be indicative of barriers such as inaccessibility that domestic work poses to attendance for smears within Hong Kong.

While there is no data on health service up- take rates including the use of cervical smear services available in respect to Filippino women residing in Hong Kong, a low smear up-take rate has been reported in South Asian women residing in Australia (Donovan et al 1992).

Evident here is the importance of acknowledging the role of healthcare professionals in promoting cervical smears, in particular the role of doctors as high status practitioners within Asian societies.

What is also of note is that despite the high motivation levels regarding particular aspects of health and lifestyle reported in other regional studies of Filipino domestic workers this cohort did not exhibit the same levels regarding smear attendance. High levels of anxiety regarding attendance for health services have been identified in immigrant female populations due to a perception of stigmatization arising from language differences, multiple pressures in the face of the changing political situations and the burden of isolation and adjustment (Meleis 1990). In addition, it is possible that the nature of domestic labour with its associated isolation, low pay multiple roles, low status, long and erratic hours may contribute to poor cervical cancer attendance rates (Sarason et al, 1983). Issues of modesty and embarrassment may lead to cultural minorities under utlising healthcare care even when cervical screening in particular tends to be a high priority for this population (Flaskerud 1987).

While a sizeable number of women felt that cervical cancer could be cured even when detected early, the majority of women had not attended for a smear and many women were not receiving regular smears suggesting a pervasive element of fatalism. Cervical cancer screening is a self-directed activity that requires women to have a strong self-belief in their self- efficacy to exercise personal control over life events. When perceived self-efficacy is low, self-doubt overrides knowledge and self-protective actions. One cause of low self-efficacy in cancer screening is the notion of fatalism suggesting Fillipino women are not likely to participate in screening tests since they believe that there is very little they can do to change their fate (Straughan & Seow, 1998).

The suggestion of a pervasive element of fatalism draws out the concept of risk being central to Filippino domestic workers respond to health promotion. Davison et al (1992) contends that low self – efficacy and fatalism may rise from two components including a lack of knowledge about potential harm and the secondly related to an external locus of control in which modern beliefs about lifestyles juxtapose within the culture of fatalism. Within these contradictory belief systems it is possible that Filippino women actively assess the personal benefit of behavioral change (including issues of modesty) not only the health risk. This notion of fatalism frequently carries it origin in the relationship of health to heredity, social conditions and environment while acknowledging what an individual has control over an what she does. In general in societies where self-efficacy is low fatalism tend to be more established.

Low social support and the lack of a regular medical provider are commonly found to be associated with fatalism (Davison et al, 1992). Mo (1992) has reported a fatalistic view of reproductive cancer in Chinese-American populations. A similar belief that cancer is fatal and notions of pre- destination has been reported among Chinese populations residing in the Asian region (Dibble et al., 1997; Hoeman et al., 1996; Lu, 1995; Salazar, 1996; Seow et al., 1995).

Stern (1981) in a study of US dwelling Filipino women's health beliefs cites a cultural avoidance of intimate examinations by male doctors. Stern (1981) goes on to cite the cultural importance of avoiding shame in social interactions by pretending to understand. Low levels of health related behaviors would not be so alarming if they were not associated with such life threatening illness and if these illnesses were not preventable to some extent or curable if diagnosed at an early stage.

It is noteworthy that previous studies (Weitzman & Berry 1992) have documented that the lack of formal education acted as a barrier towards health preventative behaviors whereas domestic workers in this study had high levels of education and consequentially engaged in a large number of health related behaviors. This again tends to point to certain possible structural and cultural barriers inherent within Hong Kong healthcare system. These may include limited clinic opening hours, lack of attention to the issue of modesty and the provision of female providers, lack of opportunistic screening and lack of material in written Tagalong (national language of the Philippines).

Such findings as reported here are in keeping with the international literature, which identifies societies with high group cohesion and strong religious beliefs as exhibiting a more externally operated locus of control (Helman 1994). Holroyd et al (2001) had previously documented a relationship between preventive screening practices and a low locus of control, or the belief that health was influenced by powerful others in a population of Filipino women. A target of future health promotion strategies involving foreign domestic helpers may be to target the role cancer plays in interpreting fertility, family and social life, all highly prized within Asian women's populations. Thus the efficacy of smears for Filipino women and the reliability of women's reports of smear checks may both need further investigation to effectively address cervical cancer mortality.

Practitioners' Views on Cervical Screening in South East Asia

A total of 16 practitioners who provided reproductive screening were further interviewed in order to influence of professional interactions on Chinese women s decision to attend for screening. More of the practitioners interviewed were female and most worked in the private sector.

Education and Social Class

The practitioners described how they felt that low educational attainment and poverty caused women to exhibit a sense of fatalism and contributed to misconceptions about etiology and treatment outcomes. This lack of correct and current knowledge has been shown limit choice of health seeking behavior (Loeher, Gregar, and Weinberger, 1991) The international literature suggests that women's level of knowledge is a particularly important factor prompting both attendance and reattendance in a range of cultural groups (Arevian et al., 1997, Fylan, 1998). Practitioners also described how, in their view, Hong Kong women lacked knowledge about health services in comparison to their counter parts in the west. This was seen to be due to magazines in the west having a strong emphasis on health and Hong Kong education levels in general being low.

Fatalism

Practitioners described women not wanting to look for a problem and the fatalistic notion of avoidance of bad news as strategies that woken due on to excuse attendance as seen in the following testimony:

> The Asian mentality is that you have got something and you must look for treatment. If you don't have anything problem you don't bother about it.

Modesty

In addition, practitioners, in particular female practitioners, thought that modesty was a barrier in Chinese women who a fear being exposed to a stranger. These are well exemplified in the following;

> I think most women would mind to consult a male doctor especially when it's necessary to undress the bottom for examination. If I were the layperson, I would mind to do that.

Modesty and embarrassment was seen by doctors to be more common in women of the older generation, exemplified in the following quote from a female practitioner;

> For some older women over fifty or sixty, they never had a Pap smear and said they don't think it's necessary, Or some said they're afraid, They're afraid if they go to see the doctor, they're afraid of the private part is being examined.

Lack of Knowledge of Risk Factors

Practitioners also described how older women in particular did not consider themselves at risk due to their perception of no longer being sexually active as well as due to a lack of knowledge of the risk factors associated with cervical cancer. This is well summed up in the following testimony;

> I don't think many Chinese know what is a risk factor. For the patients whom I know, when I talk with them I don't think they know there is a risk factor for cervical cancer. Actually very few of them know.

Female Practitioners

All the practitioners interviewed cited a female doctor as being an important in order to encourage Chinese women to attend for cervical screening, describing how many effective clinics had either all-female staff or made a female doctor available for cervical screening. Being examined by a female practitioner was seen to be preferred in that they were considered more sensitive to the needs of other women and issues of sexual inappropriateness did not arise. However, irrespective of gender a high level of skill was also seen as critical, for example:

> I'm the only female doctor here. The others are male doctors. I find that in Hong Kong still women like female doctors to perform Pap smears.

Lack of Time

Lack of time was considered an important social barrier in preventing women's attendance with four practitioners citing that women lacked time to wait for services. This is illustrated by one practitioner saying:

> Many women have to wait for 1-2 hours, and they would not have come in the next visit, as obviously time-factors are a barrier for them er.

Comparing Lay and Professional Perceptions of South East Asian Women's Barriers to Attendance for Cervical Screening

Similarities between women's and practitioners perceptions of social and cultural barriers to attendance included low education level, lack of awareness of the need for a smear, cost of the smear and embarrassment created by the procedure. In addition, acknowledgement by both professionals and women of the importance of a female smear taker is encouraging given a historical domination of males in the medicine discipline.

Differences in perceptions of barriers to attendance for cervical screening between practitioners and women were evident in the areas of risk factors and pain. It is possible that Asian women do not tend to personalize risk factors due to a cultural tendency to resort to fatalism in contrast to their practitioners who espouse a bio-medical approach (Mo, 1992). The contrast between women and practitioners in perceptions of pain is less surprising given that male practitioners were undertaking the screening as well as a cultural tendency for Chinese populations to somatise (Kleinman, 1980). The latter suggesting that it may be culturally inappropriate for Chinese women to show pain in lay professional encounters. In respect to somatisation it is possible that there is a cultural tendency to not admit pain as this may indicate a "loss of face" associated with letting go in front of a health care professional (Kleinman, 1980). What is of interest is that despite the considerable barriers to attendance outlined by both practitioners and women (both screened and unscreened) that a sizeable proportion of Chinese women do attend for regularly screening.

The women's specific culture and social barriers towards cervical screening were both complimentary and contradictory to those of practitioners. That both practitioners and women were congruent about the more tangible aspects of women's attendance barriers such as cost and education suggests a common framework from which to target screening campaigns.

However, it is possible that a large segment of women in particular these occupying marginalsied positions or holding illegal immigrant statuses may be either systematically deprived of the benefits of early detection or are receiving confusing messages about appropriate and acceptable practices. It then follows that both South East Asian women and practitioners attending these women need more knowledge of how each other perceives cancer, its prevention, and factors influencing attendance. Only with this mutual understanding as a foundation can healthcare professionals and women cooperative to improve cancer screening rates (Gregg & Curry, 1994; Johnson, et al b1999). In respect to practitioners role the incongruence of data between women and practitioners perceptions suggests that more emphasis needs to be placed on the pivotal role of cultural authority that practitioners can play in influencing cervical screening attendance in South East Asian women. In addition, the importance of promoting opportunistic screening needs to be highlighted given the cultural reluctance of women to attend for preventive health practices.

CONCLUSION

Culturally sensitive health education is needed for women, practitioners and public in promoting cervical cancer screening for South East Asian women. The emphasis on such programs should be on the importance for early diagnosis of a cervical cancer and how it can provide major advantages even for marginalised women. Community centers, both within the Asian region and internationally need to ensure that the philosophy of the staff and the approach and materials used must be culturally relevant if the programs are to be successful. The additional effort and time required by these programs to structuring reproductive screening in a way that there is congruity between women and practitioners explanations of risk and perceptions of barriers and facilitators to attendance needs to be addressed.

South East Asian migrant women workers who may not present themselves at cervical cancer screening clinics due to specific beliefs and to structural barriers in their host country such as the relative costs of the services and the need to take time off employment and face the possibility of losing their job. Promoting cervical screening for this sub-population of immigrant workers, may be more effective if it focused on changing ideas such as the value of cancer screening behavior rather than beliefs about the susceptibility to cancer. Given the economic contribution that these women make to South East Asian economies it follows that more culturally acceptable and affordable mass screening programmers are provided. Services need to be acknowledging the limited free time these women have to attend healthcare should ideally be on open on Sundays. In addition, sources of cancer preventative information need to be made available in their native languages. The content of health messages provided by the mass media and health professionals should include an explanation of each cancer screening test, describing how it is performed and the means for performing it. Doctors and nurses ideally of the same ethnic origin as the women should be used to deliver health messages and services crediting the importance of regular smears given the sizeable number of South East Asian women working as domestic labor both regionally and internationally.

Opportunistic screening should be provided every time a women accesses a health service In addition, it is important that health promotion campaigns target the protection of self through screening by emphasizing the prizing of the cultural importance of family and fertility. Health education should incorporate screening programs into settings that reflect mechanisms needed to attempt to increase perceptions of self-efficacy by stressing the benefits and the relative ease with which they can be obtained.

Future research is needed to identify predictors of cancer screening among other Asian populations, in particular illegal immigrants and those women working in the entertainment industry to assist maximize health outcomes. In addition, further studies are needed to investigate indigenous folk beliefs and practices, which would contribute to a broader picture of culturally specific health screening behavior and beliefs.

REFERENCES

Adab, P., & Hedley, A. J. (1997). Preventing avoidable death: The case of cervical cancer in Hong Kong. *Hong Kong Medical Journal, 3*(4), 427-432.

Adab, P., & McGhee, S. M. (2001). *The pattern of cervical screening in Hong Kong health services.* Unpublished manuscript.

Arevian, M., Noureddine, S., & Kabakian, T. (1997 Jan-Feb). A survey of knowledge, attitude, and practice of cervical screening among Lebanese/Armenian women. *Nursing Outlook, 45*(1), 16-22.

Aroian, K. J. (1990). A model of psychological adaptation to migration and resettlement. *Nursing Research, 39*(1), 5-10.

Bagley, C., Madrid, S., & Bolitho, F. (1997). Stress factors and mental health adjustment of Filipino domestic workers in Hong Kong. *International Social Work, 40*, 373-382.

Baldwin, D. (1996 Dec). A model for describing low-income African American women's participation in breast and cervical cancer early detection and screening. *Advances in Nursing Science, 19*(2), 27-42.

Bernal, P., & Meleis, A. I. (1995). Self care actions of Colombian Por Dia domestic workers: On prevention and care. *Women and Health, 22*(4), 77-95.

Bilimoria, M. M., & Morrow, M. (1995). The woman at increased risk for breast cancer: Evaluation and management strategies. *Canadian Cancer Journal of Clinic, 45*, 263-278.

Boffetta, P., & Parkin, D. M. (1995). Cancer in developing countries. *Canadian Cancer Journal of Clinic, 44*, 81.

Burgess, C. C., Ramirez, A. J., Richards, M. A., & & Love, S. B. (1988). Who and what influences delayed presentation in breast cancer? *British Journal of Cancer, 77*(8), 1343-1348.

Coates, R., Bransfield, D. D., Wesley, M. N., Hankey, B. F., Eley, J. W., & Greenberg, M. D. et al. (1992). Differences between black and white women with breast cancer in time from symptom recognition to medical consultation. *Journal of the National Cancer Institute, 84*, 938-950.

Constable, N. (1997). *Maid to order in Hong Kong: Stories of Filipino workers.* New York: Cornell University Press.

Davison, C., Frankel, S., & Smith, G. D. (1992). The limits of lifestyle : Re- assessing ' fatalism" in the popular culture of illness prevention. *Social Science and Medicne, 34*(6), 675-685.

Delgado, D. J., & Cabrera, D. (1989). The relationship of racial/ethnic and socioeconomic factors with the cancer experience. in L. E. Irwin, J. stern, & J. Steinfeld (eds.), *cancer and the underserved: An agenda for change in the 1990s*. Oakland: American Cancer Society California Division, 113-157.

Dibble, S. L., Vanoni, J. M., & Miaskowski, C. (1997 Jan-Feb). Women's attitudes toward breast cancer screening procedures: Differences by ethnicity. *Womens Health Issues, 7*(1), 47-54.

Donovan, J. W. (Ed.). (1992). *Immigrants in Australia: A health profile*. Canberra: Australian Government Publication.

Facione, N. C., & Dodd, M. J. (1995). Women's narratives of help-seeking for breast cancer. *Cancer Practice, 3*, 219-226.

Facione, N. C., Dodd, M. J., Holzemer, W., & Meleis, A. I. (1997). Helpseeking for self-discovered breast symptoms, implications for early detection. *Cancer Practice, 5*(4), 220-227.

Facione, N. C., Giancarlo, C. A., & Chan, L. (in press). *Seeking help for symptoms and breast cancer risk: A Chinese American perspective.* Unpublished manuscript.

Facione, N. C., Giancarlo, C., & Chan, L. (2000 Aug). Perceived risk and help-seeking behavior for breast cancer. A Chinese-American perspective. *Cancer Nursing, 23*(4), 258-267.

Facione, N. C., & Giancarlo, C. A. (1998 Dec). Narratives of breast symptom discovery and cancer diagnosis: Psychologic risk for advanced cancer at diagnosis. *Cancer Nursing, 21*(6), 430-440.

Facione, N. C., & Katapodi, M. (2000 Aug). Culture as an influence on breast cancer screening and early detection. [review] [98 refs]. *Seminars in Oncology Nursing, 16*(3), 238-247.

Family Planning Association of Hong Kong. (1999). Press conference on the report of the knowledge, attitude, and practice of family planning survey in Hong Kong. Hong Kong.

Feldman, P. H., Sapienze, A. M., & Kane, N. M. (1999). On the home front: The job of the home aide. *Generations, 18*(3), 16-19.

Flaskerud, J. H. (1987). A proposed protocol for culturally relevant psychotherapy. *Clinical Nurse Specialist, 1*(40), 150-157.

Frank-Stromborg, M., Wassner, L. J., Nelson, M., Chilton, B., & Wholeben, B. E. (1998). A study of rural Latino women seeking cancer-detection examinations. *Journal of Cancer Education, 13*(4), 231-241.

Freeman, H. P. (1989). Cancer in the socio-economically disadvantaged. *Canadian Cancer Journal Clinic, 39*, 266-288.

Freemen, H. P., & Wasfie, T. J. (1989). Cancer of the breast in poor black women. *Cancer, 63*, 2562-2569.

Fylan, F. (1998 Aug). Screening for cervical cancer: A review of women's attitudes, knowledge, and behaviour.[see comment]. [review] [83 refs]. *British Journal of General Practice, 48*(433), 1509-1514.

Gregg, J., & Curry, R. H. (1994). Explanatory models for cancer among African-American women at two Atlanta neighborhood health centers: The implications for a cancer screening program. *Social Science and Medicine, 39*(4), 519-626.

Hattar-Pollara, M., & Meleis, A. I. (1995). The stress of immigration and the daily lived experiences of Jordanian immigrant women in the united states. *Western Journal of Nursing Research, 17*(5), 521-539.

Helman, C. G. (Ed.). (1994). *Culture,health and illness.* (3rd ed.). New York: Butterworth Heinemann.

Hiatt, R. A., Pasick, R. J., & Perez-Stable, E. (1996). Pathways to early cancer detection in the multiethnic population of the San Francisco bay area. *Health Education Quarterly, 23*, 10-27.

Hoeman, S. P., Ku, Y. L., & Ohl, D. R. (1996 Oct). Health beliefs and early detection among Chinese women. *Western Journal of Nursing Research, 18*(5), 518-533.

Holroyd, E., Taylor-Pillae, R., & Twinn, S. (2003). Investigating Hong Kong's Filippino domestic workers' healthcare behavior, knowledge, beliefs and attitudes towards cervical cancer and cervical screening. *Women and Health, 38*(1), 69-82.

Holroyd, E., Twinn, S. F., & Shiu, A. T. Y. (2001). Chinese women's experiences and images of the pap smear examination. *Cancer Nursing, 24*(1), 68-75.

Hong Kong Cancer Registry. (2006). *Cancer of the cervix uteri.* Retrieved Mar/1, 2006 from http://www3.ha.org.hk/canereg/data/cx.pdf

Hong Kong General Household Survey. (1996). *Social data collected by the general household survey special topics report* No. 14). Hong Kong: Social Analysis and Research Section Census and Statistics Department. Social.

Johnson, J. L., Bottorff, J. L., Balneaves, L. G., Grewal, S., Bhagat, R., & Hilton, B. A. et al. (1999 Jul). South Asian womens' views on the causes of breast cancer: Images and explanations. *Patient Education & Counseling, 37*(3), 243-254.

Johnston, G., Orbell, S., Crombie, I., Robertson, A., & Kenicer, M. (1996). Women's preferences for cervical screening: Who, where, and when. *Health Education Journal, 55*, 84-91.

Kagawa-Singer, M. (1995). Socioeconomic and cultural influences on cancer care of women. *Seminars in Oncology Nursing, 11*(2), 109-119.

Kagawa-Singer, M. (1997 Nov-Dec). Addressing issues for early detection and screening in ethnic populations. [review] [49 refs]. *Oncology Nursing Forum, 24*(10), 1705-1711.

Katz S.J., Hislip G., Thomas D.B. & Larson E.B. (1993). Delay from symptom to diagnosis and treatment of breast cancer in Washington state and British Columbia. *Medical Care, 31*, 264-268.

Kleinman, A. (1980). *Patients and healers in the context of culture.* Berkeley: University of California Press.

Larsen, L. P., & Olesen, F. (1998). Women's knowledge of and attitude towards organized cervical smear screening. *Acta Obstetricia Et Gynecologica Scandinavica, 77*, 988-996.

Lauver, D., & Chang, A. (1991). Testing theoretical explanations of intentions to seek care for a breast cancer symptom. *Journal of Applied Social Psychology, 21*, 1440.

Lauver, D., Coyle, M., & Panchmatia, B. (1995). Women's reasons for and barriers to seeking care for breast cancer symptoms. *Women Health International, 5*, 27-35.

Lierman, L. (1988). 'Discovery of breast changes: Women's responses and nursing implications.' *Journal of Cancer Nursing, 11*(6), 352-361.

Lipson, J. G., & Meleis, A. I. (1989). Methodological issues in research with immigrants. *Medical Anthropology, 12*(1), 103-115.

Loehrer, P. J. S., Greger, H. A., Weinberger, M., Musick, B., Miller, M., & Nichols, C. et al. (1991). Knowledge and beliefs about cancer in a socio-economically disadvantaged population. *Cancer, 68*, 1665-1671.

Lu, Z. J. (1995). Variables associated with breast self-examination among Chinese women. *Cancer Nursing, 18*, 29-34.

Marcus, A. C., & Crane, L. A. (1998). A review of cervical cancer screening intervention research: Implications for public health programs and future research. *Preventive Medicine, 27*, 13-31.

Marin, G., & Marin, B. V. (1991). *Research with hispanic populations.* Newbury Park, CA: Sage Publications.

Masi, R., Mensah, L., & McLeod, K. (1993). *Health and culture: Exploring the relationships.* Oakville, Ontario, Canada: Mosaic Press.

Maxwell, A. E., Bastani, R., & Warda, U. S. (2000 Jan). Demographic predictors of cancer screening among Filipino and Korean immigrants in the united states. *American Journal of Preventive Medicine, 18*(1), 62-68.

McDonald, P. A., Thorne, D. D., & Pearson, J. C. (1999). Perceptions and knowledge of breast cancer among African–American women residing in public housing. *Ethnicity and Disease, 9*, 81-93.

McKenzie, J. L., & Chrisman, N. J. (1977). Healing herbs, gods and magic. *Nursing Outlook, 225*, 326-329.

Meleis, A. I. (1990). Between two cultures: Identity, roles, and health. *Healthcare for Women International, 12*, 365-377.

Million-Underwood, S., & Hoskins, D. (1993). Increasing nursing involvement in cancer prevention and control among the economically disadvantaged: The nursing challenge. *Seminars in Oncology Nursing, 10*, 89-95.

Mo, B. (1992). Modesty sexuality and breast health in Chinese American women. *Western Journal of Medicine, 157*(3), 260-264.

Morgan, C., Park, E., & Cortes, D. E. (1995). Beliefs, knowledge, and behavior about cancer among urban hispanic women. *Journal of the National Cancer Institute Monographs, 18*, 57-63.

Naish, J., Brown, J., & Denton, B. (1994). Intercultural consultations: Investigation of factors that deter non-english speaking women from attending their general practitioners for cervical screening. *British Medical Journal, 309*(6962), 1126-1128.

National Statistics Office & Department of Health. (2005). *National demographic and health survey,1998.* Retrieved 3/1, 2006 from http://www.census.gov.ph/data/technotes/notendhs.html

Navon, L. (1999). Cultural views of cancer around the world. *Cancer Nursing, 22*, 39-45.

Pritchard, D. A., Straton, J. A., & Hyndman, J. (1995). Cervical screening in general practice. *Australian Journal of Public Health, 19*(2), 167-172.

Rajaram, S. S., & Rashidi, A. (1998). Minority women and breast cancer screening: The role of cultural explanatory models. *Preventive Medicine, 27*, 757-764.

Salazar, M. K. (1996). Hispanic women's beliefs about breast cancer and mammography. *Cancer Nursing, 19*, 437-446.

Seow, A., Wong, M. L., Smith, W. C. S., & Lee, H. P. (1995). Beliefs and attitudes as determinants of cervical cancer screening: A community-based study in Singapore. *Preventive Medicine, 24*, 134-141.

Skinner, C. S., Sykes, R. K., & Monsees, B. S. (1998). Learn, share, and live: Breast cancer education for older, urban minority women. *Health Education Behavior, 25*, 60-78.

Stern, P. N. (1981). Solving problems of cross-cultural health teaching. *Image, 13*(2), 47-50.

Stern, P. N. (1985). A comparison of culturally approved behaviors and beliefs between filipino immigrant women, American-born dominant culture women, and western female nurses of the San Francisco bay area: Religiosity of health care. *Health Care for Women International, 6*, 123-124.

Straughan, P. T., & Seow, A. (1998). Fatalism reconceptualized: A concept to predict health screening behavior. *Journal of Gender, Culture, and Health, 3*, 85-100.

Temple-Smith, M. J., Banwell, C. L., Gifford, S. M., & Presswell, N. T. (1995). Promoting health beyond recruitment: Beliefs and attitudes to breast and cervical cancer screening services among Italian-born women in Melbourne. *Health Promotion Journal of Australia, 5*(2), 31-36.

Thompson, B., Montano, D. E., & Mahloch, J. (1997). Attitudes and beliefs toward mammography among women using an urban public hospital. *Journal of Health Care Poor Underserved, 8*, 186-201.

Twinn, S., & Cheng, F. (2000). Increasing uptakes rates of cervical cancer screening amongst Hong Kong Chinese women: The role of the practitioner. *Journal of Advanced Nursing, 32*, 335-342.

Twinn, S., Holroyd, E., & Adab, P. (2001). *The influence of extrinsic and extrinsic factors on uptake rates for cervical screening: A comparison of Hong Kong Chinese women and practitioners. health services research committee.* Unpublished manuscript.

Twinn, S., Holroyd, E., & Shui, A. (1999). *An investigation of the extent to which service provision for the screening of cervical cancer meets the needs of Hong Kong women.* Unpublished manuscript.

Van der Stuyft, P., De Muynck, A., Schillemans, L., & Timmerman, C. (1989). Migration, acculturation, and utilization of primary health care. *Social Science and Medicine, 29*, 53-60.

Ward, J., D'Este, C., & Sanson-Fisher, R. (1993). Beyond opportunistic pap smears in general practice: Women's view of strategies to promote regular screening. *Family Physician, 22*(11), 2032-2034.

Weitzman, B. C., & Berry, C. A. (1992). Health status and health care utilization among New York city home attendants: An illustration of the needs of working poor, immigrant women. *Women and Health, 19*(2/3), 87-105.

Wolf, M. (1968). *The house of Lim: The study of a Chinese farm family.* New York: Appleton Croft.

Yu, C. K., & Rymer, J. (1998 Jan). Women's attitudes to and awareness of smear testing and cervical cancer. *British Journal of Family Planning, 23*(4), 127-133.

In: New Research on Cervical Cancer
Editor: George Z. Rolland, pp. 217-232

ISBN 1-60021-300-6

Chapter 9

CERVICAL CANCER IN NORTHEASTERN THAILAND

Wannapa Settheetham-Ishida[1,*] and Takafumi Ishida[2]

[1]Department of Physiology, Faculty of Medicine, Khon Kaen University, Khon Kaen 40002, Thailand;

[2]Department of Biological Sciences, Graduate School of Science, The University of Tokyo, Tokyo 113-0033, Japan.

ABSTRACT

Cervical cancer remains the most common cancer among Thai women even though its incidence has decreased according to the age-standardized rate. Contrariwise, other data suggest the incidence rate of this cancer gradually increased in Northeast Thailand between 1992 and 2000. HPV infection is the major cause of cervical cancer and has been confirmed as a critical risk factor for the development of cancer in this region. The prevalence of HPV-16 infection was prominent, followed by HPV-18. The number of sexual partners and passive smoking history were identified as risks for HPV infection. As for passive smoking, tobacco specific carcinogens/mutagens may exist in the cervical mucus through smoking and/or in the semen of tobacco smoking partners. Cervical exposure to such carcinogens can reduce cervical immunity resulting in the persistence of HPV infection and also generating DNA lesions. It is hypothesized that certain genetic backgrounds, such as chemical metabolizing enzyme genes, may play roles in the development of this cancer.

Keywords: Cervical cancer, Northeastern Thailand, Risk factors, Cancer susceptibility.

---

* Correspondence concerning this article should be addressed to Wannapa Settheetham-Ishida Departmet of physiology, Faculty of Medicine, Khon Kaen University, Khon Kaen, 40002 Thailand. Tel/fax: +66-43-348394. E-mail address: wannapa@kku.ac.th

Introduction

Cancer is an important national health problem in Thailand. The incidence rates vary by region (*i.e.,* in the North, Northeast, South and Central (see Figure 1)) with the age-standardized incidence rates (ASR) being 149.2 in males and 125.0 in females between 1995 and 1997 (Martin and Patel, 2003). However, in Khon Kaen, Northeast Thailand, over the same period the ASR were 182.5 in males and 125.3 in females (Martin and Patel, 2003).

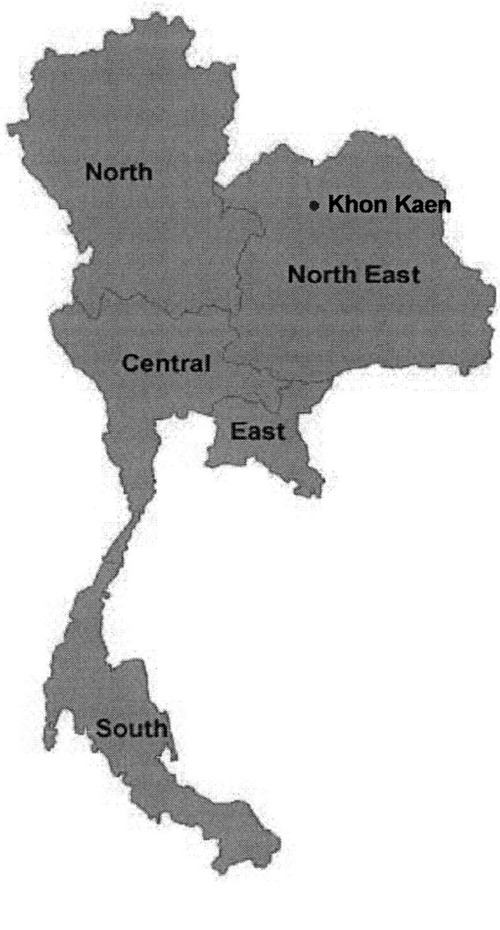

Figure 1. Map of Thailand.

Among cancers, cervical cancer is one of the most common in Thai women even though the age-standardized incidence rates indicate a decrease with 19.5 in 1995-1997 (Pengsaa and Jindawijak, 2003). The incidence rate of this cancer gradually increased in Northeastern Thailand between 1992 and 2000 (Pengsaa and Jindawijak, 2003), and remains the highest cause of mortality among females in the region (Vatanasapt *et al.,* 1998). Cervical cancer comprised one-fifth of new female cancer cases in the last two years. Two-thirds of patients with cervical cancer receive radiotherapy, while one-seventh underwent surgery at our regional University Hospital in Khon Kaen (Cancer Unit, 2004; 2005).

Cervical cancer can be detected at an asymptomatic stage using the Pap smear test; however, the test is not well accepted because of limited public health awareness. Thus, women attend hospital only after cervical cancer symptoms manifest, when they are difficult to treat so the prognosis is poor. This situation prompted us to carry out a survey to search for the risk factors for cervical cancer in Northeast Thailand to develop tools for early diagnosis and prevention of cervical cancer.

Human Papillomavirus Infection

Most cancers are multi-factorially developed through genetic background, environmental factors and lifestyle; all of which exert independently or in combination to cause cancer (Bishop, 1995; Hunter, 1991; Weinberg, 1991; 1989). Large series of molecular and epidemiological studies conducted over the last twenty years have indicated that cervical infection by certain human papillomavirus (HPV) types is a precursor event in the genesis of cervical cancer (zur Hausen, 1991; Schiffman and Castle, 2003).

The human papillomavirus is a virus sized 50-55 nm in diameter with small double-stranded DNA as its genome, which encodes a small number of genes (Doorbar and Strerling, 2001). The basic structure consists of a regulatory region, an early gene (E) region and a late gene (L) region. HPV types are identified by variation of E6, E7 and L1 parts of the HPV genome. A similarity of at least 90% in the nucleotide sequence in these three genes permits HPV to be classified as identical types.

To date, there are 100 known different types of HPV: 1) a low-risk group (such as HPV-6, -11, -26, -42 and -44); and, 2) a high-risk group (such as HPV-16, -18, -31, -33, -35, -39, 45, -51, -52, -56 and -58) (Minaguchi *et al.*, 1998). Cervical infection with certain subtypes of HPV, particularly of the high-risk group, closely correlates with the development of cervical cancer (Scheffner *et al.*, 1990; Schiffman and Castle, 2003; zur Hausen, 1991).

Strong evidence suggests that E6 and E7 HPV proteins contribute to the development of cervical cancer. They act together to stimulate keratinocytes and facilitate HPV DNA replication (Munger *et al.*, 2001). Once integration of the HPV genome into the host cells occurs, there is uncontrolled gene expression, which drives the cell cycle. In HPV-infected cells, the E7 protein binds with pRB turning E2F into an active form resulting in transcription of DNA replicated genes. Another HPV protein, E6 binds with p53 protein, which leads to degradation of the p53 protein (Scheffner *et al.*, 1990).

Epidemiological evidence indicates that infection with HPV is the major cause of cervical cancer (Monoz *et al.*, 1992; zur Hausen, 1991), such that worldwide HPV prevalence in cervical cancer is 99.7% (Walboomers *et al.*, 1999). Additionally, HPV infection was confirmed as a critical risk factor for the development of cervical cancer in Northeast Thailand. The prevalence of the high-risk group of HPV infection sub-strains -16, -18, -31, -33, -35, -52b and -58) was identified among 86.7% of squamous cell cervical cancers (SCCA) and increased the risk for development of SCCA by as much as 43.5-fold (Settheetham-Ishida *et al.*, 2005).

As expected, genotyping of HPV among SCCA patients in Northeast Thailand confirmed the high prevalence of HPV-16 infection (70.5%) followed by HPV-18 infection (23.1%), but a relatively low prevalence of HPV-33 was noted (Settheetham-Ishida *et al.,* 2005). Moreover, HPV-16 is a critical risk factor for cervical squamous intraepithelial lesions (SIL) progression in this region (Settheetham-Ishida *et al.,* 2006). Compared to other populations vis-à-vis invasive SCCA, HPV-16 is the most prevalent genotype (Iwasawa *et al.,* 1996; Thomas *et al.,* 2001a), whereas preferential distribution of HPV genotype has been suggested causative for certain types of cervical cancer. HPV-18 is more closely associated with cervical adenocarcinoma and a poor prognosis (Kjaer and Brinton, 1993). Since female subjects of the study in Northeast Thailand were patients with SSCA, the high prevalence of HPV-16 is conceivable; however, the relatively high prevalence of HPV-18 in SCCA patients compared to the low prevalence in the controls should be emphasized. The difference in HPV genotype distribution between the controls and the patients was not statistically significant, indicating any high risk subtype may have potential for SCCA development. The accumulation of HPV-18 suggests a role for HPV-18 in the development of SCCA in Northeast Thailand.

The prevalence of a high-risk group for HPV infection varies in each region of Thailand; for example, in central and southern Thailand where the infection rate ranged between 3 and 14% among controls and between 74 and 89% among patients with cervical abnormalities (Lertworapreecha *et al.,* 1998; Sukvirach *et al.,* 2003; Thomas *et al.,* 2001a). In Northeast Thailand, prevalence was 13% for controls and 87% for patients (Settheetham-Ishida *et al.,* 2005), which is comparable to the other Thai populations (Lertworapreecha *et al.,* 1998; Sukvirach *et al.,* 2003; Thomas *et al.,* 2001) and strongly suggests the involvement of other risk factor(s) in the high incidence of cervical cancer in Northeast Thailand.

Genetic Polymorphism of *p53*

A substantial series of epidemiological evidence has indicated that infection with certain types of HPV is the major cause of cervical cancer (Monoz *et al.,* 1992; zur Hausen, 1991). However, only a small fraction of women infected with these virus strains develop the cancer indicating that HPV infection is necessary but not a sufficient condition for the cancer to develop, and that the presence of other risk factors – such as genetic backgrounds and lifestyle – is suspected.

The human p53 protein comprises 393 amino acids, which can be divided into several structural and functional domains, many of which contribute to the ability of p53 to function as a transcription factor (Levine, 1997; Haffner and Oren, 1995). The p53 acts as a tumor suppressor protein and cellular growth regulator: whereas p53 is not essential for basal cellular growth and development (Donehower *et al.,* 1992), it does play a critical role in the response of cells to stress; mediating a G1/S cell-cycle arrest and/or apoptosis following damage to the DNA. When the DNA is damaged, p53 levels rise and induce G1 cell-cycle arrest (Kastan *et al.,* 1991; Lowe *et al.,* 1993).

p53 protein is one of the most important proteins in the defense system against tumor development (Levine, 1997). Participation of the *p53* alterations including somatic mutations and germ-line polymorphisms in tumor development has been well documented (Andersson *et al.,* 2001; Zehbe *et al.,* 1999). A base substitution at codon 72 of the *p53* resulting in either arginine (Arg) or proline (Pro) was identified as polymorphic in human populations (Beckman *et al.,* 1994). Codon 72 polymorphism (*Arg/Pro* allele) of the *p53* is widely distributed in various human populations (Helland *et al.,* 1998). One of the striking features of this polymorphism is efficient degradation of the Arg type of p53 by HPV E6 oncoprotein, and that carriers of the Arg type of p53 were about seven times more susceptible to the cervical cancer (Storey *et al.,* 1998).

After HPV infection, viral E6 protein binds to the cellular protein (Scheffner *et al.,* 1990) and causes dysfunction of the p53 protein activity. As recently reported, biological and biochemical differences – between the p53 protein with Arg or Pro at amino acid position 72 – indicate the possible presence of a different interaction pattern between either the p53 protein variant and the E6 protein of HPV property (Storey *et al.,*1998; Thomas *et al.,* 1999a, 1999b).

Thus, the *p53* codon 72 polymorphism has been nominated as a genetic risk factor for cervical cancer. However, the association was not significant and the susceptibility of the *Arg/Arg* genotype to cervical cancer was limited in Northeastern Thai women. This result is thus comparable to the studies of Korean, Japanese and Peruvian population which have Mongoloid background (Minaguchi *et al.,* 1998; Baek *et al.,* 2000; Klug *et al.,* 2001). The controversial results may be due to differences in ethnic background and in allele frequency. The allele frequency in Northeastern Thailand, shown in the present study, is similar to those reported in Central and Southern Thailand (Tiwawech *et al.,* 2003; Kietthubthew *et al.,* 2003).

The development of cervical cancer correlates with the presence of the high risk HPV E6 protein of the virus. It binds to and inactivates the tumor suppressor protein p53 and directs its degradation (Scheffner *et al.,* 1990; Werness *et al.,* 1990). Although inactivation of p53 by HPV is probably important for tumor development, no genetic factors have been conclusively identified that might predispose an infected individual to develop cervical carcinoma.

Thus, several studies evaluated the association between p53 and HPV in the development of cervical cancer. P53 protein is mutated in many human tumors; however, in cervical cancer, this mutation is rarely detected (Crook *et al.,* 1991; Scheffner *et al.,* 1991). Many mutated p53 proteins are not susceptible to E6-mediated degradation, while the wild type of p53 is susceptible (Marston *et al.,* 1994; Medcalf and Milner, 1993; Thomas *et al.,* 1995).

p53 is a tumor suppressor protein that modifies its cancer suppressing property (Storey *et al.,*1998; Thomas *et al.,* 1999a, 1999b), and the *p53* codon 72 polymorphism is observed with various allele frequencies worldwide. Storey *et al.* (1998) also suggested that women homozygous for the *Arg* allele were about seven times more susceptible to cervical cancer than *Arg/Pro* heterozygous women and concluded that the polymorphism is involved in the development of cervical cancer, especially in the presence of HPV infection.

Storey *et al.* (1998) showed that the *p53* polymorphism at codon 72 *p53* affects protein susceptibility to HPV-16 and 18 E6-induced degradation *in vivo*; Arg type is more susceptible than Pro type. In cell lines transfected with E6 expressing plasmids, E6-mediated degradation of the p53 with Arg was more effective than the one carrying Pro.

The high risk type of p53 with Arg for cervical cancer was supported by several epidemiological studies for European (Makni *et al.,* 2000; Yang *et al.,* 2001; Zehbe *et al.,* 1999); however, this finding was contradicted by British (Rosenthal *et al.,* 1998), Japanese

(Minaguchi *et al.,* 1998), Korean (Kim *et al.,* 2001) and Black South African (Pegoraro *et al.,* 2000) studies. In addition, the distribution of the two p53 variants in healthy women and women with HPV positive cervical cancer suggests that women with the *Arg/Arg* are at a higher risk of HPV-associated cervical cancer than *Pro/Pro* or *Arg/Pro* (Storey *et al.,* 1998), although several studies found no statistically significant differences in the distribution of *p53* codon 72 genotypes between normal women and patients with cervical cancer (Minaguchi *et al.,* 1998; Yamashita *et al.,* 1999; Beak *et al.,* 2000; Kim *et al.,* 2001; Gustafsson *et al.,* 2001). Since the distribution of the *p53* codon 72 genotype varies according to ethnicity (Helland *et al.,* 1998), it is thus difficult to generalize from conclusions obtained for a given population.

In our study in Northeast Thailand, no significant association was found between the genotype distribution of the *p53* codon 72 polymorphism and the HPV infection; even though it seems that the odds ratio (OR) were increased in individuals homozygous for the *Arg* allele compared with those homozygous for the *Pro* allele, in particular after being adjusted for other risk factors. There was no significant association between genotype distribution of the *p53* codon 72 polymorphism and the HPV infection. Since polymorphism of the *p53* itself – as well as in combination with HPV infection – may not be a genetic risk for cervical cancer of women in Northeastern Thailand, more attention should be paid to other risk factors such as sexual behaviors and smoking.

Lifestyle

Although human papillomavirus (HPV) infection is a major risk – in particular for squamous cell cervical cancer – most infected women do not develop invasive cervical cancer. This means HPV infection is not a sufficient factor, and cofactors must therefore play roles in developing cancer. Transformation of lifestyle can also modify prevalence of leading cancers. This kind of public health approach has reached Northeast Thailand; however, the high incidence of cervical cancer in the region persists.

Epidemiologic evidence suggests that other factors such as sexual behaviors are risk factors for cervical cancer in Thailand (Punyaratabunduh *et al.,* 1982; Thomas *et al.,* 1996). In our study of Northeast Thai women, we confirmed that the nominated risks for cervical carcinoma in other studies (Tachezy *et al.,* 1999; Sriamporn *et al.,* 1997; Monoz, 2002; Skegg, 2002) – number of sexual partners, age at the first sexual intercourse and number of parities (Settheetham-Ishida *et al.,* 2004a) – also increased the risk. These parameters related to sexual behaviors increased the risk of cervical cancer between 2.18 and 2.76-fold. If the first sexual intercourse occurs in a young girl – in whom the cervix is vulnerable because of inadequate production of cervical mucus that acts as a protective barrier against infectious agents – HPV infection occurs easily and leads to a higher risk of cervical cancer (Apter *et al.,* 1993).

Sexually transmitted diseases (such as syphilis, herpes simplex type 2 and chlamydia infection) are associated with the development of invasive cervical cancer (Williams *et al.,* 1994; Kahn *et al.,* 2002), as are contraceptives, particularly the pill (Skegg, 2002; Moreno,

2002); however, none of these factors were confirmed in women living in Northeast Thailand (Settheetham-Ishida *et al.,* 2004a).

Smoking has also been thought to be a risk factor for cervical cancer (Prokopczyk *et al.,* 1997); however, the OR was not increased among smoking groups in Northeastern Thai women (Settheetham-Ishida *et al.,* 2004a). A weak association of smoking and risk of invasive cervical cancer was reported from Central Thailand (Thomas *et al.,* 2001). Thomas *et al.* (2001) suggested that even if smoking is a cofactor for cervical cancer development, it operates prior to the development of *in situ* disease and is not an important determinant of risk in Thailand. This is especially so because smoking is culturally unacceptable for Thai women. Increased risks were observed when the partner smoked or had smoking history, confirming that secondary smoking is a risk factor for cervical cancer, especially among high-risk HPV positive women (Coker *et al.,* 2002). Smoking directly promotes the development of lung cancer in males, while it does the same indirectly for cervical cancer in females (National Cancer Institute, 2001).

As mentioned above, cervical infection with certain HPV types is a precursor event in the genesis of cervical neoplasia (zur Hausen, 1991; Schiffman and Castle, 2003). Oncogenic high-risk group of HPV infection was identified among 86.7% of patients with SCCA and increased the risk for cervical cancer development as high as 43.5-fold in Northeastern Thai women (Settheetham-Ishida *et al.,* 2005). Multiple sexual partners and partner's smoking habit were nominated as the risks for HPV infection. Having multiple sexual partners increased the risk for high-risk type HPV infection 3.94-fold (Settheetham-Ishida *et al.,* 2004b). This is comparable to the data obtained in Central, Northern and Southern Thailand (Thomas *et al.,* 1996; Sukvirach *et al.,* 2003). Women who have multiple sexual partners easily contract HPV from their partners (Thomas *et al.,* 2001a). Moreover, extramarital sexual contact of the husband causes HPV infection in women who are monogamous (Thomas *et al.,* 2001b).

Any smoking experience of the partner was confirmed as a risk for cervical cancer in Thai women living in the Northeast (Settheetham-Ishida *et al.,* 2004a). As for the HPV infection, an increased risk was observed when the subject had (a) current smoking partner(s) (Settheetham-Ishida *et al.,* 2004b). This confirms that passive or secondary smoking (Coker *et al.,* 2002) as a risk factor for high-risk type HPV infection. The association between sexual partner's smoking and HPV infection is explained by either inhalation of environmental smoke or exposure to smoke-related mutagens/carcinogens in semen (Tokudome, 1997) and also smoke-related agents have been detected in cervical mucus (Prokopczyk *et al.,* 1997). Smoking, thus, might cause a local immunological depletion and smoke components could favor HPV persistence (Poppe *et al.,* 1995; Lazcano-Ponce *et al.,* 2001). Moreover, smoking results in persistence of cervical HPV infection and lowers potential for clearing oncogenic infection (Giulian *et al.,* 2002). Since women in Northeast Thailand rarely smoke, most of the exposure to smoke is passive but the cancer promotion is still active.

Some other factors such as sexual behaviors (particularly, having more than one sexual partner and younger age at the first sexual intercourse) and smoking also increased risk for malignant types of HPV infection and cervical squamous intraepithelial lesions (SIL) development. These risk factors may enhance the effects of HPV infection on cervical hyperplasia and transformation (Settheetham-Ishida *et al.,* 2006).

Increased risk for age at the first sexual intercourse, number of parities, long-term use of oral contraceptives and sexual partner's smoking habit was observed even though they did not statistically increase the risk for HPV infection. Since these factors are associated with risk for cervical cancer (Settheetham-Ishida *et al.,* 2004a, 2004b), together with multiple sexual partners and partner's smoking habit, they may all contribute to the development of cervical cancer. To decrease the incidence of cervical cancer, prevention of HPV infection is essential as is limiting the number of sexual partners, especially those with a smoking habit.

Polymorphisms in Detoxification Enzymes

It has been suggested that tobacco smoking is associated with the risk of HPV infection and cervical cancer, including in Northeastern Thai women (Settheetham *et al.,* 2004a, 2004b). The presence of carcinogens – such as nicotine, cotinine and tobacco-specific nitrosamines – have been detected in the cervical mucus of smokers. Inhaled tobacco-derived components are transported to cervical site(s) where they can damage cellular DNA (Prokopczyk *et al.,* 1997; McCann *et al.,* 1992). The tobacco smoke constituents are modified by metabolizing enzymes and may promote malignant cellular growth (Prokopczyk *et al.,* 1997). Even though smoking is a risk for cervical cancer, not all smokers develop cervical cancer. Molecular studies have identified polymorphic gene products that are associated with the metabolism of tobacco smoke pro-carcinogens and possibly with susceptibility to cancer.

Glutathione S-transferase (GST) is related to human phase II detoxification enzymes, and at least five classes (alpha, mu, pi, sigma and theta class) of cytosolic GST have been identified. However, only enzymes in three classes – including GSTM (mu), GSTP (pi) and GSTT (theta) – play key roles in the detoxification of carcinogenic electrophiles of aflatoxin and polycyclic aromatic hydrocarbons (PAHs) in tobacco smoke (*i.e.,* benzo[*a*]pyrene and other procarcinogens of PAHs). The mode of action is through the activation and detoxification of tobacco carcinogens, thus one might expect the relation of polymorphism and risk to be stronger among smokers.

GSTM1 facilitates the excretion of a wide range of carcinogens, reactive oxygen species and chemotherapeutic agents with a variety of substrate specificities (Rebbeck, 1997). The absent of the homozygous allele of the *GSTM1* gene (*GSTM*-null genotype) results in a complete loss of enzyme activity to bind with genotoxic substrates including epoxides derived from aflatoxin and PAHs (Hayes and Pulford, 1995). It is believed that individuals with *GSTM1*-null genotype are more prone to develop nasopharyngeal carcinoma than those with the *GSTM1*-present genotype because of the lack of function to detoxify the ultimate form of carcinogens (Tiwawech *et al.,* 2005).

Accumulative data from molecular epidemiological studies demonstrated that individuals with *GSTM1*-null genotype are susceptible to cancer in various organs including lung, bladder, skin, oral, liver, gastric, colorectal, prostrate, breast, ovary, cervix and nasopharynx (Nazar-Stewart *et al.,* 1999; Sweeney *et al.,* 2003; Lee *et al.,* 2002; Heagerty *et al.,* 1994; Kietthubthew *et al.,* 2001; Deng *et al.,* 2001; Setiawan *et al.,* 2000; Gawronska-Szklarz *et al.,* 1999; Autrup *et al.,* 1999; van der Hel *et al.,* 2003; Spurdle *et al.,* 2001; and Sierra-Torres *et al.,* 2003). However, results of many other studies dealing with the association between

GSTM1 polymorphism in some of these cancers have been contradictory (Kelsey, *et al.*, 1997; Kim *et al.*, 2002; Zheng *et al.*, 2003; Lallas *et al.*, 2000; and Cheng *et al.*, 2003).

We then screened for the *GSTM1* polymorphism in our case-control subjects. *GSTM1*-null genotype did not significantly increase the susceptibility to cervical cancer development but just showed a tendency; this was also confirmed among women exposed to passive smoking (Table 1). It is thus presumed that specificity and inter-individual variation in the expression level of metabolizing enzymes in cervical tissue may be involved in certain genetic backgrounds, of the chemical metabolizing enzyme genes, related to the development of cervical cancer. Other phase II detoxifying enzymes, such as GSTP and GSTT as well as phase I detoxifying enzymes namely P450 (CYP) family that are responsible for the metabolic activation of carcinogens will be our next target genes. Some of these genes are known to be polymorphic in Thai population and a polymorphic locus or combinations of polymorphic loci may have potentials to play critical roles in inter-individual genetic diversity relating to cervical cancer susceptibility.

Table 1. Frequency of GSTM1 Genotypes

	GSTM1 Genotypes, (n)		OR [95% CI]
	Normal	null	
Subjects			
Controls	32	54	
Cases	34	44	1.3 [0.67-2.56]
Passive Smokers			
Controls	19	30	
Cases	28	34	1.3 [0.57-2.99]

CONCLUSION

HPV infection is identified as a critical risk factor for the development of cervical cancer in Northeast Thailand. Among high-risk HPV types, HPV-16 as well as other malignant types have more or less equal potential for the development of SCCA. Multiple HPV infection was observed in a total of 18 out of 91 individuals; however, only one-third of them had declared to have multiple sex partners. Evidently, a partners' sexual behavior is critical in the dissemination of HPV in women. The polymorphism of the *p53* itself – as well as in combination with HPV infection – may not be a genetic risk for cervical cancer.

Regarding the other risk factors such as sexual behaviors and smoking, more attention should be paid. Since sexual behaviors, sexually transmitted diseases, the use of contraceptives and smoking may serve as cofactors to increase the risk for cervical carcinoma in the presence of HPV. In order to achieve eradication of HPV infection and the prevention of cervical cancer in this region, more attention should be paid to the presence of other risk factors such as sexual behavior and smoking habit.

Acknowledgments

This work received grant support from Khon Kaen University, Faculty of Medicine, Khon Kaen University, Grant-in-aid for Scientific Research from MEXT, Japan and JSPS-NRCT Core-University Programme. The authors thank Drs., Yuenyao P, Kanjanavirojkul N and Tassaneeyakul W, Faculty of Medicine, Khon Kaen University, for their valuable contribution to fulfill this study, and Mr. Bryan Roderick Hamman for the editorial assistance of the manuscript.

References

Andersson, S., Rylander, E., Strand, A., Sallstrom, J. & Wilander, E. (2001). The significance of *p53* codon 72 polymorphism for the development of cervical adenocarcinomas. *Br. J. Cancer 85*, 1153-1156.

Apter, D., Butzow, T.L., Laughlin, G.A. & Yen, S.S. (1993). Gonadotropin-releasing hormone pulse generate activity during pubertal transition in girls: pulsatile and diurnal patterns of circulating gonadotropins. *J. Clin. Endocrinol. Metab. 76*, 940-949.

Autrup, J.L., Thomassen, L.H., Olsen, J.H., Wolf, H. & Autrup, H. (1999). Glutathione S-transferases as risk factors in prostate cancer. *Eur. J. Cancer Prev. 8*, 525–532.

Baek, W.K., Cho, J.W., Suh, S.I., Suh, M.H., Shin, D.H., Cho, C.H., Lee, T.S. & Cha, S.D. (2000). p53 codon 72 polymorphism and risk of carcinoma in Korean women. *J. Korean Med. Sci. 15*, 65-67.

Beckman, G., Birgander, R., Sjalander, A., Saha, N., Holmberg, P.A., Kivela, A. & Beckman, L. (1994). Is p53 polymorphism maintained by natural selection? *Hum. Hered. 44*, 266-270.

Bishop,J.M. (1995) Cancer: the rise of the genetic paradigm. Genes. Dev. 9, 1309-1315.

Cancer Unit (2004). Khon Kaen University Tumor Registry 2003: *Statistical Report. Khon Kaen University*, Khon Kaen, Thailand.

Cancer Unit (2005). Khon Kaen University Tumor Registry 2004: *Statistical Report, Khon Kaen University*, Khon Kaen, Thailand.

Cheng, Y.J., Chien, Y.C., Hildesheim, A., Hsu, M.M., Chen, I.H., Chuang, J., Chang J., Ma, Y.D., Luo, C.T., Hsu, W.L., Hsu, H.H., Huang, H., Chang, J.F., Chen, C.J. & Yang, C.S. (2003). No association between genetic polymorphisms of CYP1A1, GSTM1, GSTT1, GSTP1, NAT2, and nasopharyngeal carcinoma in Taiwan. *Cancer Epidemiol. Biomarkers Prev. 12*,179-80.

Cho, N.H., Lim, S.Y., Kim, Y.T., Kim, D., Kim, Y.S. & Kim, J.W. (2003). G2 checkpoint in uterine cervical cancer with HPV 16 E6 according to p53 polymorphism and its screening value small star, filled. *Gynecol. Oncol. 90*, 15-22.

Coker, A.L., Bond, S.M., Williams, A., Gerasimova, T. & Pirisi, L. (2002). Active and passive smoking, high-risk human papillomaviruses and cervical neoplasia. *Cancer Detect. Prev. 26*, 121-128.

Crook, T., Wrede, D. & Vousden, K.H. (1991) p53 point mutation in HPV negative human cervical carcinoma cell lines. *Oncogene 6*, 873-875.

Deng, Z., Wei, Y. & Ma, Y. (2001). Glutathione-S-transferase M1 genotype in patients with hepatocellular carcinoma. *Zhonghua Zhong Liu Za Zhi. 23*, 477-479.

Donehower, L.A., Harvey, M. & Slagle, B.L. (1992). Mice deficient for p53 are developmentally normal but susceptible to spontaneous tumors. *Nature 356*, 215-221.

Doorbar. J., & Strerling, J. (2001). The biology of human papillomaviruses. In J.C. Sterling & S.K. Tyring (Eds), *Human papillomaviruses clinical and scientific advances*. (pp. 10-23). London: Arnold.

Gawronska-Szklarz, B., Lubinski, J., Klandy, J., Kurzawski, G., Bielicki, D., Wojcicki, M., Sych, Z. & Musial, H.D. (1999). Polymorphism of GSTM1 gene in patients with colorectal cancer and colonic polyps. *Exp. Toxicol. Pathol. 51*, 321–325.

Giuliano, A.R., Sedjo, R.L., Roe, D.J., Harri, R., Baldwi, S., Papenfuss, M.R., Abrahamsen, M. & Inserra, P. (2002). Clearance of oncogenic human papillomavirus (HPV) infection: effect of smoking (United States). *Cancer Causes Control. 13*, 839-846.

Gustafsson, A.C., Guo, Z., Hu, X., Ahmadian, A., Brodin, B., Nilsson, A., Ponten, J., Ponten, F. & Lundeberg, J. (2001). HPV-related cancer susceptibility and p53 codon 72 polymorphism. *Acta Derm. Venereol. 81*, 125-129.

Haffner, R. & Oren, M. (1995). Biochemical properties and biological effects of p53. *Curr. Opin. Genet. Dev. 5*, 84-90.

Hayes, J.D. & Pulford, D.J. (1995). The glutathione S-transferase supergene family: regulation of GST and the contribution of the isoenzymes to cancer chemoprotection and drug resistance. *Crit. Rev. Biochem. Mol. Biol. 30*, 445-600.

Heagerty, A.H., Fitzgerald, D., Smith, A., Bowers, B., Jones, P., Fryer, A.A., Zhao, L., Alldersea, J. & Strange, R.C. (1994). Glutathione S-transferase GSTM1 phenotypes and protection against cutaneous tumours. *Lancet 343*, 266-268.

Helland, A., Langerod, A., Johnsen, H., Olsen, A.O., Skovlund, E. & Borresen-Dale, A.L. (1998). *p53* polymorphism and risk of cervical cancer. *Nature 396*, 530-531.

Hunter T. Cooperation between oncogenes. *Cell* 1991; 64: 249-70.

Iwasawa, A., Nieminen, P., Lehtinen, M. & Paavonen, J. (1996). Human papillomavirus DNA in uterine cervix squamous cell carcinoma and adenocarcinoma detected by polymerase chain reaction. *Cancer 77*, 2275-2279.

Kahn, J.A., Rosenthal, S.L., Succop, P.A., Ho, G.Y. & Burk, R.D. (2002). Mediators of the association between age of first sexual intercourse and subsequent human papillomavirus infection. *Pediatrics. 109*, E5.

Kastan, M.B., Onyekwere, O., Sidransky, D., Vogeltein, B. & Craig, R.W. (1991) Participation of p53 protein in the cellular response to DNA damage. *Cancer Res. 51*, 6304-6311.

Kelsey, K.T., Spitz, M.R., Zuo, Z.F. & Wiencke, J.K. (1997). Polymorphisms in the glutathione S-transferase class μ and θ genes interact and increase susceptibility to lung cancer in minority populations (Texas, United States). *Cancer Causes Control. 8*, 554–559

Kietthubthew, S., Sriplung, H. & Au W.W. (2001). Genetic and environmental interactions on oral cancer in Southern Thailand. *Environmental & Molecular Mutagenesis 7*, 111-116.

Kietthubthew, S., Sriplung. H., Au, W.W. & Ishida, T. (2003) The p53 codon 72 polymorphism and risk of oral cancer in Southern Thailand. *Asian Pac. J. Cancer Prev. 3*, 209-214.

Kim, J., Roh, J., Park, N., Song, Y., Kang, S. & Lee. H. (2001). Polymorphism of TP53 codon 72 and the risk of cervical cancer among Korean women. *Am. J. Obstet. Gynecol. 184*, 55-58.

Kim, W.J., Kim, H., Kim, C.H., Lee, M.S., Oh, B.R., Lee, H.M. & Katoh, T. (2002). GSTT1-null genotype is a protective factor against bladder cancer. *Urology 60*, 913-918.

Kjaer, S.K. & Brinton, L. (1993). Adenocarcinomas of the uterine cervix: The epidemiology of an increasing problem. *Epidemiol. Rev. 15*, 486-498.

Klug, S.J., Wilmotte, R., Santos, C., Almonte, M., Herrero, R., Guerrero, I,, Caceres, E., Peixoto-Guimaraes, D., Lenoir, G,, Hainaut, P., Walboomers, J.M. & Munoz,N. (2001). TP53 polymorphism, HPV infection, and risk of cervical cancer. *Cancer Epidemiol. Biomarkers Prev. 10*, 1009-1012.

Lallas, T.A., McClain, S.K., Shahin, M.S. & Buller, R.E. (2000). The glutathione S-transferase M1 genotype in ovarian cancer. *Cancer Epidemiol. Biomarkers Prev. 9*, 587-90.

Lazcano-Ponce, E., Herrero, R., Munoz, N., Cruz, A., Shah, K.V., Alonso, P., Hernandez, P., Salmeron, J. & Hernandez, M. (2001). Epidemiology of HPV infection among Mexican women with normal cervical cytology. *Int. J. Cancer 91*, 412-420.

Lee, S.J., Cho, S.H., Park, S.K., Kim, S.W., Park, M.S., Choi, H.Y., Choi, J.Y., Lee, S.Y., IM, H.J., Kim, J.Y., Yoon, K.J., Choi, H., Shin, S.G., Park, T.W., Rothman, N., Hirvonen, A. & Kang, D. (2002). Combined effect of glutathione S-transferase M1 and T1 genotypes on bladder cancer risk. *Cancer Lett. 177*, 173-179.

Lertworapreecha, M., Bhattarakosol, P. & Niruthisard, S. (1998). Detection and typing of human papillomavirus in cervical intraepithelial neoplasia grade III in Thai women. Southeast Asian J. *Trop. Med. Public Health 29*, 507-511.

Levine, A.J. (1997). P53, the cellular gatekeeper for growth and division. *Cell 88*, 323-333

Lowe, S.W., Schmitt, E.M., Smith, S.W., Osborne, B.A. & Jacks,T. (1993). p53 is required for radiation-induced apoptosis in mouse thymocytes. *Nature 362*, 847-849.

Makni, H., Franco, E.L., Kaiano, J., Villa, L.L., Labrecque, S., Dudley, R., Storey, A., & Matlashewski, G. (2000). P53 polymorphism in codon 72 and risk of human papillomavirus-induced cervical cancer: effect of inter-laboratory variation. *Int. J. Cancer 87*, 528-533.

Marston, N.J., Crook, T. & Vousden, K.H. (1994). Interaction of p53 with MDM2 is independent of E6 and does not mediate wild type transformation suppressor function. *Oncogene 9*, 2707-2716.

Martin, N. & Patel, N. (2003). Cervix incidence and leading sites. In H. Sriplung, S. Sontipong, N. Martin, S. Wiangnon, V. Vootiprux, A. Cheirsilpa, C. Kanchanabat & T. Khuhaprema. *Cancer in Thailand. Vol.III*, 1995-1997, pp. 9-18. Bangkok: National Cancer Institute, Ministry of Public Health.

Medcalf, E.A. & Milner J. (1993). Targeting and degradation of p53 by E6 of human papillomavirus type 16 is preferential for the 1620+ p53 conformation. *Oncogene 8*, 2847-2851.

Minaguchi, T., Kanamori, Y., Matsushima, M., Yoshikawa, H., Taketani, Y. & Nakamura, Y. (1998). No evidence of correlation between polymorphism at codon 72 of *p53* and risk of cervical cancer in Japanese patients with human papillomavirus 16/18 infection. *Cancer Res. 58*, 4585-4586.

Monoz, N., Bosch, F.X., de Sanjose, S., Tafur, L., Izarzugaza, I., Gili, M., Viladiu, P., Navarro, C., Martos, C., Ascunce, N., Gonzalez, L.C., Kaldor, M., Gerrero, E., Lorincz, A., Santamaria, M., de Ruiz, P.A., Arisizabal, N. & Shah, K.V. (1992). The causal link between human papillomavirus and invasive cervical cancer: a population-based case-control study in Colombia and Spain. *Int. J. Cancer 52,* 743-749.

Monoz, N. (2002). Role of parity and human papillomavirus in cervical cancer. *Lancet 359,* 1093-1101.

Moreno, V. (2002). Effect of oral contraceptives on risk of cervical cancer in women with human papillomavirus infection. *Lancet 359,* 1085-1092.

Munger, K., Basile, J.R., Duensing, S., Eichten, A., Gonzalez, S.L., Grace, M. & Zacny, V.L. (2001). Biological activities and molecular targets of the human papillomavirus E7 oncoprotein. *Oncogene. 20,* 7888-7898

National Cancer Institute (2001). *Cancer Resistry 2000.* Department of Medical Services, Ministry of Public Health.

Nazar-Stewart, V., Vaughan, T.L., Burt, R.D., Chen, C., Berwick, M, & Swanson, G.M. (1999). Glutathione S-transferase M1 and susceptibility to nasopharyngeal carcinoma. Cancer Epidemiol. *Biomarkers Prev. 8,* 547-451.

Pegoraro, R., Moodley, J., Nailker, S., Lanning, P. & Rom, L.(2000). The *p53* codon 72 polymorphism in black South African women and the risk of cervical cancer. *Br. J. Obst. Gynecol. 107,* 1164-1165.

Pengsaa P, Jindawijak S (2003). Cervix uteri. In H. Sriplung, S. Sontipong, N. Martin, S. Wiangnon, V. Vootiprux, A. Cheirsilpa, C. Kanchanabat & T. Khuhaprema. *Cancer in Thailand. Vol.III,* 1995-1997, pp. 49-50. Bangkok: National Cancer Institute, Ministry of Public Health.

Pillai, M.R., Sreevidya, S., Pollock, B.H., Jayaprakash, P.G. & Herman, B. (2002). Polymorphism at codon 72 of p53, human papillomavirus, and cervical cancer in South India. *J. Cancer Res. Clin. Oncol. 128,* 627-623

Poppe, W.A., Ide, P.S., Drijkoningen, M.P., Lauweryns, J.M. & Van Assche, F.A. (1995). Tobacco smoking impairs the local immunosurveillance in the uterine cervix. An immunohistochemical study. *Gynecol. Obstet. Invest. 39,* 34-38.

Prokopczyk, B., Cox, J.E., Hoffmann, D. & Waggoner, S.E. (1997). Identification of tobacco-specific carcinogen in the cervical mucus of smokers and non-smokers. *J. Natl .Cancer Inst. 89,* 868-873.

Punyaratabunduh, P., Supanvanich, S., Tirapat, C. & Podhipak, A. (1982). Epidemiologic study of risk factors in cancer of the vervix uteri in Thai women. *J. Med. Assoc. Thailand 65,* 231-239.

Rebbeck, T.R. (1997). Molecular epidemiology of the human glutathione S-transferase genotypes GSTM1 and GSTT1 in cancer susceptibility. *Cancer Epidemiol Biomarkers Prev. 6,*733-743.

Rosenthal, A.N., Ryan, A., Al-Jehani, R.M., Storey, A., Harwood, C.A. & Jacobs, I.J. (1998). *p53* codon 72 polymorphism and risk of cervical cancer in UK. *Lancet 352*, 871-872.

Scheffner, M., Werness, B.A., Huibregtse, J.M., Levine, A.J. & Howley, P.M. (1990). The E6 oncoprotein encoded by human papillomavirus types 16 and 18 promotes the degradation of p53. *Cell 63*, 1129-1136.

Scheffner, M., Munger, K., Byrne, J.C. & Howley, P.M. (1991). The state of the p53 and retinoblastoma genes in human cervical carcinoma cell lines. *Proc. Natl. Acad. Sci. U.S.A. 88*, 5523-5527.

Schiffman, M. & Castle, P.E. (2003). Human papillomavirus: epidemiology and public health. *Arch. Pathol. Lab. Med. 8*, 930-934

Setiawan, V.W., Zhang, Z.F., Yu, G.P., Li, YL., Lu, M.L., Tsai, C.J., Cordova, D., Wang, M.R., Guo, C.H., Yu, S.Z. & Kurtz, R.C. (2000). GSTT1 and GSTM1 null genotypes and risk of gastric cancer: a case-control study in a Chinese population. *Cancer Epidemiol. Biomarkers Prev. 9*, 73–80.

Settheetham-Ishida, W., Singto, U., Yuenyao, P., Kanjanavirojkul, N., Tassaneeyakul, W. & Ishida, T. (2004a). Contribution of epigenetic risk factors but not p53 codon 72 polymorphism to the development of cervical cancer in Northeastern Thailand. *Cancer Letters 210*, 205-211.

Settheetham-Ishida, W., Singto, Y., Kanjanavirojkul, N., Chatchawan, U., Yuenyao, P., Settheetham, D. & Ishida, T. (2004b). Co-risk factors for HPV infection in Northeastern Thai women with cervical cancer. *Asian Pacific J. Cancer Prev. 5*, 383-386.

Settheetham-Ishida, W., Kanjanavirojkul, N., Kularbkaew, C., & Ishida, T. (2005). Human papillomavirus genotypes and the p53 codon 72 polymorphism in cervical cancer of Northeastern Thailand. *Microbiol. Immunol. 49*, 417-421.

Settheetham-Ishida, W., Yuenyao, P., Tassaneeyaku, W., Kanjanavirojkul, N.,Thawmor, A., Kularbkaew, C., Hahvajanawong, C., Settheetham, D., Wattanathorn, J., Kashima, T. & Ishida, T. (2006). *Asian Pacific J. Cancer Prev. 7*, 113-118.

Sierra-Torres, C.H., Au, W.W., Arrastia, C.D., Cajas-Salazar, N., Robazetti, S.C., Payne, D.A., & Tyring, S.K. (2003). Polymorphisms for chemical metabolizing genes and risk for cervical neoplasia. *Environ. Mol. Mutagen 41*, 69-76.

Skegg, D.C.G. (2002). Oral contraceptive, parity and cervical cancer. *Lancet 359*, 1080-1081.

Spurdle, A.B., Webb, P.M., Purdie, D.M., Chen, X., Green, A. & Chenevix-Trench, G. (2001). Polymorphisms at the glutathione S-transferase GSTM1, GSTT1 and GSTP1 loci: risk of ovarian cancer by histological subtype. *Carcinogenesis 22*, 67-72.

Sriamporn, S., Pengsaa, P., Yuenyao, P., Parkin, D.M., Suwanrungrunang, K., Kamsa-ard, S. & Vatanasapt, V. (1997). Risk factors for cervical cancer in Thai women: a case-control study. *Thai cancer Journal 23*, 58-63.

Storey, A., Thomas, M., Kalita, A., Harwood, C., Gardiol, D., Mantovani, F., Breuer, J., Leigh, I.M., Matlashewski, G. & Banks, L. (1998). Role of a *p53* polymorphism in the development of human papillomavirus-associated cancer. *Nature 393*, 229-234.

Sukvirach, S., Smith, J.S., Tunsakul, S., Munoz, N., Kesararat, V., Opasatian, O., Chichareon, S., Kaenploy, V., Ashley, R., Meijer, C.J., Snijders, P.J., Coursaget, P., Franceschi, S., & Herrero, R. 2003. Population-based human papillomavirus prevalence in Lampang and Songkla, Thailand. *J. Infect. Dis. 187*, 1246-1256.

Sweeney, C., Nazar-Stewart, V., Stapleton, P.L., Eaton, D.L., and Vaughan, T.L. (2003). Glutathione S-transferase M1, T1, and P1 polymorphisms and survival among lung cancer patients. *Cancer Epidemiol. Biomarkers Prev. 12*, 527-533.

Tachezy, R., Mikyskova, I., Salakova, M. & Van Ranst, M. (1999). Correlation between human papillomavirus-associated cervical cancer and p53 codon 72 arginine/proline polymorphism. *Human Genet. 105*, 564-566.

Thomas, M., Massimi, P., Jenkins, J. & Banks, L. (1995). HPV-18 E6 mediated inhibition of p53 DNA binding activity is independent of E6 induced degradation. *Oncogene 10*, 261-268.

Thomas, D.B., Ray, R.M., Pardthaisong, T., Chutivongse, S., Koetsawang, S., Silpisornkosol, S., Virutamasen, P., Christopherson, W.M., Melnick, J.L., Meirik, O., Farley, T.M. & Riotton, G. (1996). Prostitution, condom use and invasive squamous cell carcer in Thailand. *Am. J. Epidemiol. 143*, 779-786.

Thomas, M., Kalita, A., Labrecque, S., Pim, D., Banks, L. & Matlashewski, G. (1999a). Two polymorphic variants of wild-type p53 differ biochemically and biologically. *Mol. Cell Biol. 19*, 1092-1100.

Thomas, M., Pim, D. & Banks, L. (1999b). The role of the E6-p53 interaction in the molecular pathogenesis of HPV. *Oncogene 18*, 7690-7700.

Thomas, D.B., Ray, R.M., Koetsawang, A., Kiviat, N., Kuypers, J., Qin, Q., Ashley, R.L. & Koetsawang, S. (2001a). Human papillomaviruses and cervical cancer in Bangkok. I. Risk factors for invasive cervical carcinomas with human papillomavirus types 16 and 18 DNA. *Am. J. Epidemiol. 153*, 723-731.

Thomas, D.B., Qin, Q., Kuypers, J., Kiviat, N., Ashley, R.L., Koetsawang, A., Ray, R.M., & Koetsawang, S. (2001b). Human papillomaviruses and cervical cancer in Bangkok. II. Risk factors for in situ and invasive squamous cell cervical carcinomas. *Am. J. Epidemiol. 153*, 732-739.

Tiwawech, D., Srivatanakul, P., Karalak, A. & Ishida, T. (2003). The p53 codon 72 polymorphism in Thai nasopharyngeal carcinoma. *Cancer Letters 198*, 69-75.

Tiwawech, D., Srivatanakul, P., Karalak, A. & Ishida, T. (2005). Glutathione S-transferase M1 gene polymorphism in Thai nasopharyngeal carcinoma. *Asian Pac. J. Cancer Prev. 6*, 270-275.

Tokudome, S. (1997). Semen of smokers and cervical cancer risk. *J Natl Cancer Inst, 89*, 96-97

Van der Hel, O.L., Peeters, P.H., Hein, D.W., Doll, M.A., Grobbee, D.E., Kromhout, D. & Bueno de Mesquita, H.B. (2003). NAT2 slow acetylation and GSTM1 null genotypes may increase postmenopausal breast cancer risk in long-term smoking women. *Pharmacogenetics 13*, 399-407.

Vatanasapt, V., Sriamporn, S., Kams-aard, S., Suwanrungruang, K., Pengsaa, P., Charoensiri, D.J., Chaiyakum, J. & Pesee, M. (1998). Cancer survival in Khon Kaen, Thailand, *In* R. Sankaranarayanan, R.J. Black, & D.M. Parkin (Eds.), *Cancer survival in developing countries*, IARC Scientific Publication No.145. pp. 123-134. Lyon:WHO International Agency for Research on Cancer.

Walboomers, J.M., Jacobs, M.V., Manos, M.M., Bosch, F.X., Kummer, J.A., Shah, K.V., Snijders, P.J., Peto, J., Meijer, C,J. & Munoz, N. (1999). Human papillomavirus is a necessary cause of invasive cervical cancer worldwide. *J. Pathol.* 1891,12-19.

Weinberg, R.A. (1989). Oncogenes, antioncogenes, and the molecular bases of multistep carcinogenesis. *Cancer Res, 49*, 3713-3721.

Weinberg, RA. (1991). Tumor suppressor genes. *Science 254*, 1138-1146.

Werness, B.A., Levine, A.J. & Howley, P.M. (1990). Association of human papillomavirus types 16 and 18 E6 proteins with p53. *Science 248*, 76-79.

Williams, M.A., Kenya, P.R., Mati, J.K. & Thomas, D.B. (1994). Risk factors for invasive cervical cancer in Kenyan women. *Int. J. Epidemiol. 23*, 906-912.

Wong, Y.F., Chung, T.K., Cheung, T.H., Nobori T, Hampton, G.M., Wang, V.W., Li , Y.F. & Chang. A.M. (2000). p53 polymorphism and human papillomavirus infection in Hong Kong women with cervical cancer. *Gynecol. Obstet. Invest. 50*, 60-63.

Yamashita, T., Yaginuma, Y., Saitoh, Y., Kawai, K., Kurakane, T., Hayashi, H. & Ishikawa, M. (1999). Codon 72 polymorphism of p53 as a risk factor for patients with human papillomavirus-associated squamous intraepithelial lesions and invasive cancer of the uterine cervix. *Carcinogenesis 20,* 1733-1736.

Yang, Y.C., Chang, C.L. & Chen, M.L. (2001). Effect of *p53* polymorphism on the susceptibility of cervical cancer. *Gynecol. Obstet. Invest. 51*, 197-201.

Zehbe, I., Voglino, G., Wilander, E., Genta, F. & Tommasino, M. (1999). Codon 72 polymorphism of *p53* and its association with cervical cancer. *Lancet 354*, 218-219.

Zheng, T., Holford, T.R., Zahm, S.H., Owens, P.H., Boyle, P., Zhang, Y., Zhang, B., Wise, J.P.Sr., Stephenson, L.P. & Ali-Osman, F. (2003). Glutathione S-transferase M1 and T1 genetic polymorphisms, alcohol consumption and breast cancer risk. *Br. J. Cancer 88*, 58-62.

zur Hausen, H. (1991). Human papillomaviruses in the pathogenesis of anogenital cancer. *Virology 184*, 9-13.

INDEX

A

B

C

D

F

G

H

I

J

K

L

M

N

O

P

Q

R

T